Advancing Responsible Adolescent Development

Series Editor
Roger J.R. Levesque
Indiana University, Bloomington, IN, USA

For further volumes, go to
http://www.springer.com/series/7284

Kaveri Subrahmanyam · David Šmahel

Digital Youth

The Role of Media in Development

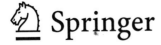 Springer

Kaveri Subrahmanyam
Department of Psychology
California State University
Los Angeles, CA 90032-8227, USA
ksubrah@calstatela.edu

David Šmahel
Institute for Research on Children, Youth
and Family
Faculty of Social Studies
Masaryk University
Jostova 10
602 00 Brno, Czech Republic
smahel@fss.muni.cz

ISBN 978-1-4419-6277-5 (hardcover)   e-ISBN 978-1-4419-6278-2
ISBN 978-1-4614-2737-7 (softcover)
DOI 10.1007/978-1-4419-6278-2
Springer New York Dordrecht Heidelberg London

Library of Congress Control Number: 2010937762

Printed on acid-free paper

Springer is part of Springer Science+Business Media (www.springer.com)

Preface

Digital media, such as computers, the Internet, video games, and mobile phones, have come to occupy a central place in the lives of today's youth. For those of us in contact with them – parents, teachers, physicians, researchers, and others – evidence of this is plentiful. Consider the teen doing homework while instant messaging several friends at the same time or one furiously texting during a family outing, in bed, or even at school. Such scenarios are becoming commonplace and many parents and teachers have encountered them at one point or another. Remarkably, most young people use interactive technologies and seem to be living their lives online.

It is important to consider the implications of young people's online living, especially for their development and well-being. In 2006, the journal *Developmental Psychology* published a special section on children, adolescents, and the Internet. It was one of the first attempts to bring together high-quality developmental research to understand youth and their digital worlds and a new field of inquiry was born. Since that special section was published, the digital landscape has changed dramatically. Chat rooms were joined by instant messaging and then social networking sites. Computers became sleeker and portable, and mobile phones took on the capabilities of computers as they got smaller and smaller. Not surprisingly, as the technologies changed, so did their use by youth.

As research in this new line of study began to accumulate, we felt that the time was ripe to write a book that would present a nuanced account of adolescents and their digital worlds. Much of the public discourse about media and youth has taken a more fearful perspective – Do new media make youth lonelier and more depressed? Does stranger contact put them at risk? Do online peer interactions weaken family relationships? Although we had no doubt that interactions with new media carried some risks for youth, we also wanted to highlight the more positive aspects of new technologies. We also felt that it was important to use a developmental approach and connect adolescents' media use to key developmental processes in order to understand their digital worlds.

Thus began our journey in early 2008. Being the neophyte authors that we were, we had no idea how much time and effort it would involve. Complicating matters, new online environments appeared, technologies such as mobile phone and text messaging came to the fore, and new research results emerged during the time that it took us to write and polish the book. In January 2010, as we finally finished and were writing this preface prior to sending the manuscript to the publishers, the latest Kaiser report on media in the lives of 8- to 18-year-olds was released. We also came across more recent studies on youth and mobile phones, and we seriously pondered whether we should go back to our manuscript and incorporate the results and issues that they raised. But any book, if it is to be published, must eventually be concluded. We had to accept that digital media will keep changing and that we would not be able to include all the research on this topic. However, we are optimistic that our developmental approach is timeless and will enable readers to connect adolescents' online behavior to offline themes, even as their online behaviors change with the technology. Our goal was to help researchers, as well as graduate and undergraduate students, formulate a better understanding of digital youth and their online worlds. We are also hopeful that this book will be useful for parents, teachers, school psychologists/counselors, physicians, and anyone working with youth as they seek to promote safe digital worlds for them.

Acknowledgments

This book would not have been possible without the help and assistance from many different people. First, we wish to thank our editor at Springer, Judy Jones, for her enthusiastic response when we approached her with our proposal and subsequently for her enormous patience and continued encouragement, as we missed deadline after deadline. We are deeply indebted to Professor Roger Levesque, our series editor, for his many readings of our manuscript, for his prompt and very insightful feedback that helped us revise the manuscript, and most importantly for his confidence and support throughout.

We acknowledge the contributions of the following research centers and universities, which collected data for the World Internet Project, the results of which are sprinkled throughout the book: the Canadian Internet Project/Recherche Internet Canada; Chinese Academy of Social Sciences, China; The Institute for Research on Children, Youth and Family, Masaryk University, the Czech Republic; ITHAKA – Information Society and Network Research Center, Hungary; the Singapore Internet Research Centre, Nanyang Technological University, Singapore; and the USC Annenberg School Center for the Digital Future, USA. Thanks are due to Professors Brad Brown, Charles Ess, and Patricia Greenfield for reading a draft of our manuscript and for their very helpful comments. David acknowledges the support of the Czech Ministry of Education, Youth, and Sports (MSM0021622406) when writing this book. We are greatly indebted to Miriam Bartsch for her help with the proofs. We also wish to thank Lukas Blinka and Stepan Konecny for their help in creating some of the illustrations that we have used in the book. Both of us also acknowledge our collaborators as well as the many students who have worked in our laboratories over the last several years. Although we do not list them individually by name, their efforts have contributed immensely to helping us study adolescents' digital worlds.

Finally, each of us would like to express our gratitude to our families and friends. David thanks his wife Lucy, his daughters Rozára and Marjána, and also his parents for their support and encouragement. Kaveri is grateful to her husband, Subra, for his unfailing encouragement and especially for his patience toward the end as the writing process dragged on forever. She is most thankful to her children who grew up in the very digital worlds that this book focuses on – Divya, a senior in college, very generously let her take a peek into some of them and Jayant, a senior in high school, taught her that every youth uses these spaces in his or her unique way! She also thanks her parents and her in-laws for their support, faith, and assistance over the years.

Brno, Czech Republic
Los Angeles, USA
January 30, 2010

David Šmahel
Kaveri Subrahmanyam

Contents

1 **Adolescents' Digital Worlds: An Introduction** 1
Emerging Media: Blurring of the Lines Between Hardware
and Content 2
The World Internet Project 3
Online Applications and Digital Contexts Used by Adolescents . . . 4
   Social Networking Sites (SNSs) 6
   Text Messaging 6
   Blogs and Microblogs 7
   Online Phoning Applications 8
   Instant Messaging (IM) 8
   Online Gaming 9
   Chat Rooms 10
   Virtual Worlds 11
   Bulletin Boards 11
   Downloading Music and Videos 12
Characteristics of Digital Communication Environments 13
   Disembodied Users 13
   Anonymity 14
   Text-Based Communication 14
   Self-Disclosure and Disinhibition 15
   Use of Emoticons 16
   Media-Multitasking and Multitasking 17
Studying Young People's Digital Worlds 19
   Logistical Considerations 19
   Methodological Considerations 20
Goals and Organization of the Book 21
References 23

2 **Connecting Online Behavior to Adolescent Development:**
A Theoretical Framework 27
Lessons from Developmental Psychology 27
   Changes During Adolescence 27
   Developmental Tasks and Issues 28
   The Role of the Context in Adolescent Development 31

Digital Media and Adolescent Development 32
A Theoretical Framework for Conceptualizing Adolescents'
Online Behavior: The Co-construction Model 33
Conclusions 36
References 36

**3 Sexuality on the Internet: Sexual Exploration, Cybersex,
and Pornography** 41
Adolescent Sexuality 42
Characteristics of Online Environments Relevant to Sexuality 42
Online Sexual Exploration 43
Constructing and Presenting Sexual Selves Online 44
Cybersex: Sexual Conversations Online 46
Accessing Sexually Explicit Content Online 47
Sexual Minority Youth and the Internet 53
Conclusions 54
References 55

**4 Constructing Identity Online: Identity Exploration and
Self-Presentation** 59
Identity During Adolescence 60
Online Self-Presentation and Virtual Identity 62
Adolescent's Online Identity Construction 63
Tools for Online Self-Presentation 64
Identity Expression and Self-Presentation
in Blogs and Homepages 67
Identity Expression and Self-Presentation in Social
Networking Sites 69
Online Behavior and Identity Status 70
Ethnic Identity Online 72
Identity Experiments and Pretending 73
Virtual Identity 75
Conclusions 76
References 77

**5 Intimacy and the Internet: Relationships with Friends,
Romantic Partners, and Family Members** 81
Adolescents' Friendships and Peer Group Relationships 81
Theoretical Background 81
Online Contexts and Relationships with Offline Friends
and Peer Group Members 83
Benefits and Costs of Interacting Online with Peers 84
Online Contexts and Relationships with Strangers 88
Adolescents' Romantic Relationships 90
Theoretical Background 90
Online Contexts and Adolescents' Romantic Relationships 91
How "Real" Are Online Romantic Relationships? 93

The Role of Culture in Online Romantic Relationships 94
Adolescent's Relationships Within Their Families 94
    Has Technology Changed Interactions with Family Members? . . . 95
    Impact on Family Relationships 97
Conclusions 99
References 100

6   **Digital Worlds and Doing the Right Thing: Morality,**
    Ethics, and Civic Engagement 103
    Morality and Ethics Online 104
        Maintaining Privacy Online 104
        Falsifying Information Online 107
        Stealing and Cheating Online 108
        Cyber Plagiarism 109
        Software Piracy and Illegal Downloading of Digital Content 111
    Political and Civic Engagement Online 113
        The Internet, Youth, and Politics 114
        The Internet, Adolescents, and Civic Engagement 115
    Conclusions 119
    References 119

7   **Internet Use and Well-Being: Physical and Psychological Effects** . 123
    Understanding the Influence of the Internet 123
    Effects on Physical Well-Being 124
        Direct Effects 125
        Indirect Effects 126
    Effects on Psychological Well-Being 130
        It is Not All About Time 131
        Do Online Activities Matter? 132
        Do User Characteristics Matter? 134
        Short-Term Effects on Well-Being 135
        Effect of Negative Interactions on Well-Being 137
    Conclusions 138
    References 139

8   **Technology and Health: Using the Internet for Wellness**
    and Illness 143
    Adolescents' Use of Online Health Resources 144
        How Much Do Adolescents' Use Online Health Resources? 144
        Health Topics That Adolescents Seek Information About 144
        Adolescents' Health Information Seeking Behaviors 145
        Online Health Resources: Opportunities for Adolescents 147
        Online Health Resources: Challenges for Adolescents 149
    The Internet as a Tool for Treatment Delivery 152
    Conclusions 153
    References 154

**9 When Is It Too Much? Excessive Internet Use and
Addictive Behavior** 157
Is the Term "Addiction" Applicable to Internet Use? 158
Prevalence of Addictive Behavior on the Internet 159
Identifying Youth Who May Be Addicted to the Internet 161
Correlates of Addictive Behavior on the Internet 164
Common Areas of Online Addictive Behavior 165
Online Games and Addictive Behavior 165
Cyber Relationship Addictive Behavior 168
Sexual Compulsive Behavior and Sexual Addictive
Behavior on the Internet 170
Online Gambling 171
Treatment of Addictive Behavior on the Internet 172
Cognitive Behavioral Therapy 173
Reality Therapy 173
Conclusions 174
References 175

**10 The Darker Sides of the Internet: Violence, Cyber
Bullying, and Victimization** 179
Effects of Violent Media Content 180
Violence in Web Sites and Other Online Content 181
Adolescents and Violence-Themed Web Sites 183
Adolescents and Online Hate 185
Violence in Online Games 188
Adolescents and Violence in Online Games 189
Aggressive Interactions in Online Contexts 190
Cyber Bullying 190
Sexual Solicitation 195
Conclusions 196
References 197

**11 Promoting Positive and Safe Digital Worlds: What Parents
and Teachers Can Do to Empower Youth** 201
The Role of Government and Industry 202
Safeguarding Youth from Inappropriate Content 202
Safeguarding Youth from Online Victimization 203
The Role of Parents 204
Safeguarding Youth from Inappropriate Content 204
Safeguarding Youth from Online Victimization 208
The Role of Schools 210
Safeguarding Youth from Inappropriate Content 210
Safeguarding Youth from Online Victimization 210
Conclusions 211
References 212

12 Adolescents' Digital Worlds: Conclusions and Future Steps 215
    Media in Adolescents' Lives 215
    Understanding the Role of Digital Media in Development 216
        Online and Offline Worlds Are Psychologically Connected 216
        Psychological Connectedness Does Not Mean Identical 217
        Implications of Connectedness for Development 219
    Youth Digital Worlds: Opportunities and Risks 221
    Promoting Positive and Safe Online Digital Worlds 223
    Digital Worlds and Development: Future Steps for Research 224
    References 227

Index 231

About the Authors

Kaveri Subrahmanyam is a professor of psychology at California State University, Los Angeles, and the associate director of the Children's Digital Media Center at Los Angeles. She received her Ph.D. in developmental psychology from UCLA in 1993. She uses developmental theory to understand young people's interactions with digital media. Using both quantitative and qualitative techniques, she has studied young people's digital worlds, including video games, chat rooms, blogs, and social networking sites such as MySpace and Facebook. She has published several research articles on youth and digital media and has co-edited a special issue on social networking for the *Journal of Applied Developmental Psychology* (2008).

David Šmahel is an associate professor on the Faculty of Social Studies, Masaryk University – Czech Republic. He received his Ph.D. in social psychology in 2003. His main interests are adolescents and their behavior on the Internet. David's research focuses on online risks, identity development and its consequences in the virtual world, online communication, virtual romantic relationships and friendships, as well as addictive behavior on the Internet. He is the project head of the "World Internet Project: the Czech Republic," which is a part of the identically titled worldwide project and is head of the Czech team for the EU Kids Online II project. David is currently the editor of *Cyberpsychology: Journal of Psychosocial Research on Cyberspace.*

Chapter 1
Adolescents' Digital Worlds: An Introduction

Whether at school, at home, or on the go, today's adolescents are surrounded by digital media such as computers and the Internet, video games, mobile phones, and other handheld devices (Roberts & Foehr, 2008). The writer and game-designer, Marc Prensky, calls them digital natives (Prensky, 2001) – they were born in digital worlds and have lived their entire lives surrounded and immersed within them. Compared to their parents, who tend to be digital immigrants, these digital natives are early adopters of technology, do not need an instruction manual to figure out how to use a cell phone or digital camera, and have no conception of life without Google or Wikipedia.

Remarkably, a majority of young people use these new digital technologies. In 2004, the Kaiser report indicated that 74% of 8- to 18-year olds in the USA had Internet access in their homes (Roberts, Foehr, & Rideout, 2005). More recently, in 2009, 93% of US children between 12 and 17 were online (Jones & Fox, 2009). Across several countries, young people report similar rates of Internet access. The 2008 World Internet Project survey of 13 countries revealed that among 12- to 14-year-old youth, the percentages of Internet users were 76% in Singapore, 88% in the USA, 98% in Israel, 95% in Canada, 96% in the Czech Republic, and 100% in the UK (Lebo et al., 2009). While young people use the Internet for both informational and communication purposes, the latter uses are especially popular in this demographic group, an issue we address shortly (Subrahmanyam & Greenfield, 2008a). Mobile phones are another technology that has become ubiquitous among adolescents: in market research in the USA, 79% of 13- to 19-year olds reported having a mobile device, and 15% reported having a smart device such as an iPhone or BlackBerry (Harris Interactive, 2008). In the European Union, 50% of 10-year olds, 87% of 13-year olds, and 95% of 16-year olds reported having a mobile phone (Europa Press-Release, 2009).

Digital technologies are undoubtedly popular among adolescents, and just as radio, film, and television before them were treated with suspicion, and seen as corrupting youth, these newer technologies are frequently viewed as having a negative influence on young people. Which new technologies do teens use and what to they do with them? Should we be concerned about their use of these media? Does adolescents' use of technology help them navigate the challenges of adolescence or

K. Subrahmanyam, D. Šmahel, *Digital Youth*, Advancing Responsible
Adolescent Development, DOI 10.1007/978-1-4419-6278-2_1,
© Springer Science+Business Media, LLC 2011

does it only complicate matters? Are digital worlds giving rise to new behaviors or are adolescents' transferring traditional adolescent behaviors onto them? What are some of the opportunities, challenges, and dangers that come with technology use? How can we ensure that young people use technology safely? We tackle some of these questions in this book in order to leave the reader with an understanding of how youth influence and are influenced by newer forms of interactive technologies.

To do this we have to start at the very beginning, and in this chapter, we describe adolescents' digital worlds. We begin by examining the blurring of the distinction between hardware (e.g., computers, cell phones) and the content (e.g., software such as word processing or online applications like e-mail or instant messaging) that they support. Then we describe the various technologies and online applications used by adolescents, including social networking sites, text messaging, blogs and microblogs, online phoning, online gaming (e.g., Massively Multiplayer Online Role Playing Games such as World of Warcraft), chat rooms, virtual worlds (e.g., Second Life), bulletin boards, and online music and videos. Where available, we draw on usage data from the World Internet Project[1] so the reader can get a sense of both the similarities as well as differences in how adolescents living in different parts of the world use online applications and virtual spaces. Next, we examine some salient aspects of the communication environment inherent to most new media: anonymity and disembodied users, disinhibited behavior, self-disclosure, and multi-tasking as well as media multitasking. The chapter concludes with the specific goals and organization plan of the book.

Emerging Media: Blurring of the Lines Between Hardware and Content

As we will show in the next sections, adolescents use a variety of hardware tools to find information, access entertainment, play games, and most of all, to interact and communicate with each other. The hardware they use include cell phones, smart mobile devices (e.g., the BlackBerry with multiple capabilities such as browsers, e-mail, navigation tools), iPods, Sidekicks (a mobile device with a Qwerty keyboard), video games (i.e., Nintendo or Xbox), interactive (digital) TV, navigation tools (GPS systems) as well as computers, desktops, and smaller or larger notebooks. In the early years of new media, hardware and the content (software or applications) they supported were largely separate. Thus, the Internet and consequently e-mail or instant messaging were generally accessed via desktops and then laptops, games were the province of game systems, and texting or short-message systems (SMS) were the purview of cell phones. Increasingly, these different hardware can connect to the Internet and we can use them for a variety of capabilities such as to download information (e.g., updating of software), rank players of video

---

[1] The World Internet Project is described in greater detail later on in this chapter.

games, download video games, play against other (live) players, download music, videos, and television programs, and even listen online to radio broadcasts.

The Internet has now become a network, wherein the previously separate hardware tools are able to come together. Activities that were exclusive to an online PC or notebook can now be performed via cell phones and other smart devices that are also portable as they are getting smaller and smaller (Roberts & Foehr, 2008). The Internet is consequently moving from static places (desks with PCs) into our pockets and adolescents, who tend to be early adopters of technological innovations (Greenfield & Subrahmanyam, 2003), are using them to be "always online," "always connected," and some even say "never alone" (C. Nass, personal communication, July 15, 2009). Adolescents are thus able to access e-mails, instant messages, and even their social networking site profiles from their cell phones and smart devices, at home, at school, or while on the move. The type of hardware is less important than the particular type of application and the communication that occurs within it. Reflecting this reality, our descriptions of the various applications in the next sections focus on their function rather than the particular hardware tool/s used to access them.

The World Internet Project

Where relevant, in this chapter, as well as elsewhere in the book, we present results based on data from seven countries that are a part of the World Internet Project (WIP; see www.worldinternetproject.net). The WIP is a global international survey on the impact of the Internet on individuals and societies, coordinated by the Center for the Digital Future at the USC Annenberg School for Communication. As one of us (David) is responsible for collecting the data from the Czech Republic, we are able to provide this unique international perspective. More than 20 partner countries and regions from North America, South America, Europe, Asia, the Middle East, and Oceania participated in the survey. Most of the WIP results reported in this book are based on the data from the following seven countries, for which the 2007 sample included a sufficient number of adolescents: the USA, Canada, Singapore, New Zealand, Hungary, the Czech Republic, and China. All samples were representative of the countries from which they were collected, except for the Chinese data, which was only representative of urban areas. The surveys were conducted via the telephone and face-to-face interviews. Table 1.1 presents descriptive information about the samples.

The results we report here are drawn from sub-samples of adolescents up to 18 years of age. The age ranges of the respondents varied and participants were as young as 12 in some countries whereas in others, they were 14, 15, or even 16 years old. Whenever possible, we tested the data from the USA, Canada, Hungary, the Czech Republic, and Singapore for age effects. We divided the participants into two groups: younger (12–15 years) and older (16–18 years) adolescents and developmental differences, if found, are reported.

Table 1.1 Descriptive Information about the Samples Drawn from Some of the Countries Participating in the 2007 WIP

Country	Number of all respondents (all ages)	Number of respondents aged up to 18 years	Age range of adolescents in the sample (in years)
Canada	3,150	417	12–18
China	2,035	161	15–18
The Czech Republic	1,586	217	12–18
Hungary	3,059	206	14–18
New Zealand	1,430	115	16–18
Singapore	886	167	13–18
USA	2021	156	12–18
Total	14,167	1,439	

Online Applications and Digital Contexts Used by Adolescents

At the outset, we remind the reader that the online applications and digital spaces described in this section were popular among youth at the time when we wrote this chapter in 2009, and there is no telling how long they are likely to remain so. In addition, we selected these particular applications based on trends in the USA and the Czech Republic as well as our own work in these two countries. Not included in our description are familiar and staple applications, such as e-mail or web sites that most adolescents use.

Figure 1.1 allows us to compare the amount of time spent on media (television, radio, newspapers, and the Internet) with face-to-face socializing for youth from five countries on the WIP 2007. Watching television, face-to-face interactions, and time online were the three most frequent activities. Notably, youth in all of the countries reported spending more time face-to-face with their peers than on the Internet.

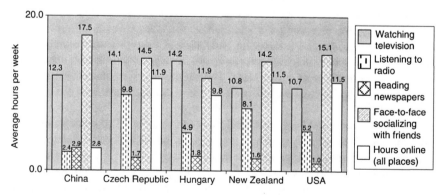

Fig. 1.1 Media use and face-to-face socializing with friends among adolescents in the 2007 WIP (12- to 18-year olds)

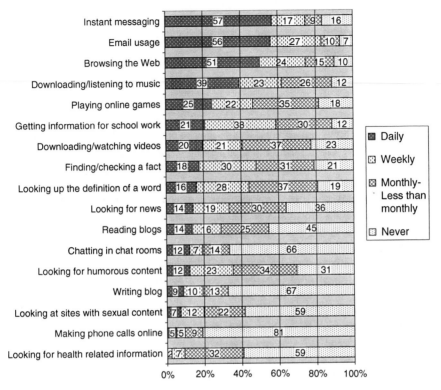

Fig. 1.2 Overview of online activities (WIP 2007 – Canada and USA) among 12- to 18-year olds

Figure 1.2 shows the frequency of various online activities that youth (12- to 18-year olds) in the USA and Canada reported engaging in on the WIP 2007, it does not include information about the use of the currently popular social networking sites such as MySpace, Facebook, as they were not included in the World Internet Project.[2] The activities are sorted according to daily use, and those at the top of the graph are the most frequent and those at the bottom are less so.

From Fig. 1.2, we see that American and Canadian youth use communication applications, such as instant messaging and e-mail most frequently followed by entertainment activities, such as downloading and listening to online music and playing online games. Ironically, parents reported that they bought these tools to help their children with school, but school-related uses were infrequent relative to the communication and entertainment activities. Adolescents in the other WIP countries used different online applications similarly. Communication tools are the most frequent, attesting that young people in a range of countries use the Internet

---

[2] Keeping up with rapidly changing technologies is a huge challenge for researchers studying adolescents' digital worlds and is addressed later on in this chapter.

primarily for communication; nonetheless, as we shall see, there are group differences (e.g., based on gender, ethnic group, and country of residence) in the use of particular online applications.

Social Networking Sites (SNSs)

As of Summer 2009, social networking sites or SNSs were the newest and more extensively used communication tool among youth (Reich, Subrahmanyam & Espinoza, 2009; Subrahmanyam, Reich, Waechter, & Espinoza, 2008). They allow users to create public or private profiles and form networks of "friends" with whom they can interact publicly (e.g., status updates or wall posts) and privately (e.g., private messages). SNS users can also post user-generated content (e.g., written notes, photos, and videos), which often elicit comments and result in further interaction.

Facebook and to a much lesser extent MySpace are the most widely used SNSs, but there are interfaces that are popular in other parts of world, such as Friendster, hi5, Orkut and Tagget.com (Wikipedia, 2009). As of September 2009, Facebook reported having more than 300 million users (Oreskovic, 2009). On large sample surveys of US youth, 55% (Lenhart & Madden, 2007) to 65% (Jones & Fox, 2009) reported that they used SNSs, and girls, particularly older ones, dominate the sites (Lenhart & Madden, 2007). In research studies with much smaller samples, 88% of high school students and 82% of college students used SNSs (Subrahmanyam et al., 2008). Within the USA, there are inter-group differences in the use of particular SNSs – more White youth report using Facebook compared to Latino youth, who tend to cluster on MySpace (Hargittai, 2007; Subrahmanyam et al., 2008), indicating that youth tend to gravitate to online venues that are also accessed by the other people in their lives. Evidence to date indicates that young people use SNSs to connect and reconnect with friends and family members (Subrahmanyam et al., 2008) (see Chapter 4).

Text Messaging

Text messaging or texting consists of short text messages up to 160 characters in length, usually exchanged between two cell/mobile phones or between the web and a mobile phone. In a recent survey conducted for The Wireless Trade Association, 14- to 19-year-old US youth reported that they spent equal amounts of time texting and talking; many (54% of the females and 40% of the males) claimed that their social life "would end or be worsened" without texting (Harris Interactive, 2008). Texting is mostly used to exchange messages with peers and centers around chatting (discussing activities and events, gossip, and homework help), planning (coordinating meeting arrangements), and coordinating communication (Grinter & Eldridge, 2001).

Blogs and Microblogs

Webblogs or blogs are personal web pages, which can be easily updated and where the entries are organized in reverse chronological order, such that newer entries are displayed before older entries (Herring, Scheidt, Bonus, & Wright, 2004). There are three basic kinds of blogs: filter blogs (content external to the bloggers such as links to world events), personal journals (content internal to the blog author such as his/her "thoughts and internal workings") and k(nowledge)-logs, which contain information and observations, generally with a technological focus (Herring et al., 2004). Although blogging was initially quite the rage among youth, the 2007 WIP data shown in Fig. 1.3 reveals that blogging, especially blog writing, is not that frequent in this age group. At the time when research was conducted, blogs were popular, we know that English language bloggers who presented themselves as teens[3] were also overwhelming female (87%) (Subrahmanyam, Garcia, Harsono, Li, & Lipana, 2009). Compared to adult blogs, which tend to have content external to the blogger (filter-type blogs and k-logs), youth blogs are typically personal journal-type blogs, are narrative and reflective in style, and contain themes related

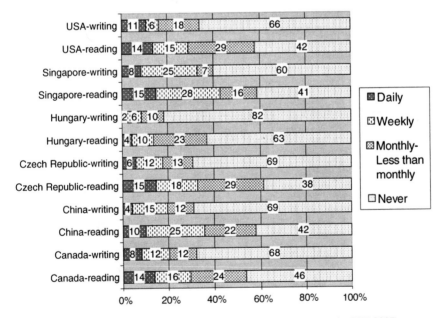

Fig. 1.3 Frequency of reading and writing blogs among 12- to 18-year olds (WIP 2007)

---

[3] Since the researchers only analyzed the blogs and did not actually contact the blog authors themselves, we have no way of knowing whether the bloggers were actually adolescents or not. This is another methodological concern that we tackle later on in this chapter.

to adolescents' peers and everyday lives implying that adolescent bloggers project offline narratives and themes onto their online blogs.

Microblogging is the latest entrant in this genre and essentially consists of very brief updates of text and multimedia (audio and video) sent via text messaging or the Internet. Twitter, the leading microblogging platform, allows users to update via "tweets," which are brief (140 characters) text-based updates sent via the Internet or text messaging to either a public or a private network of subscribers. At the time when we wrote this book in 2009, teens did not use twitter very much (TechCrunch, 2009), but we included it here since it is very much in the public eye and is very similar to the status updates on SNSs such as Facebook.

Online Phoning Applications

Adolescents also use the Internet to make phone calls or to audio chat using programs such as Skype and tools within Instant Messengers. From Fig. 1.4 we see that depending on their country of residence, between 5 and 29% of adolescents make online phone calls on a weekly basis. However, comparing Figs. 1.2 and 1.5, we see that adolescents use text-based chat such as instant messaging more often than audio chat. Many newer laptops have built-in web cams, and it is an open question whether use of voice and video chat will overtake older text-based communication formats.

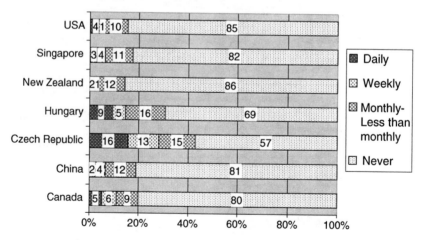

Fig. 1.4 Frequency of online phone calls among 12- to 18-year olds (WIP 2007)

Instant Messaging (IM)

Instant messaging is the synchronous exchange of a private message with another user; one can engage in multiple activities such as private messages simultaneously, switching back and forth between different conversation windows. Initially,

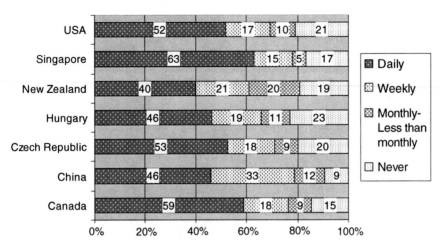

Fig. 1.5 Frequency of instant messaging among 12- to 18-year olds (WIP 2007)

messages used only text, but nowadays they allow attachments, voice or video calls, and even simple online games. Messenger services that are used the most by youth include AOL's Messenger or AIM, Microsoft Instant Messenger, Gchat (part of gmail), and BlackBerry Messenger. Figure 1.5 shows the frequency of instant message use among adolescents in the seven WIP countries. At least in the USA, teens use instant messaging to connect with offline friends to talk about "ordinary yet intimate topics" such as friends and gossip (Gross, 2004).

Online Gaming

According to the 2009 Pew Report, online gaming was the most frequent online activity among US teens with 78% reporting that they played them (Jones & Fox, 2009). Compared to stand-alone games played on a game system or computer, where one actually plays against the computer, online gamers play against several other online players, known or unknown to them. There are many different genres of online games including action games (e.g., Counter-Strike), strategy games (e.g., Civilization series), sports and simulators (i.e., NBA, NHL, soccer, F1, flight simulators etc.), role playing games (RPGs) (e.g., Perfect World, Maple Story), and logic or other games (i.e., chess, Tetris etc.).[4] A special category of RPGs are the Massively Multiplayer Online Role-Playing Games or MMORPGs such as World of Warcraft (WoW) and Everquest; set in online fantasy worlds, players assume game avatars or personas to explore the game world, interact and maybe fight with other players, and engage in other game-specific activities and quests. MMORPGs have

---

[4]Thanks to Roy Cheng, a youth gamer, for compiling this list.

been the subject of the most research, likely because of their potential for addiction, a topic we address in Chapter 9. Gaming research suggests that offline (Durkin & Barber, 2002) and online game playing (Griffiths, Davies, & Chappell, 2004) are the province of adolescent males compared to females. Figure 1.6 shows the frequency of online gaming among youth in the seven WIP countries.

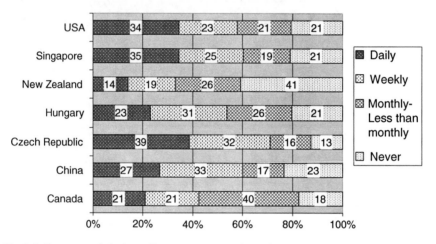

Fig. 1.6 Frequency of playing online games among 12- to 18-year olds (WIP 2007)

Chat Rooms

Chat rooms are online spaces where users interact with each other in real time; they can be either public or private. Typically, multiple-users participate in several simultaneous conversations occurring at the same time in the chat space (Greenfield & Subrahmanyam, 2003); users can also engage in "whispering", in which pairs of chat users engage in private IM conversations with each other. Early chat rooms were text-based, but subsequently, they incorporated audio and video chat. Participants in public chat rooms were often strangers to each other, unlike social networking sites, where most users interact with people they already know. Chat rooms were immensely popular when they first became available; however, safety concerns stemming from the potential to interact with strangers, especially adult predators, and the subsequent emergence of instant messaging and social networking sites led to their decline, at least among youth in some countries (see Fig. 1.7). Within chat rooms, participants adopt user names or nick names, which serve to identify their utterances in the public space. Often young users' nicknames contain information about the self, such as gender, interests, sexual personas (Subrahmanyam, Greenfield, & Tynes, 2004) and seem to be used for identity presentation (Subrahmanyam, Šmahel, & Greenfield, 2006) and partner selection (Šmahel & Subrahmanyam, 2007), which are important developmental issues and are discussed in Chapters 4 and 5.

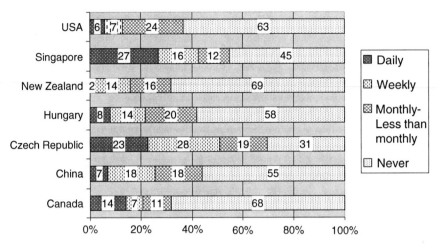

Fig. 1.7 Frequency of visiting chat rooms among 12- to 18-year olds (WIP 2007)

Virtual Worlds

Virtual worlds are three-dimensional spaces, where users assume *avatars* and engage in a variety of activities, depending on the particular environment in which they are immersed. Relatively new in the lives of young people, it is estimated that 20 million or 53% of online youth between 3 and 17 years will visit virtual worlds by 2011 (eMarketer, 2007). At the time of writing, virtual worlds were much more popular among younger children than older youth (Subrahmanyam, 2009). Examples of worlds designed for younger children are *Webkinz* and *Club Penguin*, whereas those for adolescents include *Second Life Teen Grid* and *Whyville*. The virtual world that has received the most press is *Second Life*, a three-dimensional virtual world for adult users 18 and older. A "Teen Grid" is separate form the main grid and is only open to teens between 13- and 17 years of age. Second Life residents can explore the world, meet other people and socialize with other residents by taking part in varied activities, such as concerts, classes, theaters, as well as creating and trading virtual property and services with each other. Whyville, a very different kind of virtual world for 8- to 16-year olds, allows users to engage in science and social activities (Fields & Kafai, 2007).

Bulletin Boards

Bulletin boards are public spaces, where users post messages asynchronously and there may or may not be a time lag between messages. However, unlike instant messaging or chat rooms, messages are not exchanged in real time, and are available for viewing long after they have been posted. In addition to actively exchanging information on bulletin boards, users can also passively "lurk," where they read but do not post any messages. Bulletin boards tend to be organized around a focal topic, such as college admissions, computer use, health, politics, and religion and interactions involve both the exchange of information, advice, as well as emotional support and encouragement. We do not know the extent to which adolescents' use bulletin boards, but research and anecdotal observations suggest that they do view and post on those focused on topics and issues central to their lives. For instance, we know that they use bulletin boards to find out information about general health and sexuality as well as about quintessentially adolescent problem behaviors such as cutting and anorexia – topics that we address in Chapters 8. As a parent of two teens, Subrahmanyam has observed young people participating in several US-based boards focused on college admissions, a very central issue in the lives of older adolescents. Bulletin boards based on sports are another example, and again she has observed her teen son, a sports-fanatic, spending hours on them.

Downloading Music and Videos

Downloading and listening to music and watching videos online are popular adolescent pastimes. The WIP data indicate that among 12- to 18-year-olds, it is the second most frequent online activity after the communication-based activities (see Fig. 1.2). From Figs. 1.8 and 1.9, we see that among youth in seven WIP countries, 80% or more download and listen to music on the Internet and 60% or more download and watch videos. Music, movies, and television are an integral part of youth sub-culture and college students report that downloading is an entertaining and convenient way to acquire music (Kinnally, Lacayo, McClung, & Sapolsky, 2008). Today, with more sophisticated computers and broadband technology, downloading is not limited to

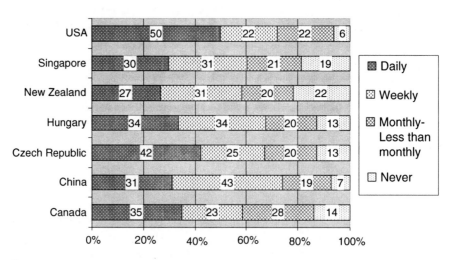

Fig. 1.8 Frequency of downloading/listening to music among 12- to 18-year olds (WIP 2007)

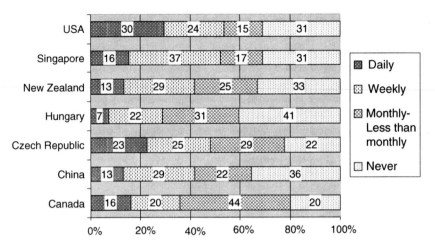

Fig. 1.9 Frequency of downloading/watching videos among 12- to 18-year olds (WIP 2007)

music and videos, and includes any kind of content, including movies, television shows, games, and podcasts; moreover, small and portable devices such as iPods ensure that this content can be accessed virtually anywhere and we expect these activities to become even more pervasive in the near future. There is of course the thorny issue of illegal downloading, a topic that we cover in Chapter 6.

Characteristics of Digital Communication Environments

Communication features prominently in young people's use of digital media such as computers and mobile phones. Yet by their very nature, these technologies provide a communication environment that is very different from that of face-to-face settings. Some important characteristics of digital communication contexts that we consider next include, disembodied users, text-based communication, disinhibited behavior, self-disclosure, use of emoticons, and multitasking as well as media-multitasking; keep in mind that each characteristic is present to different degrees in different communication forms, and even within a particular form, as it changes and evolves.

Disembodied Users

An important characteristic of most digital communication that occurs via a screen is that users are disembodied – in other words, information about their face and body is not always available as in face-to-face communication. This was particularly true for the early communication applications such as chat rooms, bulletin boards, and instant messaging. However, with web cams and the easy uploading of digital images, this is less true as users can upload digital representations of the self to convey basic identifying information such as their age and sex. Still there are differences relative to face-to-face settings. First, users can upload any representation that may or may not resemble their true selves. Second, even when such representations are available, other important real-time communication cues such as gaze, gestures, and body language remain missing. Such missing information presents both opportunities as well as challenges, and throughout the book, we will show how users, particularly young ones, have adapted to take advantage of the opportunities and circumvent the challenges that they present.

Anonymity

Because users are fundamentally disembodied when communicating via digital media, they also have the potential to be as anonymous as they wish to be. Indeed, the Internet was originally touted as a place where one could leave one's body behind (Kendall, 2003; Stallabrass, 1995; Wakeford, 1999). To some extent, this was true during the early days of the Internet. Because of the nature of technology (lower bandwidths, no images or video), the nature of the applications that were available (e.g., chat rooms, bulletin boards), and the fact that the Internet was not very diffuse, one was not as likely to meet and interact with friends and acquaintances while online. Anonymity on the Internet is much more complex today – users can choose to be anonymous on applications, such as bulletin boards and virtual worlds such as Second Life. However, anonymity may be virtually impossible on applications like social networking sites, where cues about the body and the self are readily available, and where teens may be more likely to interact with people whom they already know offline. Nevertheless, even when one is supposedly not anonymous, users can nonetheless fabricate their online identity or embellish parts of an otherwise true offline identity. Finally, online anonymity is hard to achieve, as every device on an online network has a Public IP address, and one needs to be technologically sophisticated to hide or mask an IP address.

Text-Based Communication

Most forms of digital communication are visual and text-based; they use alphanumeric characters, icons, pictures, and other visual representations and contain features of both written and oral language. Consider the conversations that occur in a chat room. Greenfield and Subrahmanyam (2003) have proposed that chat "takes place in the written medium (typing words on a keyboard and reading words on a screen), but like spoken language, particularly unplanned speech, it generally consists of shorter, incomplete, grammatically simple and often incorrect (grammar and typographical errors) sentences." Figure 1.10 shows an extract of an online teen chat room that illustrates these features.

15	Al commands:	WHAT HAPPENED MORN?
16	BLAKPower1413:	14
17	Agreatonefeb74:	kew1
18	Al commands:	HAHAHH
19	Al commands:	I AM WHAT?
20	SwimteamBabe:	a/s/l
21	SuddenReaction:	who is f*** dany
22	Al commands:	THE GREATEST?
23	Al commands:	YA, I KNOW
24	MORN8SUN:	*fuckdany?*
25	MORN8SUN:	*lol*
26	MORN8SUN:	*what?*
27	MizRose76:	AL DID I GIVE U PERMISSION TO TALK TO NE ONE?
28	PinkBabyAngel542:	WHO BELIEVE'S SPEEDO'S (ON GUYS) AREN'T RIGHT
29	PinkBabyAngel542:	TYPE 3
30	Al commands:	WHAT!!!
31	PinkBabyAngel542:	3
32	DustinKnosAll:	3
33	SwimteamBabe:	3
34	BrentJyd:	any fine ladies want to chat press 69 or im me
35	Al commands:	ARE YOU TRYING TO TALKBACK TO YOUR MASTER
36	Al commands:	??
37	Sportyman04:	hey

Fig. 1.10 Extract of a transcript from an online teen chat room analyzed by Greenfield and Subrahmanyam (2003)

This remains true of much of the interactions on other electronic communication applications such as e-mail, text messaging, instant messaging, and social networking sites, and we are seeing the emergence of a new electronic register (Greenfield & Subrahmanyam, 2003), variously called netspeak or textspeak (Crystal, 2004, 2006). A big part of Netspeak is the slang words and acronyms that users have created, teens are adept at using, and parents may have difficulty comprehending. Examples include, POS (parent over shoulder), BRB (be right back), GTG (got to go), IDK (I don't know), NIFOC (naked in front of computer), P911 (parent emergency), TDTM (talk dirty to me) (Ray, 2009). There are several online resources for those who wish to decode this register; for instance, the site www.noslang.com has both a slang dictionary and a slang translator.

Self-Disclosure and Disinhibition

There is considerable anecdotal and also experimental evidence that people behave in a disinhibited fashion and/or have high levels of self-disclosure on the Internet (Joinson, 2007). The decisive factor is probably the degree of anonymity one can experience on the Internet, as high anonymity often means greater self-disclosure, and vice versa. Research confirms that self-disclosure is higher in interactions occurring via text communication on the Internet than in the physical realm (Joinson, 2001); among undergraduate college students, spontaneous self-disclosure was higher in visually anonymous virtual discussions compared to face-to-face discussions. Within the context of computer-mediated communication, visually anonymous participants disclosed more than non-visually anonymous participants.

Regardless, youth may behave differently in different online environments, as some virtual contexts may be highly interconnected to their offline selves, whereas others may be less connected, and entail more experimenting with identity. Consequently, the level of self-disclosure and disinhibited behavior may vary in anonymous chat rooms as opposed to less anonymous social networking sites. Thus, when considering findings about self-disclosure, we should take into account the research method and the particular online context that was studied.

We will see in Chapters 2 and 5 that an important adolescent need is to develop intimate relationships that are based on openness, honesty, and self-disclosure (Brown, 2004). Research has found that during early and middle adolescence, there is an increase in self-disclosure to friends; this trend starts in early adolescence for girls and in middle adolescence for boys (Buhrmester & Prager, 1995). It is therefore not surprising that youth take advantage of the opportunities for self-disclosure that are available in digital contexts. In our own research, we have found that self-disclosure occurs in young people's online forays. For instance, teen bloggers self-disclosed often about their peers, families, partners as well as daily life (Subrahmanyam et al., 2009) and they report that they are mostly truthful when writing about their offline lives in their blogs (Blinka & Šmahel, 2009).

Use of Emoticons

On the face of it, text-based, disembodied online contexts, with their lack of facial cues and body language, should make it difficult to express and share emotions. Despite this, adolescents are very adept at conveying their emotions in their digital communication. In our analysis of English-language blogs written by teens, we found that 29% of entries contained explicit and strong emotions, such as anger, frustration, happiness, sadness and love. One important way that youth are able to do this is via their extensive use of emotional icons or "emoticons." Emoticons typically consist of characters that indicate a writer's mood or facial expression, e.g., :-), :-(, ;-), :-o, :-D, :D, :- P, =O, :-O; these commonly used emoticons convey a variety of emotions or states, from cheery and smiling to shock and surprise. Many online applications, such as instant messengers, chat room providers, and social networking sites also provide users with pre-formed graphic emoticons that they can easily insert into text-based communication. To adults, the meaning of the seemingly endless (and fast evolving) list of emoticons is not obvious, and many of us have probably had to look up online lists to glean their meaning. Therefore, it is fascinating to contemplate how young digital natives generate and transmit them with such apparent ease.

Given the widespread use of emoticons in electronic communication, an important question is whether they help Internet users to understand emotions in online communication (Šmahel, 2001, 2003b). Emoticons, particularly character-based ones, are much more ambiguous relative to face-to-face cues and may end up being interpreted very differently by different users. Nonetheless, research indicates that they are useful tools in online text-based communication (Derks, Bos, & von Grumbkow, 2008; Huang, Yen, & Zhang, 2008; Lo, 2008). One study of 137 IM users revealed that (Lo, 2008) emoticons allowed users to correctly understand the level and direction of emotion, attitude, and attention expression and that emoticons were a definite advantage in non-verbal communication. Similarly, another study showed that emoticons were useful in strengthening the intensity of a verbal message, as well as in the expression of sarcasm; it confirmed that they have an impact on message interpretation (Derks et al., 2008) and can thus similar serve functions as nonverbal behavior.

Media-Multitasking and Multitasking

Media multitasking is the practice of using different media (e.g., television and the Internet) at the same time. Electronic multitasking is the phenomenon of simultaneously using multiple computer applications (e.g., Internet and word processing applications), multiple windows of the same application (e.g., multiple instant message windows) (Subrahmanyam & Greenfield, 2008a), or even multiple attention targets in the same application window (as in an action video game with multiple, often simultaneous things occurring at different locations on the screen). Much of young people's technology use occurs in a multitasking context (Gross, 2004; Roberts et al., 2005); see Fig. 1.11 for a computer screen shot showing the multiple open windows on a teen's computer. In her 2006 article on the multitasking generation, Claudia Wallis described Piers, a 14-year old, in his bedroom in front of his computer at 9:30 p.m. as being "logged onto to a MySpace chat room and AOL messenger for the past 3 h." Also open were a Google Images window, several instant messaging windows, and iTunes, through which he was listening to a mix of music. All the while he was working on a Word file – an English class – and he reported that he gets "it done a little bit at time" (Wallis, 2006).

Such media multitasking is becoming the norm among young people. In the 2005 Kaiser Report, Roberts and colleagues found that 8- to 18-year olds in the USA consumed about 8.5 h of media content in approximately 6.5 h time, which incidentally held steady from the previous report. Multitasking is certainly not limited to young people. In a study of 1,319 Americans from different generations, combining of different tasks occurred frequently among all generations, especially while listening to music or eating (Carrier, Cheever, Rosen, Benitez, & Chang, 2009). However, members of the youngest generation (the Net-Generation, which the authors refer to as individuals born after the year 1978) reported more multitasking than other generations.

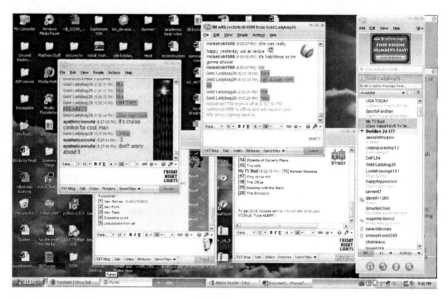

Fig. 1.11 Computer screen shot showing the multiple open windows on a teen's computer screen

We know very little about why young people are so enamored of multitasking. Consider what one young girl told us about multitasking while instant messaging: *Good net users manage about five people. They have one in one window, the second in the second window, and so on. So it's a bit different, like if you were sitting in three pubs at the same time. In three different pubs* (Šmahel, 2003a).

Another 15-year old girl told us: *It's intoxicating- you simply feel great...you're the centre of attention...that's the state when everyone is writing till you can't keep up.* Perhaps they simply like to communicate with more people simultaneously because it makes them feel important, or it enables them to obtain support from more members of their peer group, or may be even diverts them from the stresses of their own life. Alternatively, perhaps the feeling of not being able to keep up with their communication partners is intoxicating in itself; in the words of another girl: *I had the feeling that I couldn't keep up because I had so many friends that I can't even manage to talk with all of them.* These statements suggest adolescents may associate simultaneous electronic communication with multiple peers with positive feelings, feelings that may be comparable to the adrenaline rush that accompanies success in sports.

Despite its popularity, multitasking may come with some costs. In the study by Carrier et al. (2009) described earlier, participants reported that they experienced difficulties while multitasking, although those in the younger generation reported lower difficulty ratings compared to older generations. There was agreement across generations as to which tasks could be combined together (such as listening to music while eating or surfing the web while telephoning) leading the researchers to conclude that participants of all generations might share similar limitations on the ability to multitask. There are likely some social costs entailed because of multitasking as well. In our work with youth, we have heard of incidents where a youth accidentally sent a text intended for a romantic partner to a casual friend (certainly embarrassing!) or upset a peer because he/she was inattentive when interacting with them. We also suspect that multitasking very likely impacts parent–child interactions and family relationships, an issue that merits further study.

Studying Young People's Digital Worlds

We have shown thus far that the youth digital landscape is as varied as it is complex, and studying their role in development is not an easy task. Here we consider issues that arise while doing research on young people's digital worlds; when considering the role of technology in development, we must be cognizant of the logistical and methodological considerations that have hampered research on this topic.

Logistical Considerations

For researchers, one of the biggest challenges has been keeping up with the technology that teens actually use and there are several reasons for this. First, over the last decade, interactive technologies have been changing at a very rapid pace. Second, among young people, the popularity of electronic gadgets (e.g., Razr phone, i-Phone) and online applications (e.g., chat rooms and blogs) resemble fashion fads – hot and insanely popular for a while, then tapering off. Some online applications (e.g., instant messaging or social networking sites) and gadgets (mobile devices that can be used to phone, instant message, etc.) seem to have longer lasting power and may be here to stay. Third, not only do applications change, but also as we noted earlier, norms and behaviors within them are constantly in flux. Fourth, compared to adults young people are more likely to be early adopters of technology, and to become very proficient (in terms of speed and skill) at using them. Because of all of these reasons, adult researchers, generally considered digital immigrants, have the unenviable task of trying to play catch-up when it comes to studying the online behavior of young digital natives.

This has happened to us repeatedly when we first began to study young people's use of the Internet. By the time we recognized the popularity of chat rooms among youth, procured funding, designed our study, received approval from Institutional Review Boards, and conducted our study chat rooms had peaked. Even as we analyzed our data, wrote up our results, and published it, young people had moved on to instant messaging and blogs. Researchers who are interested in studying online behavior must change how they conduct their research – they have to be flexible and readily adapt their methods as the technology changes. By all indications, they are recognizing this, and we have already seen several articles and compilations about social networking site use among college students.

Another challenge is that as digital immigrants, adult researchers in effect adopt an outsider's perspective when studying adolescents' online worlds and virtual behavior; in other words, they use what the linguist Kenneth Pike called an *etic* approach. Such an approach might hinder their ability to study and understand young people's online behavior. Consider our experience when we first began to study online teen chat rooms. We could not make sense of a printed transcript of a chat conversation. Repeated examination of the transcripts gradually began to reveal some meaningful utterances, but we were still at a loss until a lab meeting, when a graduate student in her early twenties, mapped out the different conversation threads for us. We also spent a lot of time in adult chat rooms, as observers and then participants, sometimes asking other users to explain codes and conventions. All of these efforts culminated in our work on conversational coherence (Greenfield & Subrahmanyam, 2003) and on the construction of developmental processes (Šmahel & Subrahmanyam, 2007; Subrahmanyam et al., 2004, 2006) in online teen chat contexts.

Ideally, we should try to use such an *emic* approach, one where the researcher is a participant observer within the online culture under study. This was much easier when online contexts were public and we were able to gain access within them to observe and record online interactions. This is of course much harder to do nowadays as applications are either private (e.g., instant messaging) or have privacy controls that youth can use to limit access to those they choose (e.g., social networking sites such as MySpace and Facebook). Although this seems to be a challenge, creative solutions can be found, such as having teenage informants and research assistants; researchers at the Children's Digital Media Center @ Los Angeles have also used focus groups of MySpace users and have had MySpace users conduct video tours of their sites (Manago, Graham, Greenfield, & Salimkhan, 2008).

Methodological Considerations

A fundamental methodological issue is the problem of the non-existent control group; experimental and control groups are the time-honored tradition by which psychologists arrive at causal inferences when studying the effect of one variable on the other. However, because of the rapid diffusion of technology, at any given time, only small numbers of youth do not use the more popular online applications. Finding an *equivalent* control group of teens, who do not use the Internet or a particular application or use it less frequently, is well neigh impossible today, even in less-industrialized countries. Even if one did find such a group, the technology using and non-using groups would not be truly comparable, limiting what one could conclude about the Internet's effects. Longitudinal data are a way around this problem and two examples of this approach include Steinfield, Ellison, and Lampe's (2008) study of the relation between self-esteem, Facebook use, and social capital among college students and Eijnden and colleagues' s study of the relation between online communication, compulsive Internet use, and well-being among adolescents (Eijnden, Meerkerk, Vermulst, Spijkerman, & Engels, 2008).

Another methodological problem is that of operationalizing and measuring online behavior. Online time use is one of the more vexing of Internet variables to study. To highlight this problem we ask the reader to estimate the average amount of time he/she spends online every day, including a breakdown of the three most frequent online activities. Pretty soon it becomes obvious that this is a very difficult task to do – not only because the Internet has become such a big part of our every day lives, from e-mail, to health information, to movie ticket bookings, to directions, to recipes, and so on, but also because so much of this use occurs when we are multitasking. We consider the issue of time in further detail in Chapter 7, where we discuss the effect of Internet use on well-being. Other aspects of technology, such as the particular applications used, the activities within them, the people interacted with, are equally hard to measure. One option is to use software that automatically records online activities, but their use raises privacy and ethical concerns, and the interesting problem of data overload. Self-reports tend to be the most frequently used method of measuring Internet use and the reader is advised to keep in mind their limitations (e.g., memory loss, biased estimates) when we consider research that utilized such measures.

Ascertaining details about participants' identity such as their age, sex, race, and location is another important methodological challenge when studying online behavior. Greenfield and Yan (2006) point out that in developmental research, age, gender, and race are reported as a matter of course. In fact, they are important pieces of information that must be known when attempting to identify developmental trends and differences (Subrahmanyam & Greenfield, 2008b). Yet these basic pieces of information about participants are not always available in anonymous online contexts, such as chat rooms and bulletin boards; similarly, in anonymous online surveys, we do not even know if participants or respondents are correctly reporting their age, gender, and other demographic details. Even when available, such as in blog profiles, self-reported age, gender, or location information might not be accurate; in our blog study a few participants even reported that they were from "Antarctica" (Subrahmanyam et al., 2009). The challenge for researchers is to obtain both accurate age and sex information as well as ecologically valid online assessments (Subrahmanyam & Greenfield, 2008b). Some ways of accomplishing this is by recruiting subjects offline and then sending them links to online surveys (Subrahmanyam et al., 2009), or recruiting participants via e-mail in a bounded community, such as a university campus (Steinfield et al., 2008).

Goals and Organization of the Book

Our goal is to examine adolescents' use of interactive technology as well as the developmental implications of such use. Chapter 2 presents our developmental approach with an overview of adolescence (adolescent developmental tasks, such as sexuality and intimacy and the role of the context in development) and the theoretical framework that we adopt in this book. In line with this developmental treatment, Chapters 3, 4, and 5 will show how young people use digital technology in the service of core adolescent developmental issues of sexuality, identity, and intimacy. Chapter 6 does the same for the development of ethics, morality, and engagement to one's communities, a less central but nonetheless important adolescent developmental issue.

The second part of the book examines some of the practical implications of young people's technology use. In Chapters 7 and 8, we examine how technology use is related to well being – directly as an information resource and indirectly as a tool for providing interventions and treatment. Chapters 9 and 10 address the darker and more unsavory aspects of technology in young people's lives – online addictive behavior (Chapter 9) and violent and hateful content and aggressive interactions including cyber bullying by peers and sexual solicitation and victimization by predatory strangers/adults (Chapter 10). In Chapter 11, we will see what different stakeholders (e.g., parents, government) can do to protect youth from harmful online content and victimization. In Chapter 12, we present a summary and a synthesis of what it means to be an adolescent living life online in digital contexts, identify some common and enduring themes that we encountered throughout, and look ahead to the future.

Although our goal is to present a comprehensive developmental account of young people's interactions with new technologies, we do not review all the studies on this topic. Instead, we identify and highlight topics and research studies that, in our opinion, can help us to come to a better understanding of the developmental implications of adolescents' digital lives. Even though we set out to examine the different kinds of digital technologies used by youth, extant research has largely focused on the Internet and online applications accessed via computers, and so our discussion reflects this state of the field as well. However, for ease of writing, we occasionally use the terms digital media, technology, online contexts, and digital contexts interchangeably and synonymously with the term "Internet" and "Internet contexts." Similarly, at times we use the words "teens," and "youth" in place of "adolescents." Finally, we avoid the phrase "real world" to refer to offline, physical worlds, since we cannot discount the possibility that for youth, virtual worlds may be more real than even so-called real worlds.

We highlight different online applications and electronic contexts in different chapters – for instance, texting, instant messaging and social networking sites are discussed in Chapter 4, gaming in Chapters 9 and 10, web surfing in Chapter 8 and online music content in Chapter 10. As we wrote our book, we were very mindful that digital media operate like a fad, and an online application that is very much the rage at the time when we wrote this chapter, might very well be fading in popularity by the time the book was published. Therefore, we included a study on an application if the results were relevant to development, regardless of whether teens were still using it. It is our hope that a developmental approach will give the reader a timeless account of digital media in young people's lives, one that will still be relevant even when newer and more sophisticated applications have replaced the currently available ones.

References

Blinka, L., & Šmahel, D. (2009). Fourteen is fourteen and a girl is a girl: Validating the identity of adolescent bloggers. *Cyberpsychology & Behavior, 12*, 735–739.

Brown, B. B. (2004). Adolescents' relationships with peers. In M. R. Lerner & L. Steinberg (Eds.), *Handbook of adolescent psychology* (2nd ed.). Hoboken, NJ: Wiley.

Buhrmester, D., & Prager, K. (1995). Patterns and functions of self-disclosure during childhood and adolescence. In K. J. Rotenberg (Ed.), *Disclosure processes in children and adolescents* (pp. 10–56). New York, NY: Cambridge University Press.

Carrier, L. M., Cheever, N. A., Rosen, L. D., Benitez, S., & Chang, J. (2009). Multitasking across generations: Multitasking choices and difficulty ratings in three generations of Americans. *Computers in Human Behavior, 25*, 483–489.

Crystal, D. (2004). *A glossary of netspeak and textspeak*. Edinburgh: Edinburgh University Press.

Crystal, D. (2006). *Language and the internet*. Cambridge: Cambridge University Press.

Derks, D., Bos, A. E. R., & von Grumbkow, J. (2008). Emoticons and online message interpretation. *Social Science Computer Review, 26*, 379–388.

Durkin, K., & Barber, B. (2002). Not so doomed: Computer game play and positive adolescent development. *Journal of Applied Developmental Psychology, 23*, 373–392.

Eijnden, R., Meerkerk, G. J., Vermulst, A. A., Spijkerman, R., & Engels, R. (2008). Online communication, compulsive internet use, and psychosocial well-being among adolescents: A longitudinal study. *Developmental Psychology, 44*, 655–665.

Europa Press-Release. (2009). *Commission calls on mobile operators to continue to improve child safety policies* [Electronic version]. Retrieved August 14, 2009, from http://europa.eu/rapid/pressReleasesAction.do?reference=IP/09/596

eMarketer. (2007). Kids and teens: Virtual Worlds Open New Universe. Retrieved 16 July, 2009, from http://www.emarketer.com/Report.aspx?code=emarketer_2000437

Fields, D. A., & Kafai, Y. B. (2007) *Stealing from grandma or generating cultural knowledge? Contestations and effects of cheats in a tween virtual world*. Paper presented at the Situated Play, Proceedings of DiGRA 2007 conference. Retrieved March 4, 2009, from http://www.gseis.ucla.edu/faculty/kafai/paper/whyville_pdfs/DIGRA07_cheat.pdf

Greenfield, P. M., & Subrahmanyam, K. (2003). Online discourse in a teen chatroom: New codes and new modes of coherence in a visual medium. *Journal of Applied Developmental Psychology, 24*, 713–738.

Greenfield, P. M., & Yan, Z. (2006). Children, adolescents, and the internet: A new field of inquiry in developmental psychology. *Developmental Psychology, 42*, 391–394.

Griffiths, M. D., Davies, M. N. O., & Chappell, D. (2004). Online computer gaming: A comparison of adolescent and adult gamers. *Journal of Adolescence, 27*, 87–96.

Grinter, R. E., & Eldridge, M. (2001). *y do tngrs luv 2 txt msg*. Paper presented at the seventh European conference on computer-supported cooperative work ECSCW'01, Dordrecht, the Netherlands.

Gross, E. F. (2004). Adolescent internet use: What we expect, what teens report. *Journal of Applied Developmental Psychology, 25*, 633–649.

Hargittai, E. (2007). Whose space? Differences among users and non-users of social network sites. *Journal of Computer-Mediated Communication, 13, Article 14*. Retrieved November 27, 2009, from http://jcmc.indiana.edu/vol13/issue1/hargittai.html

Harris Interactive. (2008). Teenagers: A generation unplugged. Retrieved November 27, 2009 from http://files.ctia.org/pdf/HI_TeenMobileStudy_ResearchReport.pdf

Herring, S. C., Scheidt, L. A., Bonus, S., & Wright, E. (2004). *Bridging the gap: A genre analysis of weblogs*. Paper presented at the Procceedings of the 37th Hawai'i International Conference on System Sciences, Hawai.

Huang, A. H., Yen, D. C., & Zhang, X. N. (2008). Exploring the potential effects of emoticons. *Information & Management, 45*, 466–473.

Joinson, A. N. (2001). Self-disclosure in computer-mediated communication: The role of self-awareness and visual anonymity. *European Journal of Social Psychology, 31,* 177–192.

Joinson, A. N. (2007). Disinhibition and the internet. In J. Gackenbach (Ed.), *Psychology and the internet* (pp. 75–92). San Diego, CA: Academic Press.

Jones, S., & Fox, S. (2009). *Generations online in 2009.* Retrieved February 9, 2009, from http://pewresearch.org/pubs/1093/generations-online

Kendall, L. (2003). Cyberspace. In S. Jones (Ed.), *Encyclopedia of new media* (pp. 112–114). Thousand Oaks, CA: Sage.

Kinnally, W., Lacayo, A., McClung, S., & Sapolsky, B. (2008). Getting up on the download: College students' motivations for acquiring music via the web. *New Media Society, 10,* 893–913.

Lebo, H., Cole, J. I., Suman, M., Schramm, P., Zhou, L., Salvador, A., et al. (2009). *World internet project international report 2009.* Los Angeles, LA: Center for the Digital Future.

Lenhart, A., & Madden, M. (2007). Social networking websites and teens: An overview. *Pew Internet & American Life Project,* Retrieved November 28, 2009 from http://www.pewinternet.org/~/media//Files/Reports/2007/PIP_SNS_Data_Memo_Jan_2007.pdf.pdf

Lo, S. K. (2008). The nonverbal communication functions of emoticons in computer-mediated communication. *Cyberpsychology & Behavior, 11,* 595–597.

Manago, A. M., Graham, M. B., Greenfield, P. M., & Salimkhan, G. (2008). Self-presentation and gender on MySpace. *Journal of Applied Developmental Psychology, 29,* 446–458.

Oreskovic, A. (2009). *Facebook makes money, tops 300 million users.* Retrieved September 16, 2009, from http://news.yahoo.com/s/nm/us_facebook

Prensky, M. (2001). Digital natives, digital immigrants. *On the Horizon, 9*(5), 1–6.

Ray, R. (2009). *Netspeak and internet slang (Weblog).* Retrieved August 10, 2009, from http://www.wordskit.com/blog/words/netspeak-and-internet-slang-words/

Reich, S. M., Subrahmanyam, K., & Espinoza, G. E. (2009). *Adolescents' use of social networking sites - Should we be concerned?* Paper presented at the Society for Research on Child Development, Denver, CO.

Roberts, D. F., & Foehr, U. G. (2008). Trends in media use. *The Future of Children, 18*(1), 11–37.

Roberts, D. F., Foehr, U. G., & Rideout, V. (2005). *Generation M: Media in the lives of 8–18 Year-olds – report.* Retrieved December 16, 2008 from http://www.kff.org/entmedia/7251.cfm

Šmahel, D. (2001). Electronic communication and its specifics. *Ceskoslovenska Psychologie, 45,* 252–258.

Šmahel, D. (2003a). Communication of adolescents in the internet environment. *Ceskoslovenska Psychologie, 47,* 144–156.

Šmahel, D. (2003b). *Psychologie a internet: děti dospělými, dospělí dětmi. [Psychology and internet: Children being adults, adults being children.].* Prague: Triton.

Šmahel, D., & Subrahmanyam, K. (2007).'Any girls want to chat press 911': Partner selection in monitored and unmonitored teen chat rooms. *CyberPsychology & Behavior, 10,* 346–353.

Stallabrass, J. (1995). Empowering technology: The exploration of cyberspace. *New Left Review, 1/211,* 3–32.

Steinfield, C., Ellison, N. B., & Lampe, C. A. C. (2008). Social capital, self-esteem, and use of online social network sites: A longitudinal analysis. *Journal of Applied Developmental Psychology, 29,* 434–445.

Subrahmanyam, K. (2009). Developmental implications of children's virtual worlds. *Washington and Lee Law Review, 66,* 1065–1084.

Subrahmanyam, K., Garcia, E. C., Harsono, S. L., Li, J., & Lipana, L. (2009). In their words: Connecting online weblogs to developmental processes. *British Journal of Developmental Psychology, 27,* 219–245.

Subrahmanyam, K., & Greenfield, P. M. (2008a). Online communication and adolescent relationships. *The Future of Children, 18,* 119–146.

Subrahmanyam, K., & Greenfield, P. M. (2008b). Virtual worlds in development: Implications of social networking sites. *Journal of Applied Developmental Psychology, 29,* 417–419.

Subrahmanyam, K., Greenfield, P. M., & Tynes, B. M. (2004). Constructing sexuality and identity in an online teen chat room. *Journal of Applied Developmental Psychology: An International Lifespan Journal, 25*, 651–666.

Subrahmanyam, K., Reich, S. M., Waechter, N., & Espinoza, G. (2008). Online and offline social networks: Use of social networking sites by emerging adults. *Journal of Applied Developmental Psychology, 29*, 420–433.

Subrahmanyam, K., Šmahel, D., & Greenfield, P. M. (2006). Connecting developmental constructions to the internet: Identity presentation and sexual exploration in online teen chat rooms. *Developmental Psychology, 42*, 395–406.

TechCrunch. (2009). Why don't teens tweet? We asked over 10,000 of them. Retrieved September 20, 2009, from http://www.techcrunch.com/2009/08/30/why-dont-teens-tweet-we-asked-over-10000-of-them/

Wakeford, N. (1999). Gender and the landscapes of computing in an internet café. In M. Crang, P. Crang, & J. May (Eds.), *Virtual geographies: Bodies, space, and relations* (pp. 178–202). London: Routledge.

Wallis, C. (2006). The multitasking generation. *Time Magazine, 167*, 48–56.

Wikipedia. (2009). *List of social networking websites*. Retrieved January 7, 2009, from http://en.wikipedia.org/wiki/List_of_social_networking_websites

Chapter 2
Connecting Online Behavior to Adolescent Development: A Theoretical Framework

Wedged between childhood and emerging adulthood, adolescence is a period of tremendous change – biological, psychological, and social. In fact, Stanley Hall (1904) characterized it as a period of "storm and stress" and this belief remains strong in popular culture and in the minds of many parents. Although researchers have come to recognize that adolescence is not always a turbulent period (Steinberg, 2008), the storm and stress view, for better or worse, has come to frame much of the discourse about the role of interactive technologies in adolescent life. Digital worlds have become a part of adolescent life, and some see it as a threat or obstacle to an already difficult transition. Our goal in this book is to examine the role of digital media in adolescent development and this chapter presents the developmental approach that we will use to frame our discussion. The first part of the chapter will briefly review what developmental psychology has already taught us about adolescence – the challenges and the factors, particularly contextual ones that affect adolescent development. The second part of the chapter examines the role of digital media during adolescence and presents our theoretical position that adolescents' online and offline worlds are psychologically connected.

Lessons from Developmental Psychology

The psychologist John P. Hill in his now classic 1983 paper laid out a very influential research agenda for adolescence. In it, he argued that in order to understand adolescent development, researchers had to use a three-pronged approach, one which emphasized the fundamental changes, contexts, and psychosocial tasks of adolescence (Hill, 1983; Steinberg, 2008). We draw on his model of adolescence as we try to understand adolescents' digital lives.

Changes During Adolescence

Perhaps the most distinctive aspects of adolescence are the inevitable biological, cognitive, and social changes that adolescents experience, regardless of which

K. Subrahmanyam, D. Šmahel, *Digital Youth*, Advancing Responsible
Adolescent Development, DOI 10.1007/978-1-4419-6278-2_2,
© Springer Science+Business Media, LLC 2011

particular city, town, or country they live in (Steinberg, 2008). The biological changes of puberty include rapid changes in height and weight as well as in sexual maturation leading ultimately to adult body size and capabilities, including sexual reproduction (Tanner, 1978). Adolescence is also marked by tremendous cognitive advances, including the ability to think abstractly and to think and reason about hypothetical situations (Inhelder & Piaget, 1999; Steinberg, 2008). Compared to children, adolescents engage in more advanced and sophisticated thinking, but some aspects of cognitive functioning are still developing, especially those governed by the pre-frontal cortex of the brain. Recent research indicates that these areas of the brain, particularly in parts of the frontal lobe, are still developing during adolescence and are not completely developed until the early 20's or so (Sowell, Thompson, Holmes, Jernigan, & Toga, 1999; Sowell, Thompson, Tessner, & Toga, 2001). Finally, there are changes in the individual's social status, in his or her rights, responsibilities, and privileges at this time of life. In most western societies, young people are given greater freedom, are able to drive, drop out of school, take up a job, join the army, start dating, be sexually active, and even get married (Steinberg, 2008).

Developmental Tasks and Issues

Hill also pointed out the need for more research on the psychosocial issues of adolescence including, attachment, autonomy, sexuality, intimacy, achievement, and identity. He argued that research on these issues should take into account the biological and cognitive changes, as well as changes in social definition that are part of adolescence. Developmental psychologists refer to challenges or expectations that a culture has for individuals in different life phases as developmental tasks. According to Havighurst (Havighurst, 1972), "a developmental task is a task that arises at or about a certain period in the life of the individual, successful achievement of which leads to his happiness and to success with later tasks, while failure leads to unhappiness in the individual, disapproval by the society, and difficulty with later tasks." He listed the developmental tasks faced by individuals in different life stages from infancy to middle adulthood and later maturity, noting that the particular tasks could vary depending on where the individual lived. According to Havighurst, American adolescents in the 1970s had to master the following developmental tasks:

1. Achieving new and more mature relations with age-mates of both sexes – As their bodies change physically and sexually with the onset of puberty, adolescents have to learn to establish new relations with their age mates, both boys and girls. Social activities and social experimentation become pre-eminent and help them learn adult social skills leading to good social adjustment throughout their lives.
2. Achieving a masculine or feminine social role – Puberty highlights the physical differences between the sexes and adolescents have to accept and adopt societal

ideas about the approved social roles for males and females. Havighurst added that the roles themselves are changing and that adolescents, particularly girls, have more choices in front of them than ever before.

3. Accepting one's physique and using the body effectively – Changes in the body and changes in interests and attitudes go together with adolescent sexual maturation. The adolescent thus has to learn to accept as well as to protect his or her body.

4. Achieving emotional independence from parents and other adults – The adolescents' emotional ties to his or her parents changes and he/she has to become independent and autonomous from them, while at the same time developing affection for them and respect for older adults.

5. Preparing for marriage and family life – Adolescents have to develop a positive attitude toward family life; according to Havighurst, girls also had to become knowledgeable about home management and child rearing.

6. Preparing for an economic career – The adolescent has to plan and prepare for an occupation that will enable him or her to make a living and become economically independent. In our complex modern society, with its emphasis on skilled labor, most occupations require considerable preparation. Consequently, for young people, this task takes precedence over the other tasks (e.g., finding a romantic partner).

7. Acquiring a set of values and an ethical system as a guide to behavior or developing an ideology – The adolescent has to construct a coherent socio-politico-ethical ideology that will consistently orient him or her over time and space. This task is accomplished via discussions involving moral questions, reflections about the rational aspects of religion and ethics, and by appealing to moral principles when trying to solve social problems.

8. Desiring and achieving socially responsible behavior – The adolescent has to become a participating and responsible member of the social groups that he/she belongs to, such as the community and larger society. This requires that the adolescent sacrifice for the greater good and develop an ideology that is consistent with the values of his/her society.

Although adolescence has changed significantly since the 1970s and 1980s when Havighurst first wrote about these issues, most are relevant even today. Only tasks five (preparing for marriage and family life) and six (preparing for an economic career) are less central for today's adolescents. Today, most adolescents are not actively preparing for marriage and family life as in earlier times. For instance high school courses on home economics, when offered, are now often called family and consumer sciences, focus more on vocational training and making a living (Trickey, 2003), and are not exclusively for girls. Similarly, although it is now rare for adolescent dating to result in marriage and a family as it did for previous generations of adolescents (Gordon & Miller, 1984), it prepares young people for future intimate relations. With regard to task 6, young people have to spend much more time in formal education settings to get ready for future work roles (Steinberg, 2008); consequently although most adolescents today are still in high school they are not actively preparing for an economic career, in the sense that young people did 50 years ago. Still although many of today's adolescents may not be actively preparing for an economic career, they are spending more time in formal schooling, an investment that is ultimately relevant to their future career and ability to make a living.

These trends have led psychologist Jeffrey Arnett (2000, 2004) to coin the term *emerging adulthood* to describe the transitional period in human development between late adolescence and young adulthood in cultural contexts, such as in industrialized societies, where marriage and parenthood are delayed until the late twenties or beyond. According to Arnett, emerging adulthood is a "time of exploration and instability, a self-focused age, and an age of possibilities" (p. 21). Two important developmental challenges faced by individuals in this life phase are those of identity achievement and the development of intimacy. While Erikson regarded identity as a quintessentially adolescent crisis (Erikson, 1959; Kroger, 2003), we now know that emerging adults are still grappling with some aspects of their identities, such as their vocational/career, religious, and ethnic identities (Côté, 2006).

Emerging adults also have to establish intimacy via interconnections with friends, romantic partners, as well as relatives and family members. Although there is some overlap in the challenges faced by adolescents and emerging adults, the two are nonetheless distinct developmental periods with their own unique challenges and opportunities and our focus in this book is on adolescents. We operationalized adolescence as including middle and high school students up to 18 years of age and emerging adulthood as including college students, 18 years and older. Although Arnett did not specify that high school graduation signaled the end of adolescence or that the college years were synonymous with emerging adulthood, we adopted this definition since the college years in the USA and other industrialized nations offer individuals with the independence, opportunities for exploration, and self-directed focus that he envisioned for emerging adults. Consequently, we mostly drew from research on adolescents in middle and high school. Where this was not possible and we based our discussion on research with college students, we have pointed this out to the reader. In the next sub-section, we briefly describe the three adolescent developmental challenges around which the first part of this book is organized – adjusting to one's developing sexuality, formulating a coherent identity, and establishing intimate relations with peers and romantic partners (Brown, 2004; Erikson, 1950; Weinstein & Rosen, 1991).

Sexuality. Adolescents have to adjust to their developing sexuality, in particular their increased sexual drive and interest in sex and spend a lot of time using sex slang, talking about sex, exchanging sexual jokes and sex-oriented literature (Weinstein & Rosen, 1991). They are also sexually active (Mosher, Chandra, & Jones, 2005; Savin-Williams & Diamond, 2004) and the rate of sexual activity increases with age (Cubbin, Santelli, Brindis, & Braveman, 2005). Adolescents' developing sexuality and sexual behavior leads them to initiate and engage in romantic relationships (Teare, Garrett, Coughlin, & Shanahan, 1995), and these relationships come to play a central role in their lives (Furman, 2002). Their romantic relationships are a source of support to them and also contribute to other aspects of their development such as their identity, sexuality, peer and family relationships, as well as scholastic achievement and career paths (Furman & Shaffer, 2003; Furman, 2002). Romantic relationships are also a source of concern and stress for adolescents as evidenced by the finding that more than half of all the calls to a national telephone hotline dealt with relationship issues (Teare et al., 1995).

Identity. A second task facing adolescents is that of constructing a coherent and stable identity, which includes gender, sexual, moral, political, religious, and vocational components (Erikson, 1959; Kroger, 2003). A coherent sense of self is one in which the individual is comfortable with who and where the self is headed (Erikson, 1959, 1968) and includes both a "conscious sense of individual uniqueness. As well as an unconscious striving for continuity of experience" (Kroger, 2003, p. 206). Identity exploration and commitment are important and even necessary for healthy identity development. Empirical research suggests that the search for identity begins during adolescence, but a coherent identity is typically not established until late adolescence and emerging adulthood (Nurmi, Lerner, & Steinberg, 2004; Reis & Youniss, 2004; Waterman, 1999).

Interconnections and intimacy. Peers and then romantic partners become increasingly important during adolescence (Furman, Brown, & Feiring, 1999) and developing intimate relationships with them is the third important task for adolescents. These relationships should be viewed in the context of adolescents' developing autonomy and independence and distance from their families (Brown, 2004; Ryan, 2001). Research has documented adolescents' need for close friends (Pombeni, Kirchler, & Palmonari, 1990) and their desire for emotional fulfillment, intimacy, and companionship from friends and romantic partners (Connolly, Furman, & Konarski, 2000; Larson & Richards, 1991). Over the course of adolescence, these relationships acquire the hallmarks of intimacy as they come to involve openness, honesty, and self-disclosure (Brown, 2004). Self-disclosure to friends increases during early and middle adolescence and eventually adolescents self-disclose more to their friends than their parents (Buhrmester & Prager, 1995).

The Role of the Context in Adolescent Development

Hill also stressed the importance of studying the effects of adolescents' social networks, such as their peers, families, schools, churches, and job settings on their behavior and development. Indeed, research over the past few decades has shown that contexts such as peers, families, and schools mediate how youth cope with the developmental issues before them. Of particular interest to us is the role of peers as adolescents' cope with the developmental challenges that they face. For example, research suggests that when making decisions about sexual behavior, adolescents turn to their peers for support and peer communication is an important source of information about sex (Kallen, Stephenson, & Doughty, 1983; Ward, 2004). Romantic relationships are also a major topic of adolescent conversation (Furman & Shaffer, 2003). At least for heterosexual adolescents, peers play an important role in the development of romantic relationships as their initial interactions with the opposite sex occur in a group context (Furman, 2002). Similarly, peers also play an important role in the task of identity formulation. In addition to sex and romance, other popular topics in adolescent peer conversations include appearance (Giblin, 2004) and the self (Johnson & Aries, 1983), issues important to identity construction. At a broader level, adolescents are also part of crowds (e.g., "jocks", "geeks", "drammies", etc), which involve "identification of adolescents who share a similar image or reputation among peers" (Brown, 2004). According to Steinberg (Steinberg, 2008), membership in crowds is based on reputation and stereotype and so they play a role in adolescents' sense of identity. Thus, we see that contexts such as peers are important for adolescent development.

Media as a context of development. Since Hill set out the research agenda for adolescence in the 1980s, media have become an important part of young people's lives. In addition, in the last decade or so, the media landscape surrounding young people has itself changed rapidly and dramatically. Although mass media are not an organization or social network that adolescents' belong to, they have become an integral part of young people's lives.

What can we say about the role of media in adolescent development? First, let us consider older media forms such as television and print. Research tells us that just as adolescents turn to peers, they also turn to television and print media, to deal with issues in their offline lives. For instance, they get information about sex from television and magazines (Borzekowski & Rickert, 2001; Brown, Childers, & Waszak, 1990; Ward, 2004); they also use television to obtain information about aspects of their self, such as gender and sexual identity (Arnett, 1995; Brown, 2004; Ward, 2004). Many young people report having a television and a variety of other media in their bedrooms (Roberts & Foehr, 2008); they also report using the multimedia environments of their rooms to express who they are (Steele & Brown, 1995) and to learn about sexual and romantic scripts (Brown et al., 1990; Evans, Rutberg, Sather, & Turner, 1991).

Digital Media and Adolescent Development

Chapter 1 showed that adolescents are awash in various forms of digital technologies, such as computers and the Internet. Most striking about these newer interactive media is that they have brought social interaction into electronic worlds and among adolescents, communication with peers is one of the most popular uses of technology (Subrahmanyam & Greenfield, 2008). Not only have these new media become an important means of connecting adolescents to peers, they also connect them to the other contextual influences in their lives, such as their leisure activities and even their families. Thus, it is becoming increasingly clear that we must consider digital worlds as another social context for adolescent development along the lines of other familiar contexts such as families, peers, and schools. It is therefore important to consider the implications of the diffuse, pervasive, and developmentally early immersion of young people in digital worlds.

We saw earlier that self-disclosure to peers may help adolescents deal with their developmental issues and newer digital media provide opportunities for self-disclosure. We also saw that adolescents turn to older media forms for help with core developmental issues. The central premise of this book is that online communication forms, which combine peer interaction with a popular medium, may provide a promising venue for adolescents to explore the developmental challenges they face in their lives (Subrahmanyam, Greenfield, & Tynes, 2004; Subrahmanyam, Šmahel, & Greenfield, 2006). For the last 10 years, our research agenda has focused on connecting electronic media with developmental processes (Šmahel, 2003; Šmahel, Blinka, & Ledabyl, 2008; Subrahmanyam et al., 2004; Subrahmanyam et al., 2006). Using both qualitative and quantitative methods, we have shown that adolescents' online interactions in a variety of online forums (e.g., chat rooms, blogs, and social networking sites) are both a literal and a metaphoric screen for representing major adolescent developmental issues.

In this book, we adopt this approach as we try to piece together a balanced picture of digital youth and their digital worlds. We have organized the first part of the book in terms of some of the main developmental tasks and challenges faced by adolescents – sexuality, identity, intimacy, interpersonal connections, and developing an ethical and core value system. We will show that these developmental tasks or challenges are being transferred to digital worlds, and that in the process, they may be transformed, intensified, reversed, or even remain unchanged as the case may be. By linking young people's online interactions to ongoing, core developmental processes, we can arrive at a more complete understanding of their online lives, one that will endure even if the application itself does not.

A Theoretical Framework for Conceptualizing Adolescents' Online Behavior: The Co-construction Model

The theoretical framework that we adopt in this book is the co-construction model, and was first proposed by media research pioneer, Patricia Greenfield (Greenfield, 1984), and us to understand online teen chat (Subrahmanyam et al., 2004, 2006). Our attempt to connect developmental processes to adolescents' digital worlds is a departure from the media effects approach that has traditionally been used to conceptualize the role of media in human development (Anderson & Dill, 2000; Bandura, Ross, & Ross, 1961; Klapper, 1960). On the media effects model, the content of media is believed to affect children's attitudes, thoughts, and behaviors (Anderson & Dill, 2000; Bandura et al., 1961; Klapper, 1960). Proponents view media as external to the user, with its effects flowing from the outside in or from media into the user. Although not explicitly stated, the media effects approach views the user as a passive recipient of media influence. Examples of studies adopting this approach include those that examine whether television watching improves literacy or video game playing results in benefits to attentional and spatial skills. Much of the early research on adolescents' Internet use also focused on the benefits or harm to their well-being and evaluated the effects of the Internet on anxiety, depression, loneliness and other similar measures of well-being; the research on these topics is described in greater detail in Chapter 7.

Our co-construction model of new media also differs from the Uses and Gratification theory of mass media (Blumler & Katz, 1974), which suggests that different people use media for different purposes or gratifications such as escape, information, and entertainment. Compared to the media effects approach, the Uses and Gratification theory assumes that users of media have an active role both in their choice of media and consequently in the effects that media may have on them. Studies of young people's use of the Internet for peer communication (Gross, 2004), health information (Borzekowski, Fobil, & Asante, 2006; Suzuki & Calzo, 2004), and social support (Whitlock, Powers, & Eckenrode, 2006) are examples of work that have sought to understand online behavior by looking at the uses that youth may derive from them. Chapter 8 discusses young people's use of the Internet for health and well-being in detail and the Internet's avowed potential for delivering treatments and interventions.

The media effects perspective and the Uses and Gratifications theory have helped advance our understanding of young people's online behavior, but they are nonetheless limiting, as they do not take into account key features of online venues. In interactive digital environments, such as chat rooms, instant messaging, text messaging, and social networking sites, users construct and co-construct their environments. Although designers may provide the platform or the tool, in actuality, users co-construct their use and use tools in ways that the designer may have never anticipated. In fact, Greenfield and Yan (2006) refer to the Internet as a cultural tool kit consisting of an infinite series of applications. Online environments are cultural spaces, where norms are created, shared and passed on to other users. Online culture is not static, but is a cyclical dynamic entity, and users are constantly generating and passing on new norms. Therefore, it is important to move away from a picture of the adolescent Internet user as passive and mindlessly influenced by online contexts. Instead, we must see users as creating their contexts in conjunction with other users, thus influencing and being influenced by the very online culture that they are helping to create.

If adolescent users are co-constructing their online environments, then we would expect their online and offline worlds to be connected; consequently, digital worlds may serve as a playing ground for important developmental issues from offline lives. Thus, we expect that teens bring to their online haunts the issues and challenges that they face in their offline lives. As we noted earlier, for adolescents, these would include the developmental tasks of sexuality, identity, intimacy, and interpersonal connection. We expect adolescents' online and offline physical and social worlds to be linked to each other not only in terms of the topics and themes that are projected, but also in terms of the kinds of behavior engaged in, the people interacted with, and the relationships that may be sustained. Another area of connectedness is gender; for instance, gendered communication in online chat rooms suggests that offline gendered behaviors and preferences are found in online contexts (Šmahel & Subrahmanyam, 2007). Problem behaviors may also be connected and youth troubled in their offline lives might seek out trouble online.

Our thesis is that adolescents' physical, social, and digital worlds are intertwined and interconnected and have a transactional or bi-directional relationship with each other. In other words, their online and offline lives are connected to each other. Digital worlds are very real to youth – and within their subjective experiences, the "real" and "virtual" may even blend with each other. Therefore, we refrain from using the term "real world" to contrast with "online" or "digital worlds." Instead we will use the terms physical/digital and offline/online to capture both ends of the continuum representing online and offline worlds.

We expect that youth will use online contexts to extend and bootstrap their offline physical lives. We suggest that they will do so in novel and creative ways that capitalize on the opportunities and adapt to the challenges of online communicative environments, which we discussed in Chapter 1 (Greenfield & Subrahmanyam, 2003). For instance, anonymous online environments such as bulletin boards allow teens to ask questions about sensitive topics or to explore aspects of their identity that they are still exploring. In contrast, text-based applications, such as chat rooms and instant messages present special challenges to having coherent and effective communication. Users particularly, young ones, have adapted by creating, sharing, transmitting, and transforming a new chat code (Greenfield & Subrahmanyam, 2003). Consequently, although we expect virtual worlds to serve as a screen for offline behaviors and themes, we expect that they will do so with different affordances. Online contexts vary from offline ones as well as among themselves in the extent to which participants are disembodied, anonymous, and the extent to which users may interact with strangers versus known others. Consider early chat rooms that were text-based and where users were disembodied and anonymous and were more likely to interact with strangers. In contrast, social networking sites utilize text, audio, and visual images – thus, users are less likely to be disembodied; however, they have considerable freedom as to whether they are anonymous and whether they interact with strangers or known others. Because of these different affordances, we expect that even though youth may use new virtual venues to enact real-life issues, they will do so differently and with different intensities. Thus, when we find offline themes within online worlds, they may be similar, exaggerated, or reversed from their offline counterparts. Regardless of this, viewing digital worlds as continuous with physical worlds, allows us to begin to understand online behavior.

Our position that offline and online worlds are interconnected is in contrast to earlier speculation that the Internet may allow users to present online selves that are separate and from their offline ones (Byam, 1995; McKenna & Bargh, 2000; Turkle, 1995). Given the disembodied nature of most digital venues, wherein users could theoretically leave their bodies behind in their physical worlds as well their potential for anonymity, it was speculated that while online, they could be anybody they wanted to be. Online anonymity was much more likely in the early years before the diffusion of the Internet and tools such as digital cameras and web cams that made it easy to upload audio and video. These features led theorists to speculate that users would be able to leave race and gender behind as they embarked online. Turkle (1995) suggested that youth may use online environments to experiment and tinker with their identity. These speculations were consistent with the applications popular at the time such as chat rooms and Multi User Dungeons (or MUDs), where one could choose to be anonymous and more likely to interact with strangers.

As we will show in this book, the Internet and other digital tools have changed and evolved dramatically, and many of these early speculations have not borne out. Instead, young people are bringing the people and issues from their offline lives into their online worlds and interactions. Youth have at their disposal an array of online applications such as email, instant messaging, and social networking sites, which allow them to connect with people they already know. At the same time, there continue to be online contexts such as bulletin boards and MMORPG's, where one can interact with people who are not a part of one's offline life. As we consider these different applications, we will show that online worlds are connected to offline worlds, but in different ways depending on the particular context, whether users are anonymous and/or disembodied, and the activities for which they use a particular digital tool.

Conclusions

In the three decades since Hill first laid out his research agenda, we have gained tremendous insight about adolescence. We have learned more about the changes – biological, cognitive, and social – that occur, the developmental tasks such as sexuality, identity, and intimacy facing individuals in this life phase, and most importantly the role of the context (peers, families, and schools) as adolescents deal with the challenges before them. As newer interactive media have become an integral part of adolescents' lives, and allow them to connect with the other people in their lives, it is clear that they are an important social context, one that provides youth with opportunities to explore the developmental challenges before them. As a social context, digital worlds are constructed and co-constructed by adolescents themselves and consequently we propose that teens' online and offline lives are psychologically connected. In Chapters 3–5, we pursue this line of reasoning, and examine separately the role of technology in the fundamental adolescent developmental issues of sexuality, identity, and intimacy. Chapter 6 does the same for the development of ethics and civic engagement, a less central task, but nonetheless very relevant in today's society. It is our hope that such a developmental approach will help us to develop a deeper and more comprehensive understanding of the role of digital media in young people's development.

References

Anderson, C. A., & Dill, K. E. (2000). Video games and aggressive thoughts, feelings, and behavior in the laboratory and in life. *Journal of Personality and Social Psychology, 78*, 772–790.

Arnett, J. J. (1995). Adolescents' uses of the media for self-socialization. *Journal of Youth and Adolescence, 24*(5), 519–533.

Arnett, J. J. (2000). Emerging adulthood – A theory of development from the late teens through the twenties. *American Psychologist, 55*, 469–480.

Arnett, J. J. (2004). *Emerging adulthood: The winding road from the late teens through the twenties*. New York, NY: Oxford University Press.

Bandura, A., Ross, D., & Ross, S. A. (1961). Transmission of aggression through imitation of aggressive models. *The Journal of Abnormal and Social Psychology, 63*, 575–582.

Blumler, J. G., & Katz, E. (1974). *The uses of mass communications: Current perspectives on gratifications research*. Beverly Hills, CA: Sage.

Borzekowski, D. L. G., Fobil, J. N., & Asante, K. O. (2006). Online access by adolescents in Accra: Ghanaian teens' use of the Internet for health information. *Developmental Psychology, 42*, 450–458.

Borzekowski, D. L. G., & Rickert, V. I. (2001). Adolescent cybersurfing for health information: A new resource that crosses barriers. *Archives of Pediatrics and Adolescent Medicine, 155*, 813–817.

Brown, B. B. (2004). Adolescents' relationships with peers. In R. M. Lerner & L. Steinberg (Eds.), *Handbook of adolescent psychology* (2nd ed., pp. 363–394). Hoboken, NJ: Wiley.

Brown, J. D., Childers, K. W., & Waszak, C. S. (1990). Television and adolescent sexuality. *Journal of Adolescent Health Care, 11*, 62–70.

Buhrmester, D., & Prager, K. (1995). Patterns and functions of self-disclosure during childhood and adolescence. In K. J. Rotenberg (Ed.), *Disclosure processes in children and adolescents* (pp. 10–56). New York, NY: Cambridge University Press.

Byam, N. K. (1995). The emergence of community in computer-mediated communication. In S. G. Jones (Ed.), *Cybersociety: Computer-mediated communication and community* (pp. 138–163). Thousand Oaks, CA: Sage.

Connolly, J., Furman, W., & Konarski, R. (2000). The role of peers in the emergence of heterosexual romantic relationships in adolescence. *Child Development, 71*, 1395–1408.

Cubbin, C., Santelli, J., Brindis, C. D., & Braveman, P. (2005). Neighborhood context and sexual behaviors among adolescents: Findings from the National Longitudinal Study of Adolescent Health. *Perspectives on Sexual and Reproductive Health, 37*, 125–134.

Côté, J. E. (2006). Emerging adulthood as an institutionalized moratorium: Risks and benefits to identity formation. In J. J. Arnett & J. L. Tanner (Eds.), *Emerging adults in America: Coming of age in the 21st century* (pp. 85–116). Washington, DC: American Psychological Association.

Erikson, E. H. (1950). *Childhood and society*. New York, NY: W W Norton & Company.

Erikson, E. H. (1959). *Identity and the life cycle: Selected papers*. Oxford: International Universities Press.

Erikson, E. H. (1968). *Identity: Youth and Crisis*. New York, NY: W W Norton & Company.

Evans, E. D., Rutberg, J., Sather, C., & Turner, C. (1991). Content analysis of contemporary teen magazines for adolescent females. *Youth & Society, 23*, 99–120.

Furman, W. (2002). The emerging field of adolescent romantic relationships. *Current Directions in Psychological Science, 11*, 177–180.

Furman, W., Brown, B. B., & Feiring, C. (1999). *Contemporary perspectives on adolescent romantic relationships*. New York, NY: Cambridge University Press.

Furman, W., & Shaffer, L. (2003). The role of romantic relationships in adolescent development. In P. Florsheim (Ed.), *Adolescent romantic relations and sexual behavior: Theory, research, and practical implications* (pp. 3–22). Mahwah, NJ: Lawrence Erlbaum Associates Publishers.

Giblin, A. A. (2004). *Adolescent girls' appearance conversations: Evaluation, pressure and coping*. Seattle, WA: University of Washington.

Gordon, M., & Miller, R. L. (1984). Going steady in the 1980s: Exclusive relationships in six Connecticut high schools. *Sociology & Social Research, 68*, 463–479.

Greenfield, P. M. (1984). *Mind and media: The effects of television, video games, and computers*. Cambridge, MA: Harvard University Press.

Greenfield, P. M., & Subrahmanyam, K. (2003). Online discourse in a teen chatroom: New codes and new modes of coherence in a visual medium. *Journal of Applied Developmental Psychology, 24*, 713–738.

Greenfield, P. M., & Yan, Z. (2006). Children, adolescents, and the Internet: A new field of inquiry in developmental psychology. *Developmental Psychology, 42*, 391–394.

Gross, E. F. (2004). Adolescent Internet use: What we expect, what teens report. *Journal of Applied Developmental Psychology, 25*, 633–649.

Hall, G. S. (1904). *Adolescence: Its psychology and its relations to physiology, anthropology, sociology, sex, crime, religion and education, and education.* New York, NY: D Appleton & Company.

Havighurst, R. J. (1972). *Developmental tasks and education.* New York, NY: David McKay Company.

Hill, J. P. (1983). Early adolescence: A research agenda. *The Journal of Early Adolescence, 3*, 1–21.

Inhelder, B., & Piaget, J. (1999). *The growth of logical thinking from childhood to adolescence.* London: Routledge.

Johnson, F. L., & Aries, E. J. (1983). Conversational patterns among same-sex pairs of late-adolescent close friends. *Journal of Genetic Psychology, 142*, 225–238.

Kallen, D. J., Stephenson, J. J., & Doughty, A. (1983). The need to know: Recalled adolescent sources of sexual and contraceptive information and sexual behavior. *Journal of Sex Research, 19*, 137–159.

Klapper, J. T. (1960). *The effects of mass communication.* New York, NY: Free Press.

Kroger, J. (2003). Identity development during adolescence. In G. R. Adams & M. D. Berzonsky (Eds.), *Blackwell handbook of adolescence* (pp. 205–226). Malden, MA: Blackwell.

Larson, R., & Richards, M. H. (1991). Daily companionship in late childhood and early adolescence: Changing developmental contexts. *Child Development, 62*, 284–300.

McKenna, K. Y. A., & Bargh, J. A. (2000). Plan 9 from cyberspace: The implications of the Internet for personality and social psychology. *Personality and Social Psychology Review, 4*, 57–75.

Mosher, W. D., Chandra, A., & Jones, J. (2005). *Sexual behavior and selected health measures: Men and women 15–44 years of age, United States, 2002.* Retrieved October 28, 2005, from http://www.cdc.gov/nchs/data/ad/ad362.pdf

Nurmi, J.-E., Lerner, R. M., & Steinberg, L. (2004). Socialization and self-development: Channeling, selection, adjustment, and reflection. *Handbook of adolescent psychology* (2nd ed., pp. 85–124). Hoboken, NJ: Wiley.

Pombeni, M. L., Kirchler, E., & Palmonari, A. (1990). Identification with peers as a strategy to muddle through the troubles of the adolescent years. *Journal of Adolescence, 13*, 351–369.

Reis, O., & Youniss, J. (2004). Patterns in identity change and development in relationships with mothers and friends. *Journal of Adolescent Research, 19*, 31–44.

Roberts, D. F., & Foehr, U. G. (2008). Trends in media use. *The Future of Children, 18*, 11–37.

Ryan, A. M. (2001). The peer group as a context for the development of young adolescent motivation and achievement. *Child Development, 72*, 1135–1150.

Savin-Williams, R. C., & Diamond, L. M. (2004). Sex. In R. M. Lerner & L. Steinberg (Eds.), *Handbook of adolescent psychology* (2nd ed., pp. 189–231). New York, NY: Wiley.

Šmahel, D. (2003). Communication of adolescents in the internet environment. *Ceskoslovenska psychologie, 47*, 144–156.

Šmahel, D., Blinka, L., & Ledabyl, O. (2008). Playing MMORPGs: Connections between addiction and identifying with a character. *Cyberpsychology and Behavior, 11*, 715–718.

Šmahel, D., & Subrahmanyam, K. (2007). 'Any girls want to chat press 911': Partner selection in monitored and unmonitored teen chat rooms. *CyberPsychology & Behavior, 10*(3), 346–353.

Sowell, E. R., Thompson, P. M., Holmes, C. J., Jernigan, T. L., & Toga, A. W. (1999). In vivo evidence for postadolescent brain maturation in frontal and striatal regions. *Nature Neuroscience, 2*, 859–860.

Sowell, E. R., Thompson, P. M., Tessner, K. D., & Toga, A. W. (2001). Mapping continued brain growth and gray matter density reduction in dorsal frontal cortex: Inverse relationships during postadolescent brain maturation. *Journal of Neuroscience, 21*, 8819.

Steele, J. R., & Brown, J. D. (1995). Adolescent room culture: Studying media in the context of everyday life. *Journal of Youth and Adolescence, 24,* 551–576.

Steinberg, L. (2008). *Adolescence.* New York, NY: McGraw-Hill.

Subrahmanyam, K., & Greenfield, P. M. (2008). Communicating online: Adolescent relationships and the media. *The Future of Children, 18,* 119–146.

Subrahmanyam, K., Greenfield, P. M., & Tynes, B. M. (2004). Constructing sexuality and identity in an online teen chat room. *Journal of Applied Developmental Psychology: An International Lifespan Journal, 25,* 651–666.

Subrahmanyam, K., Šmahel, D., & Greenfield, P. M. (2006). Connecting developmental constructions to the Internet: Identity presentation and sexual exploration in online teen chat rooms. *Developmental Psychology, 42,* 395–406.

Suzuki, L. K., & Calzo, J. P. (2004). The search for peer advice in cyberspace: An examination of online teen bulletin boards about health and sexuality. *Journal of Applied Developmental Psychology, 25,* 685–698.

Tanner, J. M. (1978). *Growth at adolescence* (2nd ed.). Oxford: Blackwell.

Teare, J. F., Garrett, C. R., Coughlin, D. G., & Shanahan, D. L. (1995). America's children in crisis: Adolescents' requests for support from a national telephone hotline. *Journal of Applied Developmental Psychology, 16,* 21–33.

Trickey, H. (2003). *Home economics comes of age.* Retrieved June 19, 2008, from http://www.cnn.com/SPECIALS/2001/schools/stories/homeec.revolution.html

Turkle, S. (1995). *Life on the screen: Identity in the age of the Internet.* New York, NY: Simon & Schuster.

Ward, L. M. (2004). Wading through the stereotypes: Positive and negative associations between media use and black adolescents' conceptions of self. *Developmental Psychology, 40,* 284–294.

Waterman, A. S. (1999). Identity, the identity statuses, and identity status development: A contemporary statement. *Developmental Review, 19,* 591–621.

Weinstein, E., & Rosen, E. (1991). The development of adolescent sexual intimacy: Implications for counseling. *Adolescence, 26,* 331–339.

Whitlock, J. L., Powers, J. L., & Eckenrode, J. (2006). The virtual cutting edge: The Internet and adolescent-self-injury. *Developmental Psychology, 42,* 407.

Chapter 3
Sexuality on the Internet: Sexual Exploration, Cybersex, and Pornography

Several years ago when chat rooms were the rage among adolescents, we studied the culture of online teen chat rooms, analyzing chat participants' utterances and nicknames. We were struck by our finding that sexuality was as much a part of online chat (Subrahmanyam, Šmahel, & Greenfield, 2006) as we knew it to be in adolescents' offline lives (Cubbin, Santelli, Brindis, & Braveman, 2005; Rice, 2001). Approximately 5% of the conversation threads across our entire chat corpus consisted of sexual themes (e.g., ANY HOT CHICKS WANNA CHAT PRESS 69), and 3% consisted of obscene language, amounting to one sexual comment per minute and less than one obscenity (e.g., *my dick*) per minute. Equally striking was our finding that 20% of all of the nicknames were sexualized, and included implicitly sexualized (*RomancBab4U* or *Snowbunny2740*) and explicitly sexualized (*SexyDickHed* or *Da1pimp6sur*) ones. Online, the nicknames seemed to serve the same functions as offline behaviors such as dressing provocatively or wearing makeup.

Chat rooms are not unique in this regard and sexual topics were frequently found in a study of two online teen health bulletin boards (Suzuki & Calzo, 2004). Online sites with sexual content are among the most popular aspects of the web (Cooper, Delmonico, & Burg, 2000) and as a group, adolescents are the biggest consumers of pornography online (Flood & Hamilton, 2003; Lo & Wei, 2005; Mitchell, Finkelhor, & Wolak, 2003, 2005; Peter & Valkenburg, 2006a, 2006b; Ybarra & Mitchell, 2005). Sexuality is an important adolescent developmental issue and it is not surprising that it features prominently in adolescents' online lives as well. In this chapter, we show how young people use the Internet to deal with their developing sexuality. We begin by highlighting important aspects of this adolescent developmental issue and then examine the characteristics of online environments that support sexual activities more generally. Then, the bulk of the chapter will describe adolescents' online sexual exploration, from the construction of their sexual self to their access of sexually explicit content. Because most of the research on adolescents' online sexual exploration is silent on the issue of gay and lesbian youth, the potential role of the Internet for sexual minority youth is considered separately.

K. Subrahmanyam, D. Šmahel, *Digital Youth*, Advancing Responsible
Adolescent Development, DOI 10.1007/978-1-4419-6278-2_3,
© Springer Science+Business Media, LLC 2011

Adolescent Sexuality

Sexuality as a developmental issue is present throughout the life cycle, but becomes especially salient during adolescence (Steinberg, 2008, p. 13). Adolescents have to adjust to their developing sexuality, in particular their increased sexual drive and interest in sex (Chilman, 1990; Macek, 2003; Weinstein & Rosen, 1991) and are faced with the task of constructing their sexual selves. They spend a lot of time talking about sex, sharing sexually tinged jokes and sex-oriented literature, and using sex slang (Rice, 2001). Sexual exploration, finding a romantic partner, and engaging in a romantic relationship take on importance during adolescence (Buzwell & Rosenthal, 1996). In the USA and other Western countries, many adolescents engage in sexual activity (Mosher, Chandra, & Jones, 2005; Savin-Williams & Diamond, 2004) and the rate of sexual activity increases with age (Cubbin et al., 2005).

Peers and romantic partners play an important role in adolescents' construction of their sexuality (Connolly, Furman, & Konarski, 2000). Peers who are generally becoming more salient in adolescents' lives are a source of support when making decisions about sexual behavior, and peer communication is a primary source of information about sex (Ward, 2004). Dating and romantic relationships are a context for adolescent sexual exploration. In fact, in a study of Australian adolescents in various phases of dating, McCabe and Collins (1984) found that the level of sexual activity increased as dating became more serious. However, there are some gender differences. At first, males have more sexual expectations than females, but these differences diminish as the relationship develops. The social context of sexuality also differs between boys and girls (Macek, 2003). Boys tend to connect sexuality with wooing a partner; during early and middle adolescence, sexual behavior is a topic of conversation in their peer groups, and sexual competence is seen as increasing social status. In contrast, girls view sexuality in terms of their attractiveness to the opposite sex and their partner stimulates their sexuality. Although the issues of dating, romantic relationships, and sexuality are clearly interconnected, romantic and sexual relationships may also be developed independently (Miller & Benson, 1999). In fact, the Internet supports such a dissociation and research indicates that adolescents, at least those in Western countries, may develop purely online relationships, in which they talk about sexual issues and experiment with their sexuality (Šmahel, 2003). Some adolescents even report having experienced their first sexual encounter virtually (Šmahel, 2003).

Characteristics of Online Environments Relevant to Sexuality

We noted earlier in this chapter that sexual content is one of the most dominant aspects of the web. To explain this phenomenon, Cooper, Putnam, Planchon, and Boies (1999a) and Cooper, Scherer, Boies, and Gordon (1999b) have identified three characteristics of online environments that support sexuality. The *Triple A Engine* as they are called were not intended for adolescents but are relevant to our discussion and so we briefly describe them here:

(1) Accessibility – there are millions of easily accessible web pages and large numbers huge numbers of people on social networking sites, in chat rooms, and on private messaging systems, who are available for communicating about sexual matters.

(2) Affordability – pornography and sexual communication online are cheap, as one only needs a computer and Internet connection to access them.

(3) Anonymity – online it is possible to be as anonymous as one chooses to be and people perceive online sexual communication to be anonymous as well. Note that at the time that Cooper proposed the *Triple A Engine*, the web was much more anonymous than it is presently. Certainly, there remain online contexts (e.g., bulletin boards, websites with sexual content) where one can be anonymous.[1] However, many of the communication applications currently popular among teens (e.g., social networking sites) capitalize on interacting with known others (Reich, Subrahmanyam, & Espinoza, 2009) and so anonymity does not hold up as much anymore for some online communication tools.

At the same time, the Internet also presents some unique challenges for sexuality-users are disembodied and so cues for physical appeal such as age, gender, race, or physical appearance (height, weight, etc.) are not readily available. Missing also are face-to-face cues such as gesture, gaze, and other elements of body language. However, tools, such as webcams and camera phones, provide these cues directly and many applications (e.g., social networking sites) allow users to exchange such information easily via pictures and video clips.

Online Sexual Exploration

In the next sections, we examine adolescents' use of digital technologies, such as the Internet and cell phones, to deal with their changing bodies, growing interest in sex, and the developmental task of constructing their sexual selves. In general, these technologies provide quick and easy access to information stores, allows users to create content of their own, and interact with other users. Sexual content is no different, and adolescents are not only consumers of sexually themed material, but are actively engaged in constructing many aspects of the sexualized environment they are immersed in Greenfield (2004). In the next sections, we examine three ways in which adolescents engage in online sexual exploration: constructing and presenting their emerging sexual selves, engaging in sexual conversations or cybersex, and accessing pornography; a fourth section considers these issues separately for sexual minority youth. Using the Internet to search for information about health and sexuality is covered in Chapter 8. Although online sexual exploration is very similar

---

[1] Although less sophisticated computer users often do not recognize this, true anonymity on the web is elusive as computers have IP addresses and users leave digital footprints that can be traced.

in spirit to its offline counterpart, we will show that it takes on new forms as youth adapt to the characteristics of online environments.

Constructing and Presenting Sexual Selves Online

In the upcoming paragraphs we will show how youth use online contexts (e.g., chat rooms and mobile phones) and the different tools within them (e.g., nicknames, avatars, and pictures) to explore their changing sexuality as well as to construct and present their sexual selves (Subrahmanyam, Greenfield, & Tynes, 2004; Subrahmanyam et al., 2006). We start with our studies on online teen chat rooms; because the chat rooms were public and some were unmonitored, they provided a rare glimpse into adolescents' online sexual exploration. Using qualitative discourse methodology, we micro-analyzed a transcript from an online teen chat room monitored by an adult (Subrahmanyam et al., 2004). Microanalysis of the chat conversation revealed that participants discussed a broad range of sexual topics and concerns, including abortion, pre-marital sex, and birth control methods, such as condoms. The following extract of the discussion demonstrates the participants' preoccupation with sexual issues:

> 548. Immaculate ros: sex sex sex that all you think about?
> 559. Snowbunny: people who have sex at 16 r sick :-(
> 560: Twonky: I agree
> 564. OOo0CaFfEiNe: no sex until ur happily married. . .thatz muh rule
> 566. Twonky: I agree with that too
> 567. Snowbunny: me too caffine!

In this case, the anonymous teen chat room seemed to encourage the chat participants to talk frankly and openly about sex. Note that even users who were not actively participating in the conversation could nonetheless passively participate by "lurking;" in Chapter 8, we touch on research on health bulletin boards, which suggest that such "lurking" is very common when sexual topics are discussed (Suzuki & Calzo, 2004).

Lest the reader think that the conversation snippet above is an isolated example, we consider the results of a quantitative study, in which we analyzed 10 hours of conversations in online teen chat rooms in a corpus that contained more than 12,000 utterances (Subrahmanyam et al., 2006). We analyzed users' nicknames as well as their utterances. At least one sexual utterance was produced by 28% of the nicknames and 19% of nicknames were sexualized. Even though a majority (72%) of the participants did not utter a single sexual utterance, they had access to the sexual content because of the public nature of the chat window. We also coded utterances in terms of the extent to which they were sexually implicit or explicit. Examples of sexually implicit utterances are

> *all hott guys that wanna talk to a hott 13/f/nj im me or hit 5813;*
> *who wants to chat with a hot and sexy 13/f/ct press 12345?*

Examples of sexually explicit utterances are:

> *don't get your penis caught in your zipper;*
> *any hot, horny or wet ladies wanna chat with a cute 18 m from canada pic on*
> *file if so pm me or press 123.*

Three percent of the utterances in the entire corpus were sexually implicit and 3% were explicit. This means that there was about one sexual utterance every minute, a very high rate of exposure for the youth participants. While we are sure that adolescents do talk about sex and sex-related topics in their face-to-face conversations, we think it unlikely that they do so at the rate that we observed in online chatrooms.

Thus, young people's online exploration involves a core offline concern such as sexuality. Equally interesting, trends in online sexuality parallel offline developmental ones. Chat participants who self-described as older[2] produced more explicit sexual utterances (Subrahmanyam et al., 2006). Sexualized nicknames that were coded as implicit (e.g., *RomancBab4U, Snowbunny2740, innocent_angel*) were created more often by participants who described themselves as females (26%) rather than males (10%). Sexually implicit nicknames attract sexual attention passively and subtly and are reminiscent of similar patterns of offline behavior. Gender comparisons suggested that female identity (via feminine nicknames such as *Lilprincess72988*) was associated with implicit sexual communication, whereas male identity (via masculine nicknames such as *Vikingdude123*) was associated with explicit sexual communication. It appears that sexualized nicknames could very well serve as the face and body of an adolescent who wishes to convey a sexualized presence online.

Online applications, such as instant messaging, that came after chat rooms are more private and allow users to choose and limit who is privy to their communications. Youth have also become more savvy about privacy issues and most seem to use the privacy controls provided by online applications, such as blogs and social networking sites (Hinduja & Patchin, 2008; Subrahmanyam, Garcia, Harsono, Li, & Lipana, 2009). Thus, it is no longer that easy to conduct the kind of research that we did with chat rooms, and we could not find any other scientific research on adolescents' construction of their sexuality in newer digital contexts.

However, a recent survey of 13- to 19-year olds by the National Campaign to Prevent Teen and Unplanned Pregnancy and Cosmogirl.com suggests that technology continues to be used by teens for sexual exploration via the exchange of sexually suggestive content (National Campaign to Prevent Teen and Unplanned Pregnancy & Cosmogirl.com, 2008). Twenty percent of teens (22% of girls and 18% of boys) reported that they had "electronically sent or posted online nude or semi-nude

---

[2]We purposefully characterized the chat participants in this awkward, but more accurate manner. We did not ask them for their age or any other identifying information, but instead obtained it from their self-declared statements in the public space of the chat room and had no way of verifying the information.

pictures or videos of themselves;" 11% of young teen girls (between 13- and 16-years) reported that they had done so. Sexually suggestive content included explicit text, and nude or semi-nude personal pictures or videos captured on a cell phone or digital camera and sent via personal texts, emails, and instant messages. Because it is so easy to forward electronic content, many of these sexually suggestive messages may reach people, who were not the originally intended recipient.

As our research on chat rooms suggested, the exchange of sexual content electronically may simply be a manifestation of adolescents' heightened interest in exploring all things related to sex – indeed, most respondents in one survey viewed it as a harmless activity and reported that they were sending the messages either to a romantic partner or to someone they wanted to date (National Campaign to Prevent Teen and Unplanned Pregnancy & Cosmogirl.com, 2008). Adolescents' perception that it is harmless is not entirely correct, given recent incidents concerning *sexting*, which is the sending of sexually explicit text or pictures via cell phone. In the USA, some youth, who have engaged in *sexting*, have been prosecuted for various offences including possession and transmission of child pornography and felony pandering obscenities charges (Galanos, 2009). Although reports of sexting are mostly anecdotal and the aforementioned survey is not a scientific one, they illustrate that youth use electronic media to construct and present their sexual selves, and do so in ways that may not always be obvious to parents and researchers. Although the core purposes of the activities remain unchanged, the particular forms change, as users adapt to the capabilities afforded by newer technologies.

Cybersex: Sexual Conversations Online

Scholars have defined *Cybersex* in various ways, from a broad definition that it involves viewing pornographic content to a narrower one that it entails online sexual communication between people. Perhaps the most frequently used definition treats cybersex as sexual chatting/talking between two or more individuals that may or may not include role playing and masturbatory activities for one or more of them (e.g., Noonan, 2007; Saleh, 2009; Whitty & Carr, 2006). The lure of cybersex is perhaps best captured by Turkle (1997), who wrote that:

> Many people who engage in netsex say that they are constantly surprised by how emotionally and physically powerful it can be. They insist that it demonstrates that truth of the adage that ninety percent of sex takes place in the mind. This is certainly not a new idea, but netsex has made it commonplace among teenage boys, a social group not usually known for its sophistication about such matters. (p. 21)

While the word "cybersex" often carries a negative connotation, here we use the term neutrally, to describe the sexual communication that may occur between two or more Internet users.

Surprisingly, there is limited research on cybersex among adolescents and there is no hard data on the question of its prevalence in the USA. However, in a survey study of 681 12- to 20-year olds in the Czech Republic, 16% of males and 15% of females reported that they had engaged in "virtual sex" activities (Šmahel, 2006). There were no age differences and 14% of 12- to 14-year olds, 16% of 15- to 17-year olds, and 14% of 18- to 20-year olds reported engaging in cyber sex.

The *Triple A Engine* (Accessibility, Affordability, Anonymity) (Cooper et al., 1999a, 1999b) described earlier in this chapter makes online contexts a perfect venue for cybersex. Research suggests that adolescents may engage in cybersex as a means of acquiring knowledge about sex (Divinova, 2005). For example, in Divinova's study, a 15-year-old girl noted that: "... when I was 11 years old, it was a perfect way how to get sexual information, which interested me a lot." Some adolescents even report that they initiated online relationships to gain experience in cybersex activities; they also admitted that their first sexual encounter had taken place on the Internet (Šmahel, 2003). Adolescents' participation in cybersex is not surprising given their increased interest in sex (Suler, 2008). Although cybersex among adolescents might be viewed unfavorably because it is seen as superficial, artificial, or unnatural, it is probably a relatively safe way to gain sexual experience, as long as they follow basic rules, and not reveal details of their identity, such as their name, address, telephone number, etc. (Divinova, 2005). However, one concern about cybersex is its potential for compulsive or addictive behaviors, a topic that we explore in Chapter 9.

Accessing Sexually Explicit Content Online

Perhaps no other Internet-related topic has resulted in as much consternation and hand wringing as young people's access to sexually explicit material online, which again is made possible because of the Triple-A engine of accessibility, affordability, and anonymity (Peter & Valkenburg, 2006c). Commonly referred to as pornography, such material is readily available online. In 2006, it was estimated that there were 420 million pornography sites and every second, 28,258 Internet users across the world viewed pornography; worldwide, the revenue from the pornography industry reached $97 billion that year (FamilySafeMedia, 2006). Since the early days of the Internet, sites containing sexual and pornographic content have been among the most frequently visited web pages and the keywords "sex" and "pornography" are two of the most frequently searched keywords (e.g. Cooper, Delmonico, & Burg, 2000). Cooper and colleagues report that 50% of males and 50% of females searched for the keyword "sex," 96% of males and 4% of females searched the keyword "porn," and 36% of males and 64% of females searched the keywords "Adult Dating." In the upcoming subsections, we examine the extent to which adolescents are exposed to sexually explicit material as well as the correlates and outcomes of such exposure. See Chapter 11 for more on what parents, schools, and other stakeholders can do to protect youth from such inappropriate content.

Adolescents' exposure to sexually explicit content. Before we examine the research on this topic, it is worth noting that there is tremendous variation in what exactly is subsumed under the terms "sexually explicit," and different researchers have used different definitions of "sex" and "pornography." Examples of specific categories of online sexual content in one study included (a) pictures with clearly exposed genitals, (b) movies with clearly exposed genitals, (c) pictures in which people were having sex, (d) movies in which people were having sex, and (e) erotic contact sites (Peter & Valkenburg, 2006a). While this list is by no means exhaustive, it provides a sense of the kinds of content that are included under the term "sexually explicit."

On survey research, between 23% and 71% of adolescents report being exposed to sexually explicit materials (Flood & Hamilton, 2003; Lo & Wei, 2005; Mitchell et al., 2003, 2005; Peter & Valkenburg, 2006a, 2006b; Ybarra & Mitchell, 2005). The relatively high rates of exposure are consistent with adolescents' developmentally appropriate interest in sexuality and with research, which indicates that they access offline pornography (Brown & L'Engle, 2009; Lo & Wei, 2005; Ybarra & Mitchell, 2005). Despite their use of pornography and its seeming consistency with developmental demands in their life, adolescents may actually be ambivalent about it. In a Swedish study involving 15- to 25-year olds, the majority reported they had viewed pornography, yet 46% of females and 23% of males described it as "degrading." Males, particularly the youngest ones, reported more positive attitudes about pornography (Wallmyr & Welin, 2006).

It is important to distinguish between intentional and unintentional or accidental exposure to sexually explicit material; the latter has been a source of concern, particularly with regard to younger adolescents. A nationally representative survey of 1,501 10- to 17-year-olds conducted in the Fall of 1999 and Spring of 2000 revealed that 25% of adolescents had come into unwanted contact with online sexual images over the previous year (Mitchell et al., 2003). The majority of the incidents (73%) occurred when respondents were surfing the Internet and 27% occurred when they opened an e-mail or clicked on a link in an IM or in an e-mail. Although most adolescents did not experience negative reactions to the unwanted exposure, about 24% stated that they were "very/extremely upset about the exposure." Boys reported unwanted exposure more often than girls (57% vs. 42%) and older adolescents more often than younger. The probability of exposure to unwanted sexual material was higher among adolescents who used the Internet a great deal, who accessed it outside their home, joined chat rooms, and used e-mail.

The same survey also asked respondents whether they had intentionally viewed sexual material on the Internet and traditional media (e.g., magazines) in the previous year. Almost 25% of adolescent males reported intentionally viewing sexual content compared to 5% of the females (Ybarra & Mitchell, 2005). Older youth stated they had looked at sexual sites more often; they also preferred online sexual content whereas younger adolescents preferred more traditional exposures (such as X-rated videos) than those found on the Internet. Other research similarly confirms that males and older adolescents access sexually explicit content at much higher rates than females and younger adolescents (Flood & Hamilton, 2003; Lo & Wei, 2005; Wallmyr & Welin, 2006). Figure 3.1, which presents data from the Czech World Internet Project (2008), illustrates nicely how the rate of viewing online sexual content increases with age; research shows that interest in offline sexual

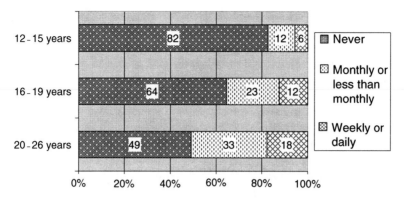

Fig. 3.1 Frequency of viewing sites with sexual content among Czech adolescents and emerging adults (Czech WIP, 2008)

materials also increases with age and this is yet another instance where online developmental trends parallel offline ones.

To examine how broader societal attitudes about sex and adolescent sexual activity in particular may influence adolescents' access to inappropriate material, we examine the 2007 WIP data (Fig. 3.2) and a longitudinal study of adolescents' exposure to sexually explicit material conducted in the Netherlands (Peter & Valkenburg, 2006a, 2006b, 2007, 2008a, 2008b). Starting in 2005, the Dutch researchers conducted an online survey on a sample of 745 Dutch adolescents between 13- and 18 years of age (Peter & Valkenburg, 2006a). In the 6-month period prior to the survey, 71% of Dutch male adolescents and 40% of female adolescents reported exposure to some kind of sexually explicit materials. On the WIP data, there was considerable

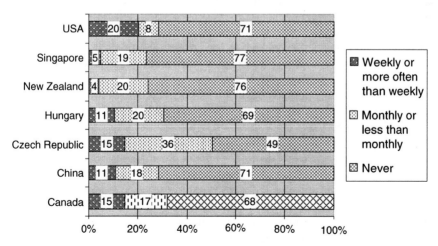

Fig. 3.2 Frequency of looking at sites with sexual content among emerging adults (18–21 years old) (WIP 2007)

variability across the countries and the greatest proportion of youth who reported viewing sexually explicit content at least once a week were from the USA, Canada, and the Czech Republic. In general these rates of access were much lower than the Dutch data, even though the WIP respondents were older and considered to be in late adolescence and emerging adulthood. The Netherlands is widely considered to be sexually very permissive and it is no surprise that the Dutch participants reported much higher rates of accessing sexually explicit content. Gender differences were also present and males generally reported greater access to sexually tinged content in the Dutch study as well as in most of the WIP countries (USA, New Zealand, Hungary and Canada). There were no gender differences in China and Singapore, and in general, young women in Western countries reported accessing sexual content less often compared to women in Asian countries. Taken together the research suggests that young people's online access of sexually explicit content parallels their offline patterns of sexual socialization.

Factors associated with access of sexually explicit material. Research on adolescents in the USA suggests that sexually explicit media are viewed more frequently by African–American adolescents (compared to White), teens of lower socio-economic status, adolescents with less-educated parents, and higher sensation-seeking adolescents (Brown & L'Engle, 2009). Such intentional exposure to pornography has been associated with delinquent behaviors and substance abuse in the previous year and online sexual material seekers more often report clinical features associated with depression and less emotional bonding with their parents and immediate family members (Ybarra & Mitchell, 2005). The Dutch study described earlier also found that adolescents were more likely to have accessed sexual material if they were sensation seekers, were less satisfied with their lives, used sexual content in other media, were more sexually interested, and had friends that were predominantly younger. Among female adolescents, greater sexual experience was associated with decreased exposure to online explicit sexual materials. However, among boys there was no relationship between sexual experience and online exposure to sexual materials (Peter & Valkenburg, 2006a). In summary, we see that in addition to demographic factors such as age, gender, and ethnicity, problem behaviors in offline life as well as psychological well-being might predict whether an adolescent seeks out pornography.

Effects of accessing sexually explicit material. It is also important to consider the effects that could accrue from adolescents' access of sexually explicit material. This is an important issue since teens are at a formative stage with regard to the development of their sexuality. Consequently a legitimate concern is that exposure to pornographic content could distort their views about among sex as well as influence their attitudes toward sex and sexual behaviors. For instance, it could lead to permissive and casual attitudes about sex or even emphasize casual sexual encounters. An alternative hypothesis that is much harder to test is whether adolescents with more permissive attitudes and greater interest in sex are simply more likely to access sexually explicit content in the first place.

A study of Taiwanese middle and high school students (14- to 17-year olds) does indeed suggest that exposure to online pornography was related to a greater acceptance of sexual permissiveness and the greater likelihood of engaging in sexually permissive behavior (Lo & Wei, 2005). Since the study was correlational, it does not control for the possibility that teens with permissive attitudes and views are more likely to access pornographic content in the first place. However, a longitudinal study of middle and high school students in the USA does provide a clearer picture. For young males, increased exposure to sexually explicit media at a young age predicted more permissive sexual norms two years later, whereas for females, greater exposure to explicit sexual media predicted less progressive gender role attitudes two years later (Brown & L'Engle, 2009). Increased exposure to sexual media predicted higher sexual harassment perpetration for males two years later, but not for females. Male and female adolescents who used all three types of sexually explicit media (Internet, video, magazines) were more likely to report engaging in oral sex and sexual intercourse two years later. The study demonstrated that exposure to sexually explicit media was one of the strongest predictors of sexual attitudinal and behavioral measures two years later.

A related question is whether adolescents' exposure to sexually explicit materials may be associated with recreational attitudes toward sex. Using data from the Dutch sample described earlier, the researchers found that adolescents' exposure to explicit online material was determined by the gender of the adolescent and that it was not directly related to recreational attitudes toward sex, but rather was mediated by the extent to which adolescents evaluate sexual material as realistic (Peter & Valkenburg, 2006b). Adolescent users, who accessed explicit material more frequently, were predominantly male, and tended to perceive this material as more realistic. This perception was associated with a recreational attitude toward sex. Therefore, more exposure to explicit online material does not directly influence the development of a recreational attitude toward sex, but rather, this attitude may implicitly stem from the perception of online sexual material as being realistic.

Another concern is whether adolescents' exposure to explicit online materials increases their preoccupation or cognitive engagement with sex. Like cybersex, such a preoccupation with sex could potentially be addictive, and so it is an important issue to address. Dutch researches analyzed data from a three-wave longitudinal study of 962 Dutch adolescents 13- to 20 years of age; the data were collected in 2006, with six months between each wave (Peter & Valkenburg, 2008a). Because of the longitudinal nature of the data, the study results are informative about the potential direction of effects. The results suggest that although respondents' exposure to sexually explicit materials online did result in preoccupation with sex, sexual preoccupation at the outset of the study did not increase exposure to sexual materials over the course of the study. It appears that subjective sexual arousal may mediate exposure effects of online sexual materials on sexual preoccupation. Exposure to sexually explicit material leads to higher sexual arousal, which in turn resulted in greater preoccupation and cognitive engagement with sex. Contrary to other results on this topic, there were no gender differences in the influence of online sexual material exposure on subjective sexual arousal. Another potential outcome of exposure to online sexual materials is sexual uncertainty or attitudes toward uncommitted sexual exploration. Data from the first wave of the Dutch longitudinal study revealed that more frequent exposure to online sexual materials was associated with higher sexual uncertainty and more positive attitudes toward uncommitted sexual exploration, such as sexual relations with casual partners or one-night stands (Peter & Valkenburg, 2008b).

Overall the research confirms the speculation that exposure to sexually explicit material is associated with more permissive attitudes, greater preoccupation with sex, and more casual sexual exploration. The Dutch researchers have argued that uncertainty is part of sexual development during adolescence and that sexually explicit materials could play an important role in the lives of adolescents. As we pointed out earlier, the Netherlands is much more liberal and much less restrictive when it comes to attitudes toward sex and sexually explicit material, and parents and public officials in other countries may not endorse this view. We also need more research to identify the direction of influence between exposure and preoccupation with sexual content. Since there are indications that some teens (e.g., sensation-seeking teens, teens who are online more) are more likely to access sexual material, it is important to study whether it has differential effects on them as well.

Accessing sexually violent materials. One category of sexually explicit material that we address separately is that of sexually violent materials that are readily accessible online. A report coming from the Australian Institute recommends distinguishing between 'mainstream' pornography (commercially available pornographic videos) and the proliferation of violent and extreme material on the Internet (Flood & Hamilton, 2003). Violent sexual content is common in the stories, images and videos circulating among some Internet newsgroups and web sites. Although the Internet provides easy access to violent pornography, research regarding its influence on youth is scarce. The Australian report describes three types of online pornography, which focus on non-consenting sexual acts: rape, bestiality and 'upskirts' web sites. The authors suggest that pornography use among adolescents and the consumption of violent portrayals are associated with sexually aggressive attitudes and behavior. This association may be particularly strong for 4–5% of Australian 16- and 17-year olds, who reported watching X-rated videos and pornographic content online every week. The researchers suggest that the regular consumption of violent and extreme pornography is a risk factor for boys and young men in the perpetration of sexual assault. Simply put, such habits may foster a greater tolerance for sexual violence.

Other researchers have similarly warned that women may experience greater incidences of sexual violence because of easily accessible online sexual violence sites (Gossett & Byrne, 2002). These author conducted a content analysis of 31 freely accessible web sites containing violent pornographic material. Four sites from their sample specifically advertise the genuineness of their rape images, with one of the sites promising, *Want a video of a real rape? This is no joke, they actually raped a girl and made this video* (p. 696). The analysis revealed that the iconography of online pornography strongly emphasized the depiction of victims and the sexual representation of unequal power relations. Gossett and Byrne suggest that the online world provides an interactive experience in which Internet users are encouraged to see through the eyes of a rapist. In contrast to offline forms of pornography, online pornography can enhance the sense of power given to the user over such images. According to the authors, violent pornography is much more easily accessible on the Internet than it is or was in offline settings, and consequently may lead to an increase of such behavior in the physical world. Although there is no research to date on this issue, it is very likely that exposure to sexually violent content may influence youth attitudes and tolerance towards such types of behavior.

Sexual Minority Youth and the Internet

Our discussion so far has presented a picture of the Internet as offering the opportunity for youth to construct and present their sexual selves, engage in cyber sex with partners and view sexually explicit content. Although not specifically stated, most of this research has focused on heterosexual youth. Yet the very same features and characteristics that allow heterosexual youth to use the Internet for sexual exploration can be even more important for sexual minorities, such as gays, lesbians, bisexuals, and transgender youth, who are often struggling with their sexual identities and may feel socially isolated as a consequence. Indeed, today the media in general and the Internet in particular, offer them a tremendous variety of resources to support their homosexual feelings and attraction. Cloud notes the various media resources that are available to teens, from television shows to books to magazines, and websites such as www.outproud.org (Cloud, 2005). Scholars have recognized the potential of the Internet both to provide information as well as opportunities for interaction. Alexander notes that: "Beyond connecting individuals and information to one another across geographic divides, Internet technologies offer individuals – and groups – revolutionary ways to represent themselves by combining texts and images, linking to other sites of interest or import, and experimenting with different modes of representation" (Alexander, 2002).

Research on sexual minority youths' use of technology for sexual identity purposes is in its infancy, and most of what we found on the topic was either in the lay press (Cloud, 2005; Egan, 2000; Silberman, 2004) or was speculative and/or based on anecdotal reports (Alexander, 2002; Driver, 2006; Harper, Bruce, Serrano, & Jamil, 2009; Maczewski, 2002). There is a small body of work with gay men and we present a few findings to give the reader a sense of the possibilities that the Internet may afford gay youth. Mostly, the Internet may serve as a gatekeeper of sorts by providing gay individuals initial and continued contact with lesbian, gay and bisexual communities (Henrickson, 2007). Conducted in New Zealand, the study revealed that the Internet was a medium of greater importance for Asian-born immigrants, who also reported being more socially isolated. Thus, the Internet may be particularly valuable for "minorities inside a minority" such as rural gay youth, gay youth in socially conservative towns, and gay youth from ethnic minority groups.

Chat rooms may be particularly valuable as a context for coming out and reducing anxieties about gay life, as well as to receive social support, enter local gay communities, and search for sexual and romantic partners (Tikkanen & Ross, 2003).

We expect that sexual minority youth can take advantage of online contexts for information about homosexuality, social support, and to enter local gay communities, and search for romantic partners (Thomas, 2003). These opportunities may very well be contributing to Savin-Williams' conclusion that youth are "coming out" or disclosing their homosexual identity at much younger ages than before (Savin-Williams, 2005).

Conclusions

From presenting their sexual selves to cybersex and accessing sexually explicit content, we have shown how adolescents use technologies such as the Internet to help them with the developmental task of establishing their sexuality. In line with our connectedness hypothesis, adolescents' online sexual explorations reflect a core offline concern. Although some age and gender trends in their online explorations are similar to offline ones, online behaviors were not identical as youth adapted to the characteristic of the online environment in question.

What are the practical implications of their online sexual exploration? Research has documented that in their offline lives, adolescents think about sex, talk about sex, and experiment with sex. Throughout this chapter, we have shown that it is no different when it comes to their digital lives as well and it is important to view adolescents' online sexual activities as a part of their sexual development. We suggest that the Internet has not really changed adolescent sexuality all that much. Certainly large amounts of information are more easily available and there are more opportunities for exploration. However, at a fundamental level, sexuality is tied to our bodies and most sexual exploration must still take place in the offline physical world. The Internet cannot substitute kissing, touching, blushing, hugging, cuddling, and the basic elements of "physical exploration" will therefore remain unchanged. At best, the Internet is a tool that can help youth to overcome their shyness, to learn to talk about sex, find a romantic partner, or learn about sexuality and sexual health. We believe that warm parent–child communication and relationships are probably the best way to ensure that teens' online sexual exploration occurs safely and positively (Greenfield, 2004).

Although we do know that youth use the Internet for online sexual exploration, we are just beginning to study the effects of such exploration, particularly as regards to pornography. Online sexual exploration and exposure to sexually related materials very likely involves both positive and negative aspects. Although it may provide a beneficial means for sexual exploration when searching for sexually-related health materials, exposure to sexual content can also be accidental, unwanted, or threatening, as in the case of sexual solicitation or victimization, topics that we consider in Chapter 10. More research is necessary to understand both the benefits and costs of accessing sexual material. Additionally, most of the research on this topic is from Western countries, particularly the USA and the Netherlands. The Netherlands in particular is considerably more sexually permissive than most. It is quite likely that the Internet plays very different roles in contexts that are more sexually conservative and we must be careful when interpreting and generalizing extant research to other contexts.

References

Alexander, J. (2002). Introduction to the special issue: Queer webs: Representations of LGBT people and communities on the world wide web. *International Journal of Sexuality and Gender Studies, 7*, 77–84.

Brown, J. D., & L'Engle, K. L. (2009). X-rated: Sexual attitudes and behaviors associated with US early adolescents' exposure to sexually explicit media. *Communication Research, 36*, 129–151.

Buzwell, S., & Rosenthal, D. (1996). Constructing a sexual self: Adolescents' sexual self-perceptions and sexual risk-taking. *Journal of Research on Adolescence, 6*, 489–513.

Chilman, C. S. (1990). Promoting healthy adolescent sexuality. *Family Relations, 39*, 123–131.

Cloud, J. (2005, October). The battle over gay teens. *Time, 2*. Retrieved August 5, 2009, from http://www.time.com/time/magazine/article/0,9171,1112856,00.html

Connolly, J., Furman, W., & Konarski, R. (2000). The role of peers in the emergence of heterosexual romantic relationships in adolescence. *Child Development, 71*, 1395–1408.

Cooper, A., Delmonico, D. L., & Burg, R. (2000). Cybersex users, abusers, and compulsives: New findings and implications. *Sexual Addiction & Compulsivity: The Journal of Treatment & Prevention, 7*, 5–29.

Cooper, A., Putnam, D. E., Planchon, L. A., & Boies, S. C. (1999a). Online sexual compulsivity: Getting tangled in the net. *Sexual Addiction & Compulsivity, 6*, 79.

Cooper, A., Scherer, C. R., Boies, S. C., & Gordon, B. L. (1999b). Sexuality on the Internet: From sexual exploration to pathological expression. *Professional Psychology: Research and Practice, 30*, 154–164.

Cubbin, C., Santelli, J., Brindis, C. D., & Braveman, P. (2005). Neighborhood context and sexual behaviors among adolescents: Findings from the national longitudinal study of adolescent health. *Perspectives on Sexual and Reproductive Health, 37*, 125–134.

Divinova, R. (2005). *Cybersex – forma internetové komunikace. [Cybersex – form of internet communication].* Prague: Triton.

Driver, S. (2006). Virtually queer youth communities of girls and birls: Dialogical spaces of identity work and desiring exchanges. In D. Buckingham (Eds.), *Digital generations: Children, young people and new media* (pp. 229–245). Mahwah, NJ: Lawrence Erlbaum Associates Publishers.

Egan, J. (2000). Lonely gay teen seeking same [Electronic version]. *New York Times Magazine, 110*. Retrieved August 17, 2009, from http://partners.nytimes.com/library/magazine/home/20001210mag-online.html

FamilySafeMedia. (2006). Pornography statistics. *Family Safe Media.* Retrieved November 17, 2008, from http://www.familysafemedia.com/pornography_statistics.html

Flood, M., & Hamilton, C. (2003). Regulating youth access to pornography. *Discussion Paper Number 53.* From https://www.tai.org.au/documents/dp_fulltext/DP53.pdf

Galanos, M. (2009). *Is 'sexting' child pornography?* Retrieved July 16, 2009, from http://www.cnn.com/2009/CRIME/04/08/galanos.sexting/index.html

Gossett, J. L., & Byrne, S. (2002). "Click here": A content analysis of Internet rape sites. *Gender & Society, 16*, 689–709.

Greenfield, P. M. (2004). Inadvertent exposure to pornography on the Internet: Implications of peer-to-peer file-sharing networks for child development and families. *Journal of Applied Developmental Psychology: An International Lifespan Journal, 25*, 741–750.

Harper, G. W., Bruce, D., Serrano, P., & Jamil, O. B. (2009). The role of the Internet in the sexual identity development of gay and bisexual male adolescents. In P. L. Hammack & B. J. Cohler (Eds.), *The story of sexual identity: Narrative perspectives on the gay and lesbian life course* (pp. 297–326). New York, NY: Oxford University Press.

Henrickson, M. (2007). Reaching out, hooking up: Lavender netlife in a New Zealand study. *Sexuality Research and Social Policy: Journal of NSRC, 4*, 38–49.

Hinduja, S., & Patchin, J. W. (2008). Personal information of adolescents on the Internet: A quantitative content analysis of myspace. *Journal of Adolescence, 31*, 125–146.

Lo, V., & Wei, R. (2005). Exposure to Internet pornography and taiwanese adolescents' sexual attitudes and behavior. *Journal of Broadcasting & Electronic Media, 49*, 221–237.

Macek, P. (2003). *Adolescence* (2nd ed.). Praha: Portál.

Maczewski, M. (2002). Exploring identities through the Internet: Youth experiences online. *Child and Youth Care Forum, 31*, 111–129.

McCabe, M. P., & Collins, J. K. (1984). Measurement of depth of desired and experienced sexual involvement at different stages of dating. *The Journal of Sex Research, 20*, 377–390.

Miller, B. C., & Benson, B. (1999). Romantic and sexual relationship development during adolescence. In W. Furman, B. B. Brown, & C. Feiring (Eds.), *The development of romantic relationships in adolescence* (pp. 99–121). Cambridge: Cambridge University Press.

Mitchell, K. J., Finkelhor, D., & Wolak, J. (2003). The exposure of youth to unwanted sexual material on the Internet: A national survey of risk, impact, and prevention. *Youth & Society, 34*, 330–358.

Mitchell, K. J., Finkelhor, D., & Wolak, J. (2005). The Internet and family and acquaintance sexual abuse. *Child Miltreatment, 10*, 49–60.

Mosher, W. D., Chandra, A., & Jones, J. (2005). *Sexual behavior and selected health measures: Men and women 15–44 years of age, United States, 2002*. Retrieved October 28, 2005, from http://www.cdc.gov/nchs/data/ad/ad362.pdf

National Campaign to Prevent Teen and Unplanned Pregnancy & Cosmogirl.com. (2008). *Sex and tech: Results from a survey of teens and young adults*. Retrieved July 16, 2009, from http://www.thenationalcampaign.org/sextech/PDF/SexTech_Summary.pdf

Noonan, R. J. (2007). The psychology of sex: A mirror from the Internet. In J. Gackenbach (Ed.), *Psychology and the internet: Intrapersonal, interpersonal, and transpersonal implications* (2nd ed., pp. 93–139). San Diego, CA: Academic Press.

Peter, J., & Valkenburg, P. M. (2006a). Adolescents' exposure to sexually explicit material on the Internet. *Communication Research, 33*, 178–204.

Peter, J., & Valkenburg, P. M. (2006b). Adolescents' exposure to sexually explicit online material and recreational attitudes toward sex. *Journal of Communication, 56*, 639–660.

Peter, J., & Valkenburg, P. M. (2007). Who looks for casual dates on the Internet? A test of the compensation and the recreation hypotheses. *New Media & Society, 9*, 455.

Peter, J., & Valkenburg, P. M. (2008a). Adolescents' exposure to sexually explicit Internet material and sexual preoccupancy: A three-wave panel study. *Media Psychology, 11*, 207–234.

Peter, J., & Valkenburg, P. M. (2008b). Adolescents' exposure to sexually explicit Internet material, sexual uncertainty, and attitudes toward uncommitted sexual exploration: Is there a link? *Communication Research, 35*, 579–601.

Reich, S. M., Subrahmanyam, K., & Espinoza, G. E. (2009, April 3). *Adolescents' use of social networking sites – Should we be concerned?* Paper presented at the Society for Research on Child Development, Denver, CO.

Rice, F. P. (2001). *Human development*. Upper Saddle River, NJ: Prentice Hall.

Saleh, F. M. (2009). *Internet pornography and cybersex*. Paper presented at the American Society for Adolescent Psychiatry. Retrieved November 20, 2009, from http://www.adolpsych.org/presentations09/Saleh-InternetPornographyandCybersex.pdf

Savin-Williams, R. C. (2005). *The new gay teenager*. Cambridge, MA: Harvard University Press.

Savin-Williams, R. C., & Diamond, L. M. (2004). Sex. In R. M. Lerner & L. Steinberg (Eds.), *Handbook of adolescent psychology* (2nd ed., pp. 189–231). New York, NY: Wiley.

Silberman, S. (2004). We're teen, we're queer, and we've got e-mail [Electronic version]. *Wired Magazine, 2.11*. Retrieved August 15, 2009, from http://www.wired.com/wired/archive/2.11/gay.teen_pr.html

Šmahel, D. (2003). *Psychologie a Internet: Děti dospělými, dospělí dětmi. [Psychology and Internet: Children being adults, adults being children.]*. Prague: Triton.

Šmahel, D. (2006, March 23). *Czech adolescents' partnership relations and sexuality in the Internet environment.* Paper presented at the Biennial Meeting of the Society for Research on Adolescence, San Francisco, CA. Retrieved August 20, 2008, from http://www.terapie.cz/materials/smahel-SRA-SF-2006.pdf

Steinberg, L. (2008). *Adolescence.* New York, NY: McGraw-Hill.

Subrahmanyam, K., Garcia, E. C., Harsono, S. L., Li, J., & Lipana, L. (2009). In their words: Connecting online weblogs to developmental processes. *British Journal of Developmental Psychology, 27,* 219–245.

Subrahmanyam, K., Greenfield, P. M., & Tynes, B. (2004). Constructing sexuality and identity in an online teen chat room. *Journal of Applied Developmental Psychology: An International Lifespan Journal, 25,* 651–666.

Subrahmanyam, K., Šmahel, D., & Greenfield, P. (2006). Connecting developmental constructions to the Internet: Identity presentation and sexual exploration in online teen chat rooms. *Developmental Psychology, 42,* 395–406.

Suler, J. (2008). *The psychology of cyberspace.* Retrieved August 20, 2008, from http://www-usr.rider.edu/~suler/psycyber/psycyber.html

Suzuki, L. K., & Calzo, J. P. (2004). The search for peer advice in cyberspace: An examination of online teen bulletin boards about health and sexuality. *Journal of Applied Developmental Psychology, 25,* 685–698.

Thomas, A. B. (2003). Internet chat room participation and the coming-out experiences of young gay men: A qualitative study (Doctoral dissertation, University of Texas, Austin, 2003). *Dissertation Abstracts International, 64,* 815.

Tikkanen, R., & Ross, M. W. (2003). Technological tearoom trade: Characteristics of Swedish men visiting gay Internet chat rooms. *AIDS Education and Prevention, 15,* 122–132.

Turkle, S. (1997). *Life on the screen identity in the age of the Internet* (1st ed.). New York, NY: Touchstone.

Wallmyr, G., & Welin, C. (2006). Young people, pornography, and sexuality: Sources and attitudes. *The Journal of School Nursing, 22,* 290–295.

Ward, L. M. (2004, March 11). *And TV makes three: Comparing contributions of parents, peers, and the media to sexual socialization.* Paper presented at the Society for Research in Adolescence, Baltimore, MD.

Weinstein, E., & Rosen, E. (1991). The development of adolescent sexual intimacy: Implications for counseling. *Adolescence, 26,* 331–339.

Whitty, M. T., & Carr, A. (2006). *Cyberspace romance: The psychology of online relationships.* Basingstoke; New York, NY: Palgrave Macmillan.

Ybarra, M. L., & Mitchell, K. J. (2005). Exposure to Internet pornography among children and adolescents: A national survey. *CyberPsychology & Behavior, 8,* 473–486.

Chapter 4
Constructing Identity Online: Identity Exploration and Self-Presentation

Since the inception of the Internet, perhaps no other topic related to it has engendered as much speculation or excitement as the potential for users to leave their bodies behind and create new and different selves or personas online (e.g. Kendall, 2003; Stallabrass, 1995; Turkle, 1997, 2005; Wakeford, 1999). For example, Turkle described one Midwestern college junior who played four different characters across three different multi-user dungeons or Dungeon or (MUDs): a seductive woman, a "macho cowboy" type, a rabbit of unspecified gender, and a furry animal. The various computer screens, or windows, made it possible to turn pieces of his mind on and off: "I just turn on one part of my mind and then another when I go from window to window ... 'rl' [real life] is just one more window, and it's not usually my best one" (Turkle, 1997, p. 13). A little over 10 years later, Manago and colleagues quote a female focus group participant in their study of the social networking site, MySpace, as saying: "Whenever you put any kind of information out there you have the intention of what you want people to think about you" (Manago, Graham, Greenfield, & Salimkhan, 2008, p. 450). Although very different in essence, both cases illustrate how users are taking advantage of technology to negotiate and present aspects of the self.

Formulating a unified sense of self, in other words constructing a coherent and stable identity, is an important adolescent developmental task, and the focus of this chapter. Identity is a relatively complex term, and differences abound in how identity is construed across different disciplines, such as psychology (and even in different schools of psychology), sociology, anthropology, and philosophy, as well as by researchers from different cultural contexts, as we (Indian-American and Czech) discovered when we began working on this chapter. Here we adopt Moshman's definition, which summarizes the elements emphasized in the most important theories, and which offers a framework for studying identity during adolescence: "*An identity is, at least in part, an explicit theory of oneself as a person*" (Moshman, 2005, p. 89). According to this view, one's identity is a sophisticated conception of the self, one which should help to answer questions such as "who am I?", "where do I belong?", and "where am I headed?"

In this chapter, we begin by examining theoretical conceptions about identity in the context of adolescence as well as explore the meaning of the terms online

K. Subrahmanyam, D. Šmahel, *Digital Youth*, Advancing Responsible Adolescent Development, DOI 10.1007/978-1-4419-6278-2_4,
© Springer Science+Business Media, LLC 2011

self-presentation and virtual identity. To show how adolescents use technology in the service of identity, we will first describe some online tools they can use for self-presentation and identity construction. Then we show how adolescents use these tools to explore identity on the Internet, particularly through blogs and social networking sites. We also describe research that will help to understand the relation between young people's online activities and their processes of identity development. In a separate section, we show how youth use the Internet to construct their ethnic identity. Last, we turn to questions surrounding adolescents' identity experiments and online pretending.

Identity During Adolescence

Erikson, who was the first to draw attention to the notion of identity (Kroger, 2006), viewed adolescence as the period when individuals have to accomplish the task of constructing an identity of the self or the ego identity. Creation of an ego identity represents the integration of existing accumulated experience, skills, talents, and opportunities offered by various social roles into one compact and complex identity of the individual. For Erikson, the issues of vocational decision making, ideological values, and sexual identity were the bases of ego identity (Erikson & Stone, 1959; Erikson, 1968). Erikson argued that adolescents are in a period of psychosocial moratorium, during which time they can explore alternative roles and identities. Those who do so are more likely to be satisfied with their identities, and adolescents' reflections about themselves, their characteristics, and social position helps them explore and construct their identity (Nurmi, 2004).

Erikson's (1968) theory about identity was subsequently elaborated by Marcia, who viewed identity as a process and developed an approach to measure an adolescent's identity status at any given point (Marcia, 1966, 1976). For Marcia, the concepts of exploration and commitment were key to identifying where an adolescent was in his or her identity development. Exploration occurs when an adolescent is drawn into the process of choice and decision making over the issues of relationships, religion, life style, or occupation/jobs. It is a process of active search and discovery. In contrast, commitment is the acceptance of a certain goal and life program, and entails an individual taking responsibility for his or her life choices and actions.

For Marcia, the presence and/or absence of the core dimensions of exploration and commitment yielded the following four distinct states of identity or identity statuses:

(1) *Foreclosed identity* is characterized by the presence of commitment and the absence of exploration. Although the adolescent is satisfied with his/her sense of identity, it is drawn from authority figures and the youth may tend to be rigid and conformist.

(2) *Identity diffusion* is a state where the adolescent experiences neither crisis nor commitment and is not actively exploring his/her sense of self. According to Marcia, youth who are in a state of identity diffusion are easily influenced by peers, and may often change opinions and behavior, in accordance with group expectations or norms.

(3) In the stage of *moratorium*, the adolescent experiences a crisis about his or her identity, but does not commit to a particular sense of self. Akin to a time-out, he or she may experience states of anxiety and doubts, explore and try out new roles without committing to them, and experiment, discover and explore new values and norms.

(4) In the stage of *identity achievement*, both crisis and commitment are present. The adolescent experiences a crisis about his or her identity, explores and experiments, and eventually commits to a particular sense of self, accepting the responsibility that goes with such a commitment. Youth in this stage of identity achievement are believed to have a positive self-image, are flexible, and independent.

On Eriskon's and Marcia's views, exploration is key to the development of a healthy identity during adolescence. Developmental research suggests that although such identity exploration may take place throughout adolescence, identity as a developmental task may be more important to older rather than younger adolescents (Nurmi, 2004; Reis & Youniss, 2004; Waterman, 1999). Identity exploration does not occur in a vacuum and is related to other aspects of an individual's life. Adolescents' search for the self is related to their pubertal status (Papini, Sebby, & Clark, 1989), as well as family variables such as satisfaction and dissatisfaction with different aspects of family functioning (e.g., decision making, affective quality of family relationships) (Papini et al., 1989) and family interaction patterns and communication styles (Grotevant & Cooper, 1985; Quintana & Lapsley, 1990; Reis & Youniss, 2004). Friends and peers (See Chapter 5) are believed to be important, as adolescents may be more likely to try out new attitudes and behaviors in their company (Akers, Jones, & Coyl, 1998) and depend on them for support and feedback and to serve as mirror when they test different aspects of their self-definition (Akers et al., 1998; Kroger, 2006). Indeed, mutual friends are similar in ego identity as well as in attitudes, behaviors and intentions related to identity (Akers et al., 1998) and problems with friends is negatively associated with adolescent identity trajectories (Reis & Youniss, 2004). As we noted in the Introduction to this chapter, the Internet is seen as providing an ideal venue for such identity exploration (Turkle, 1997; Wallace, 1999) and we will examine how digital youth take advantage of this newest context to express and construct their identities.

An alternative conceptualization of identity relevant for our purposes is that proposed by McAdams, who has argued that the development of identity is an ongoing and fluid process, during which identity is adapted to current postmodern conditions (McAdams, 1997). Identity is never "established," but instead is a process of narration that occurs in the context of several multiple selves. According to McAdams

(1999), individuals on the brink of adulthood construct narratives or dynamic internal life stories about themselves and these stories form the basis of their identities. These identity narratives draw from the adolescents' past, present, and future and contain themes related to agency (or achievement and mastery) and communion (or interrelations to others). Later in this chapter, we will describe how youth use digital media such as blogs to construct self-narratives.

Identity is a multi-dimensional construct and scholars have distinguished between different aspects of identity, such as personal, social, gender and ethnic identity. Personal identity is based on self-assessment and self-reflection (e.g., "who I am" "I am myself"), and social identity is connected to feelings of inclusion or belonging to one's social context or social group (e.g., "where I belong", "what I am part of") (Macek, 2003). Gender is important during adolescence and emerging adulthood (Arnett, 2004; Macek, 2003); males and females often have very different social roles and the identity process they undergo can vary according to these social roles. Ethnic identity is also constructed during adolescence and is defined as "an enduring, fundamental aspect of the self that includes the sense of membership in an ethnic group and the attitudes and feelings associated with that membership" (Phinney, 1996). We will show that digital contexts can support youth as they construct their personal, social, gender, and ethnic identities (Manago et al., 2008; Tynes, Giang, & Thompson, 2008; Tynes, Reynolds, & Greenfield, 2004).

Online Self-Presentation and Virtual Identity

On the Internet, the terms "virtual identity" and "online identity" can take on two different meanings (Šmahel, 2003). First, they refer to identity as an identification and self-presentation (or representation) of the individual on the Internet. Second, they refer to online identity in a psychological sense – a sophisticated conceptualization of an individual's online self or persona. The first construal derives from the fact that individuals have a "virtual representation" rather than an actual physical presence within digital contexts (Šmahel, 2003). A virtual representation is a "cluster" of digital data about a user in a virtual context and includes a name or more accurately, a nickname/username, email address, online history, and status within that virtual setting. In other words, it is simply a user's face and body within that particular digital context. Individuals can have different digital representations in different online contexts (e.g. multiple email addresses such as teacher@university.cz and stamp-collector@something.cz) or even different digital representations within the same context (e.g., multiple avatars within an online game or virtual world).

The second construal of virtual identity comprises the thoughts, ideas, visions, or fantasies that users attribute to their virtual representations. It is the transfer, perhaps unconsciously, of the thoughts, emotions, and other aspects of their self to their online selves (Šmahel, 2003). Virtual identity is also comprised of personal and social aspects. Personal virtual identity relates to "who I am" as a person in a particular virtual environment, or more precisely, to a users' representation in that virtual environment. Social virtual identity characterizes where an individual belongs in a particular virtual world, the online community or communities that he/she may be a part of, the individual's status within those communities, etc. For example, a user's avatar in World of Warcraft (aMMORPG) could be that of a strong mage[1] of the highest level and a leader of the guild. The personal identity attached to this avatar could include superiority, reinforcement of the self, and improvement of self-esteem. The social identity of this role could entail a leadership position among a group of players – it may be connected to the acknowledgment and admiration elicited from other players and a sense of responsibility for other players and for the success of common campaigns (Šmahel, Blinka, & Ledabyl, 2008). Although both meanings of the term online identity are valid, research on adolescents' online identity construction has mostly dealt with digital representation and self-presentation, as we will see in the next sections.

Adolescent's Online Identity Construction

As we noted earlier, construction of a stable and coherent identity requires exploration (Erikson, 1959), and for today's adolescents, exploration can occur in both offline and online worlds (Subrahmanyam, Šmahel, & Greenfield, 2006). As we will show in this section, online contexts offer plenty of opportunities for the questioning and searching envisioned by Erikson and Marcia. Indeed it has been suggested that the potential anonymity and relative safety of the Internet may allow for experimentation, and thus provides the perfect venue for youth to test aspects of their identities (Wallace, 1999). However, not all online venues allow users to remain anonymous, and in these contexts, adolescents interact with their peers, form relationships, and polish their social skills, activities that may help them with the task of formulating their sense of self.

Online identity construction also includes online self-presentation, which includes the different ways by which users present themselves to other online users. Keep in mind that in less anonymous but more private contexts, such as social networking sites, such information may be more readily available. But in more anonymous online contexts, such as chat rooms and bulletin boards, even basic information such as gender, age, physical appearance, physical attractiveness, and race may not be readily available (McKenna & Bargh, 2000; Šmahel, 2003; Subrahmanyam, 2003; Subrahmanyam et al., 2006; Suler, 2008). Regardless, online self-presentation is important because individuals have considerable choice with regard to which aspects of the self to reveal. It could be aspects of their self that they especially wish to highlight, such as their gender, interests, or sexual preference; but it could also be aspects that they aspire to assume, want to eschew, or even explore and experiment with to see their own and other people's reaction. Identity construction is not a monolithic activity, and in the next sub-sections, we describe

---

[1] A mage is a specialized role in WoW with specific responsibilities and abilities.

the many different ways in which it occurs online and show that it depends very much on the particular tools and affordances of the online environment in question.

Tools for Online Self-Presentation

Nicknames (usernames). In some online applications such as chat rooms, discussion forums, or textual online games, identity is often established through a nickname or username, which may convey information about a user's gender (e.g., *prettygurl245*), sexual identity (*straitangel*), as well as special interests (*soccerchick*). In our research on online teen chat rooms, we analyzed approximately 500 nicknames and found that in many ways, users' online screen names mirrored their offline selves (Subrahmanyam et al., 2006). For instance, in teen chat rooms, 48% of self-described females used a feminine nickname (e.g., *MandiCS12*, *Lilprincess72988*), while 32% of self-described males used a masculine nickname (e.g., *RAYMONI8*, *BlazinJosh55*) (Šmahel & Subrahmanyam, 2007; Subrahmanyam et al., 2006). Additionally, 26% of self-described females and 10% of self-described males used sexual nicknames (e.g., *SexyDickHed*, *angel*, *prettygirl*), a pattern suggestive of differences in the offline world. Sexualized nicknames were stand-ins for the face and body of youth, who wished to convey their interest and intentions to engage in sexualized activities. In other words, they seemed to be used to attract the interest and attention of partners (Šmahel & Subrahmanyam, 2007; Šmahel & Vesela, 2006; Subrahmanyam, Greenfield, & Tynes, 2004). Adolescents also frequently incorporated their interests in their nicknames as in *soccerboy or musicgirl* (both nicknames incorporate information about interests and gender). In text-based chat rooms, nicknames were probably the most salient aspect of users' virtual identities. However, in contexts such as blogs, social networking sites, and games, nicknames or user names are probably not very salient as more details are available about users' virtual identity, such as an avatar with clothes, equipment, and history in online games.

a/s/l code. In an effort to share basic facts about their identity in the Internet environment, young Internet users have come up with creative strategies. One such strategy that we found in our own research on online teen chat rooms is the "a/s/l" (age/sex/location) slot filler code (Greenfield & Subrahmanyam, 2003). The a/s/l code can be used as a question asking other user or users to identify themselves or with the information filled in such as 16/M/CA. The latter format signifies to others that the user is a 16-year-old male from California. It was the most frequent utterance that we encountered in the chat rooms we studied. The a/s/l code enabled chat users to share information about themselves and their identity, providing them with a basic sense of potential conversational partners within that online setting. From classic studies in social psychology, we know that age and sex are also the primary categories to which people are assigned to in face-to-face communication (Brewer and Lui, 1989). Other information that is readily apparent in face-to-face interactions (e.g., figure, clothes, face) is estimated in online chat rooms or more generally in text-based online communication (Šmahel, 2003).

Interestingly, the particular codes constructed by online users for sharing identity information seem to vary as a function of the context. The a/s/l codes we observed were in teen chat rooms hosted by US providers, where users interacted in English. However, they were absent in chat rooms that we observed in the Czech Republic. One possible reason is that Czech nicknames readily convey participants' gender, because in the Czech language, it is possible to derive gender from the grammatical suffix of the name and nickname. Location information is not very useful because the Czech Republic is not very big (with a population of about 10 million people). Therefore, Czech adolescents usually only provided their age in their chat utterances since information about gender and location was moot in this case. Even though the Internet is a global phenomenon, we can expect to see differences in the particular devices that users in different contexts come up with for self-presentation since cues that are likely to be relevant to identity may themselves vary depending on cultural and geographic specifics.

Avatars. Within computer games (e.g., MMORPGs) and complex virtual worlds (e.g., Second Life), players' online identities or personas are avatars, which are adjustable, motion-enabled graphical representations (see Fig. 4.1). Depending on the online space, avatars can assume a variety of forms, ranging from human-like to fantastical creatures, and are typically 3D and animated. Consequently, the options for creating a virtual identity are even greater, since players have complete control over their avatar and can shape it literally any way they want. Research suggests that within MMORPG games, adolescent and young adult players have a greater

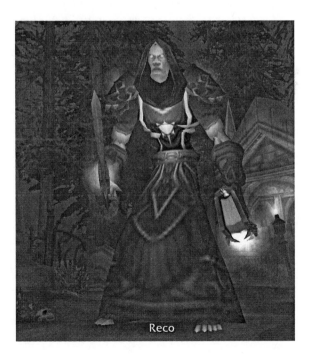

Fig. 4.1 An example of an avatar: From the online game "The World of Warcraft"

tendency to identify with their avatars than adults (Šmahel, Blinka, & Ledabyl, 2008); they more often stated that "they are the same as their avatars" and that "they possess the same skills and abilities as their avatars."

Avatars as virtual characters very likely create a better field for projection and identification than nicknames alone. If a young user can see his or her complete graphic representation, including face, figure, clothes, and equipment (such as magical powers, weapons, pets, etc.) and can change this representation, it opens up more room for identifying with the virtual representation itself. In the case of nicknames, users are connected to their virtual representations through social communication, that is, they create a social identity by communicating with others; in contrast, users' relationship to their avatars or virtual representations is more direct, as it is based on communication as well as visual aspects of the avatar and its actions. For an adolescent gamer, a virtual game character or avatar may thus serve as a means of identification with positive as well as negative aspects of offline personality (Šmahel, Blinka, & Ledabyl, 2008).

Photos and videos. Photographs and videos can be used for online self-presentation and are easy to upload in blogs, social networking profiles, and other similar user-generated sites. Our study of 195 English blogs maintained by self-declared adolescents revealed that 60% of bloggers published their user pictures and younger bloggers were more likely to post pictures than older ones (Subrahmanyam, Garcia, Harsono, Li, & Lipana, 2009) (see Fig. 4.2). It may be that using photos to present oneself is more important for younger adolescents because at this stage, public visual displays of the self may drive their sense of self (Baumeister, 1986). However, it may also be that younger teens are simply more technologically skilled and at ease with creating and publishing user pictures (Greenfield & Subrahmanyam, 2003). Although we know that youth make extensive use of visual media in their online profiles, we do not know how the details of such use, how it

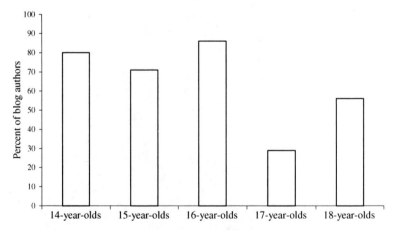

Fig. 4.2 Percentage of blog authors who adopted a userpicture as a function of age (adapted from Subrahmanyam et al., 2009)

relates to their identity development, and in particular whether it helps or hinders their emerging sense of self. There are also the issues of privacy and safety that come with displaying pictures online, and we address them in Chapters 10 and 11.

The preceding suggests that young people take advantage of the tools available within a particular online context for exploration and self-presentation. From unique chat codes (e.g., asl), nicknames, and avatars to photographs and videos, adolescents take advantage of online tools to quickly and easily reveal aspects of their self that they wish to share with their online partners and peers. Contrary to early speculation that technology makes it easy for users to leave their bodies behind and assume new and alternative identities, on the Internet, adolescent users seem to go out of their way to present their offline selves and not stay disembodied.

Identity Expression and Self-Presentation in Blogs and Homepages

Blogs and web pages present virtually constructed images of adolescent's lives, their problems, joys, and the issues with which they are dealing at the time. When their online writings and images are public, they provide researchers with a window into how youth use technology in the service of their developing identity (Huffaker & Calvert, 2005; Mazur & Kozarian, 2009; Schmitt, Dayanim, & Matthias, 2008; Subrahmanyam et al., 2009; Suzuki & Beale, 2006). Here we describe two studies – one on blogs (Subrahmanyam et al., 2009) and one on personal homepages (Schmitt et al., 2008), which have yielded a rich but complicated picture of young people's online identity construction.

In the blog study, we analyzed 195 English-language blogs written by bloggers who identified themselves as teens (usually by stating their age) (Subrahmanyam et al., 2009). The teen authors made extensive use of the previously described self-presentation tools, such as Usernames (or nick names) and Userpictures. Usernames, which are present in all blogs, conveyed the authors' gender about 40% of the time. Among such gendered Usernames, we also found agreement between bloggers' stated gender (which we found in their profile or from the content of their entries) and the gender identity presented in their usernames. In addition to their gender, bloggers frequently provided information about their age (75%) and location (70%). Although Userpictures are optional in blogs, 60% of bloggers had one, and younger bloggers were more likely to do so. Userpictures generally contained images (71%) or images and text (26%). Most of the images that we could code were self-photographs or related to pop culture. Pop culture, especially music, has always been a means for adolescents to present who they are (Thornton, 1996) and together with self-images, were frequently found in their blogs as well.

We did not see too many instances of explicit musings about identity such as the following: *I am soft spoken and I am strong, but I won't stand up for myself very often. I am naive and come off snobby a lot of the time. But when it all comes down to it, inside me there is this evil fairy who takes over at times and destructs my life.* Also infrequent in the blog entries were themes related to romance, sexuality, and problem behaviors. Perhaps the authors were conscious that their blogs were public and so avoided writing about sensitive topics; recall from Chapter 3 that they have no such inhibitions in the more anonymous chat rooms (Subrahmanyam et al., 2006). The blog entries we analyzed were narrative and reflective in style, focused on the teen authors' peers and everyday activities (e.g., school, after-school activities), and were emotional in tone about the people and events in their life. McAdams suggests that such narratives or life stories help individuals on the brink of adulthood to construct a coherent sense of their self (McAdams, 1997). We concluded that although the teen bloggers did not often write openly about identity, the narratives they constructed in their online blogs may have helped them with the task of establishing their sense of self.

The study of young people's personal homepages by Schmitt et al. (2008) utilized both a large scale survey of 500 8- to 17-year olds and a content analysis of 72 homepages created by youth in the same age range. On the survey study, youth reported feelings of mastery at being able to create homepages. Most felt that they "can make it [their] own way" and even more importantly, help others to understand who [they] are;" majority also felt that it was easier to share information about themselves on their home page than face-to-face. The content analysis corroborated these results, as there was evidence of both mastery (especially about hobbies and sports) and identity expression. Like the teen bloggers, these youth also included information about themselves, such as their age, gender, location, and a self-representation, such as photos or cartoon pictures. They also wrote about their interests, relationships, and values. Noteworthy offline parallels included the finding that girls and older adolescents provided more information about themselves. Participants' statements about their personalities and strengths nicely illustrate the latter developmental trend. Pre-adolescents simply stated what they were good at such as this 9-year old: *I am very good at playing games online and I am also good at typing.* Compare this to the more detailed description and defense of herself by a 16-year old in the same study: *If you don't like what I look like, keep it to yourself [be]cause I am who I am and I like who I am! That's what I'm all about. . .having fun and being myself*!! Because the sample of homepages analyzed was small and no details were provided as to how frequent such explicit identity statements were, we really cannot say whether they were more frequent than what we found in our analysis of adolescents' blogs, which was described in the previous paragraph.

Both studies show that teens' use of technology in the service of identity occurs not for the active identity experimentation suggested by Erikson (1968), and popularized by Turkle (1997), but for self-expression and for sharing this information with peers. Like other aspects of online behavior, adolescent' identity expression in blogs and homepages may be dependent on the context. In an ongoing Czech study using the methodology of our study of English language blogs (see Subrahmanyam et al., 2009), 203 blogs authored by 12- to 17-year olds were analyzed (Blinka, Šmahel, & Subrahmanyam, n.d.). In contrast to the English-language blogs, most Czech blogs were enhanced with pictures – about 91% of teen bloggers used pictures, mostly photographs of celebrities (music stars, actors etc.), as well as signs and subculture symbols (i.e., emo or gothic symbols). Czech adolescents seem to express their belonging to particular subcultures of music genres much more often than bloggers who maintained English-language blogs. Such online expressions of affiliation with offline cultural idols and/or belonging to offline subcultures could be an important way that adolescents use technology to explore their off-line identity.

Identity Expression and Self-Presentation in Social Networking Sites

Although social networking sites like Facebook and MySpace seem to be primarily used for connecting with peers (and this issue is described in detail in the next chapter), aspects of identity expression and presentation have been found within them (Livingstone, 2008; Manago et al., 2008; Strano, 2008; Subrahmanyam, Reich, Waechter, & Espinoza, 2008). From her interviews with 16 social networking site users, who were 13- to 16-years old, Livingstone (2008) concluded that teens' identity development "seemed to be expressed in terms of decisions regarding the style or choice of site" (p. 400). Some adolescents, for example, switched from MySpace to Facebook because they saw that there were older people on Facebook and that the profiles on Facebook appeared simpler and typically less colorful. Younger teens put more effort into 'decorating' their site profiles, wherein they provided more elaborate information about themselves, whereas older adolescents preferred plain sites that brought to the forefront their connections to other social networking sites users. In other words, younger adolescents reported presenting their identity more often on social networking sites. In fact, in our blog study, we similarly found that bloggers who reported being younger were more likely to have userpictures, although there were no age differences in their actual content (Subrahmanyam et al., 2009).

Because online profiles are typically private, it has not been possible for researchers to document the culture of social networking sites, as it was possible with the more public chat rooms and blog sites. But in-depth focus group interviews with 23 MySpace users by Manago and colleagues have shed some light on identity forays in this venue (Manago et al., 2008). Even though the participants were 18- to 23-year-old college students, very similar processes likely occur with adolescents and so we describe some interesting findings. The researchers discovered several constructions of personal, social, and gender identity and concluded that "MySpace gives emerging adults a tool to explore possible selves and express ideal selves that they may want to become" (p. 455). At the same time, an "increased pressure on young women to objectify their sexuality while also preserving their innocence may be a confusing and detrimental influence on their development" (p. 455). Remarkable to us are the parallels between young people's online gender role constructions and their offline ones: Within mainstream US culture, positive valence is associated with affiliative and attractive females and strong and powerful males and the focus group participants reported similar gendered patterns for the MySpace profiles.

Online Behavior and Identity Status

An important issue is whether adolescents' online activities relate to their overall identity development. In the next subsections, we discuss the potential role of the Internet for individuals in the four statuses proposed by Marcia that we discussed earlier. Although some of our ideas are more speculative in nature, where available, we draw on the results of two relevant studies that we conducted in the Czech Republic – a qualitative interview study of 16 participants (12- to 25-year olds) and a quantitative survey study of 681 12- to 20-year-old youth (Šmahel, 2003, 2005; Vybiral, Šmahel, & Divínová, 2004); a self-report measure of ego identity status developed by Adams, Shea, and Fitch (1979) was used to measure participants' identity status.

Foreclosed identity. Recall that adolescents who have foreclosed their identity have committed to a particular ego identity, typically one advocated by their parents and other authority figures, but without any crisis or active exploration. Such a foreclosed identity may often be the first to occur during an adolescent's identity development. However, within online contexts, such adolescents could revert to a state, where there is no commitment akin to that found in individuals with a diffused or an uncommitted identity. Online contexts and virtual identities can help with this process, allowing youth to experiment with their identity earlier than they would "dare" to in reality. The results of our quantitative study provided evidence for this possibility. Among teens who were identified as having a foreclosed identity, approximately 47% agreed with the statement that "parents know only very little of what I do on the Internet" and 20% agreed with the statement "on the Internet I am a different person than at home, my parents would evidently not recognize me there." At the same time, 62% of them stated that on the Internet they do not have to comply with the rules of everyday life that they do not agree with. Nonetheless, in comparison with other statuses, adolescents with a foreclosed identity more frequently stated that they behaved according to their parents' expectations and attitudes in virtual worlds. At least for some adolescents who had foreclosed their identities offline, the Internet had become an environment in which they did not feel the "commitment" that defined their offline life. In their cases, online and virtual identities could very well become a forerunner for changes to come in their offline identities.

Diffused identity. Individuals in a state of diffusion experience neither crisis nor commitment, are easily influenced by their peers, often change their views and behavior, and have low self-confidence and problems in interpersonal relationships. We speculate that for adolescents with diffused identities, online environments can become a safe haven, a space where they could learn to express their views, communicate with others, and break group norms without fear of group sanctions. However, there was little empirical support for these ideas in our studies. Diffused identity is hard to measure using a questionnaire as it includes characteristics of all the statuses. Moreover, there was low reliability of the scales measuring this status raising concerns about the reliability of our results.

Moratorium. Individuals in a state of moratorium are concerned about their identity but have not yet committed themselves or show weak commitment at best.

According to Marcia, adolescents in a state of moratorium try out and experiment with different roles and identities, and discover new values. As noted previously, the Internet can be an ideal venue for such identity exploration and experiments. The findings of our research also support this: While online, adolescents in a state of moratorium more frequently break rules and norms that are common in offline life, and more frequently change their self in the virtual environment in comparison with their offline life. Adolescents scoring higher in moratorium report that online they are more open and pretend more often to be better than they are in their offline life. They also state that their parents would not recognize them online, and are more likely to report using the Internet to clarify their values and attitudes. Overall, 59% of adolescents who were in a state of moratorium agreed with the statement that they clarify their attitudes and norms on the Internet, and 58% stated that they are more open online than in reality. Keep in mind that this does not mean that all adolescents in a state of moratorium use the Internet for these purposes; rather they do so more often compared to individuals in the other identity states.

Identity achievement. Individuals in this identity state have experienced both an identity crisis and commitment. However, it would simplistic to think that the search for one's identity, one's "self" and one's values ends in the period of adolescence. In fact, some have suggested that the search for the "self" is a lifelong process, one that never ends (McAdams, 1997). With regard to identity achievement, virtual environments may help by reflecting users' current goals and values via the safe "return" to the moratorium phase (Wallace, 1999). An adolescent or adult may go through the so-called "MAMA" cycle, where phases of moratorium and identity achievement are repeated one after the other. Thus digital contexts could play a role in the search for the self by providing youth with opportunities for safe experimentation with their identity. Our quantitative research also confirmed that adolescents in a state of identity achievement more frequently reported testing or diverging from the norms and rules of everyday life.

The above discussion provides preliminary support for the notion that adolescents' offline identity statuses may be related to their online behavior (Šmahel, 2003, 2005). Although adolescents' online behaviors often correspond to their offline identity status, compared to offline contexts, online contexts afford opportunities for more exploration and fewer commitments. In particular, as noted in Chapter 1, an important aspect of many online communicative environments is that they may disinhibit users and increase the potential for self-disclosure. The Internet may strengthen aspects of exploration and weaken commitment and consequently adolescents' identity statuses could be somewhat different online from offline settings. Participants in our qualitative study also seemed to recognize that some online environments, especially anonymous chat rooms, might come without commitments. A 19-year-old female commented thus about online environments: "barriers from real life are missing, you can be more open, but also more vulnerable;" A 16-year-old female said: "I do not believe people in chat rooms, you cannot see through the screen, you do not know if people are telling the truth" (Šmahel, 2003). Keep in mind that we conducted the studies in 2002 and 2003, when chat rooms were at their peak. Online contexts, such as social networking sites and text messaging, might offer different sets of opportunities for exploration and commitment and more research is needed to understand how activities in these online spaces relate to identity development.

Ethnic Identity Online

Up until this point, we have focused our discussion on aspects of the self that apply broadly to most adolescents such as age, gender, and interests. Now we shift our attention to the role of technology in one very specific aspect of the self, ethnic identity, which as we already noted, is believed to constructed during adolescence (Phinney, 1996); sexual identity (whether one is straight or gay) is also equally important during adolescence and was covered in Chapter 3. Contrary to early expectations, we now know that young people bring their race and ethnicity to digital contexts, such as teen chat rooms, on bulletin boards, and on Facebook and YouTube (Greenfield et al., 2006; Subramanian, 2010; Tynes, 2007; Tynes et al., 2004).

For example, Tynes and colleagues analyzed 30 min chat conversations recorded in monitored and unmonitored teen chat rooms during 2003 (Tynes et al., 2004). A monitored chat room is one in which an adult oversees the teen chat room and enforces the rules of conduct, such as no hate speech and harassment of fellow chatters, whereas an unmonitored chat room has no such monitor and so users are free to talk about any topic in any manner. There was a 19% chance of exposure to negative remarks directed at a racial group in a monitored chat room compared to a 59% chance in an unmonitored chat room. Racial or ethnic slurs were also recorded more often in unmonitored chat rooms, indicating that in the absence of social control (such as a monitor), negative inter-group attitudes may emerge and become prevalent. However, the researcher also observed positive instances of discussions about race and ethnicity. This study analyzed discourse found in the chat room with the unit of analysis being the chat room itself. The assumption was that such chat room snapshots would reveal the content users are most likely to encounter in online teen chat rooms.

Therefore, it is equally important to ask youth what they have learned about race and ethnicity within this context. Tynes interviewed teen (13- to 18-year olds) chat participants via instant messenger and the following excerpt illustrates the learning potential of such chat discourse (Tynes, 2007, p. 1316):

TeenTalk2: can you give an example of what you learn?
Rothrider95: i learn to see things from an oppressed persons
point of view
TeenTalk2: oh. can you say more about that
TeenTalk2: like which groups in particular
Rothrider95 rican americans mostly
TeenTalk2: and what things
Rothrider95: how it must fell to be oppressed

According to Tynes, the teen participants reported that adopting and enacting race-related identities were the primary means by which they learned about race and ethnicity online. Participants also reported adopting one of six typical racialized roles: as discussants (46%), witnesses (41%), targets (41%), friends (28%), sympathizers (18%), and advocates (15%). From the percentages, it is evident that they reported assuming more than one role. 'Witnesses' typically observed discussions without engaging in them, whereas 'Discussants' actively engaged in them. Sympathizers reported that they shared the feelings of the chat room discussants or said that they had learned to see a race-related phenomenon from another point of view. 'Advocates' reported that they had tried persuading other participants with arguments and 'Targets' stated that they had experienced racial prejudice directed at them. As 'Friends', adolescents reported that they built relationships within a diverse ethnic group and gained new knowledge about ethnic-related issues from this experience. Overall, the youth participants reported that they had acquired a wide range of information from racial or ethnic discussions, including about cultural practices and belief systems. They also reported they had learned about the ways in which racial oppression affected the lives of people of color. Racial role taking also helped teen chat participants to understand the life of people from other ethnic groups and to enrich their knowledge about race.

Social networking sites, which are more private and which offer users tools for self-presentation (e.g., photographs), offer different sets of opportunities for ethnic identity construction. Subramanian found that young South Asian American women reported feeling safe sharing pictures of themselves in traditional South Asian clothes (e.g., salwar kameez) on Facebook to both a South Asian and non-South Asian audience, but not feeling comfortable doing so face to face with the same audience (Subramanian, 2010). For young minorities within minorities, such as South Asian Muslim women, interactive forums like Facebook provide an opportunity to co-construct traditional cultural constructs, for example, acceptable gender roles. According to Subramanian, young South Asian Muslim women in college use wall posts and status messages to analyze how "one should act while wearing hijab[2] to what Bollywood movies[3] good Muslim women should and should not be watching" (Subramanian, 2010). Although elements of such discussion may be more nostalgic and not necessarily reflect the dynamic and current state of their home culture, nonetheless they help these South Asian women to develop and maintain their cultural and ethnic identity.

Identity Experiments and Pretending

This chapter began with the speculation that Internet users would take advantage of the disembodied nature of online contexts and explore alternative identities. Thus

---

[2]The traditional garb that Muslim women are supposed to wear.

[3]Hindi movies made in Bollywood, Hollywood's counterpart in Mumbai, India.

began the myth of the Internet user as frequently pretending to be someone else and changing his/her virtual representations on a day-to-day basis. The same myth exists about the adolescent Internet user as well. A popular misconception is that of adolescents sitting in front of their computers pretending to be someone else, at least in one open window on the screen. Early research referred to these actions as "identity experiments." In her now classic work on this issue, Turkle gave several examples of youth experimenting with identity or pretending online (1997), often with positive effects on their lives. The reader should keep in mind that Turkle's work was based on the environments within MUDs, which are text-best social environments, where pretending and role-playing are normative and expected.

Research to date has found contradictory support for the idea that identity experiments in the sense of pretending are commonplace among Internet users in general and adolescents in particular. Among those Internet users who report pretending, adolescents report doing so more often than adults. Only 15% of all Internet users in a representative sample of the Czech population agreed that they "sometimes pretended to be someone else on the Internet" (Šmahel & Machovcova, 2006). The greatest proportion of "pretenders" was found among 12- to 15-year olds (27%) and among 16- to 20-year olds (25%); this is also the period when the search for identity is believed to be at the forefront of development (Erikson & Stone, 1959; Erikson, 1968). Similarly Gross (2004) found that among US adolescents in 7th (12- and 13-year olds) and 10th grade (15- and 16-year olds), feigning a different identity was rare and when it occured, it was usually to make fun of friends rather than to actually create a "dreamed-of identity." Creating a virtual identity in the sense of fragmenting the real and virtual selves was not a common phenomenon among the youth in these studies; more frequently, they seemed to connect the real and virtual worlds in the sense that they test and clarify their off-line values and attitudes in the online world (Šmahel, 2003; Suler, 2008).

Different results were obtained by Valkenburg, Schouten and Peter (2005), who surveyed Dutch youth between 9- and 18 years of age. Approximately, 50% of participants who used instant messengers or chat rooms (that is 41% of the whole sample) reported using the Internet for online identity experiments. The most important motives provided for online identity experimentation were self-exploration (to see how others would react), social compensation (to overcome shyness) and social facilitation (to help relationship formation). The youngest participants (9- to 12-year olds) reported pretending to be someone else most often (72%). Girls and younger teens most often pretended to be older (50%). Less frequently, they reported pretending be a real-life acquaintance (18%), a more flirtatious person (13%), or an elaborate fantasy person (13%). Because the study only asked participants whether they had experimented with identity "at least sometimes", it is hard to know how often they actually faked their identity. Regardless of this, most of the pretending involved portraying oneself as older, something that most youth have done at some point in their lives, online and off. Therefore, it is debatable whether we can actually label their pretending as true identity experimentation.

Online pretense and lying are more likely to occur in some online contexts, such as chat rooms (Konecny & Šmahel, 2007) compared to others (Blinka & Šmahel,

2009; Huffaker & Calvert, 2005). In our survey of 120 13- to 17-year olds, who maintained blogs (Blinka & Šmahel, 2009), the majority (56%) reported never having lied on their weblogs, and only two bloggers stated that they had lied about their gender or age, a proportion which represents only 1.6% of the sample. Lying, on the few occasions that it occurred, was most often about issues of partnership (17% rarely lied, 4% sometimes lied), family situation (14% rarely, 2% sometimes), appearance (10% rarely, 1% sometimes) and sexual experience (7% rarely, 2% sometimes and 1% frequently lied). Within the context of blogs, identity experiments seem relatively uncommon among adolescents; when they do lie, they do so typically to improve their image among others, such as by presenting themselves as having more partners, greater sexual experience, and looking more attractive. These issues are very likely the very same ones that they embellish in their offline lives.

Virtual Identity

Online tools such as graphic figures (avatars) and nicknames also play a role in the construction of virtual identities or online personas, which are distinct from the online self-presentation that we described earlier. According to Thomas, virtual identities are also constructed through the feeling of belonging to a virtual group, communicating with the help of slang, and acquiring technical knowledge (Thomas, 2000). Skills, such as the ability to use certain software, control a chat room, or search for new software, are becoming an integral part of self-evaluation; these digital skills are valued highly and "belong" to the adolescent's virtual identity. Thomas also claims that children and adolescents' virtual identity is very flexible and changes in accordance with current cultural icons (fashion and music trends etc.), which may consequently help them to test various self-images. The importance of feeling part of a virtual community was evident in a survey of 548 adolescents and emerging adult MMORPG players (Šmahel, 2008); 66% of the players, who were between 12- and 19 years of age agreed that "they feel they belong somewhere" and 55% agreed that they have the feeling of being self-important. The sense of belonging to a group was the greatest for older adolescents (16–19 years). For this group of gamers, the social (group) aspects of virtual identity seemed to be at least as important as the individual one.

There remain several questions about youth and virtual identities. A basic one is whether it is even possible to have true virtual identities – given that virtual representations cannot really feel or experience anything, is it even possible to think and talk about an explicit theory of someone as "a virtual character?" Moreover, if such virtual identities do indeed exist, how stable are they, and what is their impact on young people's identity development? Turkle has claimed that creating fragmented virtual identities can help individuals to overcome difficulties in their real lives (Turkle, 1997, 2005) and has described a number of examples where virtual identity has helped people with problems in their offline lives because virtual experiences were transferred into reality. In contrast, Reid (1998) has argued that the fragmentation of identities in online contexts may prevent the development of a flexible and complete personality. She has claimed that compared to offline relationships, virtual ones lack continuity: online relationships are too easy to leave, and escape may become a major strategy for dealing with a problem. Virtual identities may become dissociated and inflexible, and consequently fragmented online identities may have a more negative influence on the individual. Research is necessary to sort through these alternative possibilities to determine whether virtual identities hinder or help adolescents' identity trajectories.

Conclusions

Constructing a stable and coherent identity is a key developmental task during adolescence. Identity itself is a multidimensional construct, and is comprised of different aspects, including personal, social, gender, and ethnic identities. The term online identity is similarly complex and can be used either to refer to users' online self-presentation or to a more psychological conception of their online personas or selves.

In this chapter, we have shown the many different ways that adolescents construct their identities using digital tools such as nicknames, avatars, profiles, photos, videos, and language/codes unique to different online communities. Much of their online identity construction entails identity exploration as well as identity expression and self-presentation: presenting and testing aspects of their self or identity within a community of peers, modifying and testing parts of their self for feedback from peers, creating narratives about themselves, and searching for partners or friends. As one female adolescent in one of our studies claimed: *I wasn't any different, but I expressed some opinions rather extremely* (Šmahel, 2003). At least for adolescents, extant research calls to question the view of online environments as one where people slip in and out of different identities all the time, supposedly bending their gender and feigning personas that are older, younger, nicer, more attractive, and taller. Adolescents only rarely pretended on the Internet, and when they did pretend online, they were more likely to do so in contexts, such as chat rooms, where anonymity was possible.

Youth seem to construct and co-construct their personal, social, gender, and ethnic identities in online environments as they are faced with the crucial questions of who they are, where they belong, and what they want to do with their lives. But these are only preliminary findings and we need more research to understand how young people's online living, and the virtual identities that follow from such living may impact their development in the long term. For instance, although we know that adolescents' use digital tools for identity construction, we do not yet understand the influence of their online self-presentation and identity expression on their development. One issue is the relation between digital contexts, users' online self-presentations, and users themselves. There is a gap or a distance between users and their online representations, which may separate them from the actions of their online representation, such as when their avatar kills another player in an online game. Future research should examine the implications of the psychological distance between adolescents' and their digital representations for their self-presentation and identity development as well as more broadly for their development (e.g., for romantic relationship formation, ethical behaviors, aggression, etc). Although the sparse evidence to date suggests connections between users' online activities and their offline identity status, we need more research to understand how adolescents' virtual selves (e.g., their avatar in a game, or their Facebook self) influence their identity development. Addressing these questions will help us understand how youth formulate their sense of self as they negotiate changing and evolving digital contexts.

References

Adams, G. R., Shea, J., & Fitch, S. A. (1979). Toward the development of an objective assessment of ego-identity status. *Journal of Youth and Adolescence, 8*, 223–237.

Akers, J. F., Jones, R. M., & Coyl, D. D. (1998). Adolescent friendship pairs: Similarities in identity status development, behaviors, attitudes, and intentions. *Journal of Adolescent Research, 13*, 178–201.

Arnett, J. J. (2004). *Adolescence and emerging adulthood: A cultural approach* (2nd ed.). Upper Saddle River, NJ: Pearson Prentice Hall.

Baumeister, R. G. (1986). *Pubilc self and private self*. New York, NY: Springer.

Blinka, L., Smahel, D., Subrahmanyam, K., & Seganti, F. R. (n.d.). Cross-Cultural Differences in the Teen Blogosphere: Insights from a Content Analysis of English- and Czech-Language Weblogs Maintained by Adolescents. *Paper under review*.

Blinka, L., & Šmahel, D. (2009). Fourteen is fourteen and a girl is a girl: Validating the identity of adolescent bloggers. *CyberPsychology and Behavior, 12*, 735–739.

Brewer, M. B., & Lui, L. (1989). The primacy of age and sex in the structure of person categories. *Social cognition, 7*, 262–274.

Erikson, E. H. (1959). *Identity and the life cycle: Selected papers*. Oxford: International Universities Press.

Erikson, E. H. (1968). *Identity, youth, and crisis* (1st ed.). New York, NY: W. W. Norton.

Erikson, E. H., & Stone, I. (1959). *Identity and the life cycle; selected papers*. New York, NY: International Universities Press.

Greenfield, P. M., Gross, E. F., Subrahmanyam, K., Suzuki, L. K., Tynes, B. M., Kraut, R., et al. (2006). Teens on the Internet: Interpersonal connection, identity, and information. In R. Kraut, M. Brynin, & S. Kiesler (Eds.), *Computers, phones, and the Internet: Domesticating information technology* (pp. 185–200). New York, NY: Oxford University Press.

Greenfield, P. M., & Subrahmanyam, K. (2003). Online discourse in a teen chatroom: New codes and new modes of coherence in a visual medium. *Journal of Applied Developmental Psychology, 24*, 713–738.

Gross, E. F. (2004). Adolescent Internet use: What we expect, what teens report. *Journal of Applied Developmental Psychology, 25*, 633–649.

Grotevant, H. D., & Cooper, C. R. (1985). Patterns of interaction in family relationships and the development of identity exploration in adolescence. *Child Development, 56*, 415–428.

Huffaker, D. A., & Calvert, S. L. (2005). Gender, identity, and language use in teenage blogs. *Journal of Computer-Mediated Communication, 10*, 1. Retrieved October 15, 2009, from http://jcmc.indiana.edu/vol10/issue2/huffaker.html

Kendall, L. (2003). Cyberspace. In S. Jones (Ed.), *Encyclopedia of new media* (pp. 112–114). Thousand Oaks, CA: Sage.

Konecny, S., & Šmahel, D. (2007). *Virtual communities and lying: Perspective of Czech adoles-cents and young adults*. Paper presented at the AOIR Conference 2007, Vancouver.

Kroger, J. (2006). *Identity development: Adolescence through adulthood*. Thousand Oaks, CA: Sage Publications, Inc.

Livingstone, S. (2008). Taking risky opportunities in youthful content creation: Teenagers' use of social networking sites for intimacy, privacy and self-expression. *New Media & Society, 10,* 393–411.

Macek, P. (2003). *Adolescence* (2nd ed.). Praha: Portál.

Manago, A. M., Graham, M. B., Greenfield, P. M., & Salimkhan, G. (2008). Self-presentation and gender on MySpace. *Journal of Applied Developmental Psychology, 29,* 446–458.

Marcia, J. E. (1966). Development and validation of ego-identity status. *Journal of Personality and Social Psychology, 3,* 551–558.

Marcia, J. E. (1976). Identity six years after: A follow-up study. *Journal of Youth and Adolescence, 5,* 145–160.

Mazur, E., & Kozarian, L. (2009). Self-presentation and interaction in blogs of adolescents and young emerging adults. *Journal of Adolescent Research, 25,* 124–144.

McAdams, D. P. (1997). The case for unity in the (post) modern self: A modest proposal. In R. D. Ashmore & L. J. Jussim (Eds.), *Self and identity: Fundamental issues* (pp. 46–78). New York, NY: Oxford University Press.

McAdams, D. P. (1999). Personal narratives and the life story. In L. A. Perwin & O. P. John (Eds.), *Handbook of personality: Theory and research* (Vol. 2, pp. 478–500). New York, NY: Guilford Press.

McKenna, K. Y. A., & Bargh, J. A. (2000). Plan 9 from cyberspace: The implications of the Internet for personality and social psychology. *Personality and Social Psychology Review, 4,* 57–75.

Moshman, D. (2005). *Adolescent psychological development rationality, morality, and identity* (2nd ed.). Mahwah, NJ: Lawrence Erlbaum Associates.

Nurmi, J.-E. (2004). Socialization and self-development: Channeling, selection, adjustment, and reflection. In R. M. Lerner & L. Steinberg(Eds.), *Handbook of adolescent psychology* (2nd ed., pp. 85–124). Hoboken, NJ: Wiley.

Papini, D. R., Sebby, R. A., & Clark, S. (1989). Affective quality of family relations and adolescent identity exploration. *Adolescence, 24,* 457–466.

Phinney, J. S. (1996). When we talk about American ethnic groups, what do we mean? *American Psychologist, 51,* 918–927.

Quintana, S. M., & Lapsley, D. K. (1990). Rapprochement in late adolescent separationindividua-tion: A structural equations approach. *Journal of Adolescence, 13,* 371–385.

Reid, E. (1998). The self and the Internet: Variations on the illusion of one self. In J. Gackenbach (Ed.), *Psychology and the Internet, intrapersonal, interpersonal, and transpersonal implica-tions* (pp. 31–44). San Diego, CA: Academic Press.

Reis, O., & Youniss, J. (2004). Patterns in identity change and development in relationships with mothers and friends. *Journal of Adolescent Research, 19,* 31–44.

Schmitt, K. L., Dayanim, S., & Matthias, S. (2008). Personal homepage construction as an expression of social development. *Developmental Psychology, 44,* 496–506.

Šmahel, D. (2003). *Psychologie a internet: Děti dospělými, dospělí dětmi. [Psychology and Internet: Children being adults, adults being children.]*. Prague: Triton.

Šmahel, D. (2005). *Identity of Czech adolescents – Relation of cyberspace and reality*. Paper presented at the 9th European Congress of Psychology, Granada, Spain. From http://www.terapie.cz/materials/granada2005-smahel.pdf

Šmahel, D. (2008). *Adolescents and young players of MMORPG games: Virtual communities as a form of social group*. Paper presented at the XIth EARA Conference, Torino, Italy. Retrieved May 5, 2009, from http://www.terapie.cz/materials/eara2008-torino.pdf

Šmahel, D., Blinka, L., & Ledabyl, O. (2008). Playing MMORPGs: Connections between addiction and identifying with a character. *Cyberpsychology and Behavior, 11,* 715–718.

Šmahel, D., & Machovcova, K. (2006). *Internet use in the Czech Republic: Gender and age differences*. Paper presented at the Cultural Attitudes Towards Technology and Communication 2006, Tartu.

Šmahel, D., & Subrahmanyam, K. (2007). "Any girls want to chat press 911": Partner selection in monitored and unmonitored teen chat rooms. *Cyberpsychology and Behavior, 10*, 346–353.

Šmahel, D., & Vesela, M. (2006). Interpersonal attraction in the virtual environment. *Ceskoslovenska Psychologie, 50*, 174–186.

Stallabrass, J. (1995). Empowering technology: The exploration of cyberspace. *New Left Review, 1/211*, 3–32.

Strano, M. M. (2008). User descriptions and interpretations of self-presentation through Facebook profile images. *Cyberpsychology: Journal of Psychosocial Research on Cyberspace, 2*. Retrieved from http://www.cyberpsychology.eu/view.php?cisloclanku=2008110402

Subrahmanyam, K. (2003). Review of youth and media: Opportunities for development or lurking dangers? Children, adolescents, and the media. *Journal of Applied Developmental Psychology, 24*, 381–387.

Subrahmanyam, K., Garcia, E. C., Harsono, S. L., Li, J., & Lipana, L. (2009). In their words: Connecting online weblogs to developmental processes. *British Journal of Developmental Psychology, 27*, 219–245.

Subrahmanyam, K., Greenfield, P. M., & Tynes, B. (2004). Constructing sexuality and identity in an online teen chat room. *Journal of Applied Developmental Psychologyn International Lifespan Journal, 25*, 651–666.

Subrahmanyam, K., Reich, S. M., Waechter, N., & Espinoza, G. (2008). Online and offline social networks: Use of social networking sites by emerging adults. *Journal of Applied Developmental Psychology, 29*, 420–433.

Subrahmanyam, K., Šmahel, D., & Greenfield, P. M. (2006). Connecting developmental constructions to the Internet: Identity presentation and sexual exploration in online teen chat rooms. *Developmental Psychology, 42*, 395–406.

Subramanian, M. (2010). New Modes of Communication: Web Representations and Blogs: United States: South Asians. *Encyclopedia of Women and Islamic Cultures*. Retrieved October 18, 2010 from http://brillonline.nl/subscriber/entry?entry=ewic_COM-0660.

Suler, J. (2008). *The psychology of cyberspace*. Retrieved August 20, 2008, from http://www-usr.rider.edu/~suler/psycyber/psycyber.html

Suzuki, L. K., & Beale, I. L. (2006). Personal web home pages of adolescents with cancer: Self-presentation, information dissemination, and interpersonal connection. *Journal of Pediatric Oncology Nursing, 23*, 152–161.

Thomas, A. (2000). Textual constructions of children's online identities. *CyberPsychology and Behavior, 3*, 665–672.

Thornton, S. (1996). *Club cultures: Music, media, and subcultural capital*. London: Wesleyan University Press.

Turkle, S. (1997). *Life on the screen identity in the age of the Internet* (1st ed.). New York, NY: Touchstone.

Turkle, S. (2005). *The second self computers and the human spirit* (20th anniversary ed.). Cambridge, MA: MIT Press.

Tynes, B. M. (2007). Role taking in online "classrooms": What adolescents are learning about race and ethnicity. *Developmental Psychology, 43*, 1312–1320.

Tynes, B. M., Giang, M. T., & Thompson, G. N. (2008). Ethnic identity, intergroup contact, and outgroup orientation among diverse groups of adolescents on the Internet. *CyberPsychology and Behavior, 11*, 459–465.

Tynes, B. M., Reynolds, L., & Greenfield, P. M. (2004). Adolescence, race, and ethnicity on the Internet: A comparison of discourse in monitored vs. unmonitored chat rooms. *Journal of Applied Developmental Psychology, 25*, 667–684.

Valkenburg, P. M., Peter, J., & Schouten, A. (2005). Adolescents' identity experiments on the Internet. *New media and Society, 7*, 383–402.

Vybiral, Z., Šmahel, D., & Divínová, R. (2004). Dospívání ve virtuální realitě – adolescenti a internet. [Growing up in virtual environment: Adolescents and the Internet.]. In P. Mares (Ed.), *Society, reproduction, and contemporary challenges* (pp. 169–188). Brno: Barrister & Principal.

Wakeford, N. (1999). Gender and the landscapes of computing in an Internet café. In M. Crang, P. Crang, & J. May (Eds.), *Virtual geographies: Bodies, space, and relations* (pp. 178–202). London: Routledge.

Wallace, P. M. (1999). *The psychology of the Internet*. New York, NY: Cambridge University Press.

Waterman, A. S. (1999). Identity, the identity statuses, and identity status development: A contemporary statement. *Developmental Review, 19*, 591–621.

Chapter 5
Intimacy and the Internet: Relationships with Friends, Romantic Partners, and Family Members

In the previous two chapters, we examined the role of digital technologies in two important developmental tasks – sexuality and identity. In this chapter, we explore the role of technology in the third task facing adolescence, that of developing intimacy and interconnections with the people in their lives (Brown, 2004; Furman, Brown, & Feiring, 1999). We saw in Chapter 1 that online communication tools, such as email, instant messaging, text messaging, games, and social networking sites are very popular among adolescents. Youth use them to interact and communicate with their peers – offline friends, online friends, romantic partners – as well as their family (Šmahel & Subrahmanyam, 2007; Šmahel & Vesela, 2006; Subrahmanyam & Greenfield, 2008; Subrahmanyam, Reich, Waechter, & Espinoza, 2008; Valkenburg & Peter, 2009; Valkenburg, Peter, & Schouten, 2006). This chapter will examine how these online tools and contexts intersect with adolescents' relationships and developing intimacy.

We consider the mediating role of technology in three important relationships in young people's lives: friendships and peer group relationships, romantic relationships (dating), and relationships within the family. First, we describe their use of online contexts to interact with their friends and other peers. Because of concerns about purely online friendships, (Subrahmanyam & Greenfield, 2008), we examine separately their online interactions with offline friends and acquaintances as well as their online relationships with peers, who are not part of their offline world, and the quality of such purely online relationships. Then we describe adolescents' online romantic relationships, and reflecting extant research, will focus on those that are purely online. The final section will describe technology and teens' relationships with their family, with a special emphasis on how teens' status as the technology expert may be altering traditional family dynamics and relationships.

Adolescents' Friendships and Peer Group Relationships

Theoretical Background

Adolescents are faced with the developmental task of establishing intimate relationships with peers and then romantic partners, individuals who are increasingly

K. Subrahmanyam, D. Šmahel, *Digital Youth*, Advancing Responsible
Adolescent Development, DOI 10.1007/978-1-4419-6278-2_5,
© Springer Science+Business Media, LLC 2011

important in their lives (Brown, 2004; Furman et al., 1999). These relationships come to take on greater weight compared to earlier years, and possibly even reach their peak in terms of importance compared to other life phases (Bee, 1994). Adolescents' relationships with their peers reflect their need to learn to communicate, to seek a position within a group, and to share their experiences. Whereas in childhood, relationships with peers serve as a platform for spending time with each other and even just playing together, over the course of adolescence, peers become salient in young peoples' lives, as they develop autonomy and become independent from their families (Brown, 2004; Ryan, 2001). Research has documented adolescents' need for close friends (Pombeni, Kirchler, & Palmonari, 1990) and in fact, it is at this point in their lives that young people develop the capacity for intimacy, openness, honesty, and self-disclosure with their friends (Brown, 2004). Self-disclosure to friends increases over the course of adolescence and is important because it enables youth to obtain the social input and provisions, which can help them deal with the issues that they face in their lives (Buhrmester & Prager, 1995). We will show in this chapter that adolescents' online lives also have the new levels of interaction and relationships typical of their offline lives.

The structure of adolescent peer relationships also changes with development. Dunphy (1963) observed the formation, dissolution, and interaction of teenage groups in a high school in Sydney. He identified two basic types of peer groups: cliques and crowds. Cliques usually involve three to nine members, are generally same-sexed, and are cohesive groups with high levels of intimacy. Clique members tend to meet more frequently on weekdays, and their most frequent activity is communication. Crowds have between 15 and 30 members, with an average of 20 members. A crowd usually consists of two to four cliques getting together, typically at parties, soirées etc. Crowds are mixed-gender as same-gendered cliques come together. The crowd's activities are more organized and takes place on weekends rather than on weekdays. For heterosexual adolescents, they provide an opportunity to meet members of the opposite sex, thus establishing their first romantic and erotic contacts. Within the social context of the Internet, we see adolescents' need for peer interaction in their use of online applications, such as social networking sites, chat rooms, and discussion groups.

Adolescents report that friends are their most important resources and source of support, even more than their parents and other family members (Brown, 2004). Most adolescents report having close friends, although in adolescence, friendships sometimes have a shorter life and close friends may change within a period of 6 months or less (Brown & Klute, 2004). Adolescents' friendships are often based on equality and reciprocity, as they choose friends who are similar to them and are usually of the same sex (Brown & Klute, 2004; Brown, 2004). A number of studies have also shown that adolescents' behavior is related to what their friends do, both with regard to positive (e.g., not using drugs) and not so positive ones (e.g., using drugs) (Brown & Klute, 2004).

Online Contexts and Relationships with Offline Friends and Peer Group Members

By now, the reader is no doubt aware that adolescents heavily use online communication applications. While we can not say for sure who they interacted with in the first generation of applications, such as chat rooms, in recent years, their online interactions seem to definitely involve peers from offline settings, such as schools, after-school settings (e.g., sports, and clubs) and neighborhoods. Gross (2004) studied the online activities of 261 7th (mean age = 12 years) and 10th graders (mean age = 15 years) from suburban California public schools, who completed four consecutive end-of-day reports on their school-based adjustment and Internet activity. Although most participants reported that they used the Internet for social and nonsocial uses, online communication was the most frequently reported online activity. Adolescents described their online interactions as occurring in more private settings (IM or e-mail), with friends who were also a part of their physical world, and their online conversations were mostly devoted to fairly ordinary, yet intimate topics (i.e., gossip). In fact, teens in the USA report using instant messenger programs, mainly because they allow them to connect to friends, to 'hang out' with a group of friends, and therefore feel part of a group (Boneva, Quinn, Kraut, Kiesler, & Shklovski, 2006).

US youth report very similar uses with regard to social networking sites. One the Pew Internet Project, an overwhelming majority of teens who used social networking sites (91%) reported that they used the sites to keep in touch with friends they see frequently; a slightly smaller group (82%) reported that they used them to stay in touch with friends they rarely see in person. However, there were gender differences as teen girls reported that they used social networking sites mostly to reinforce preexisting friendships, and boys reported that they used them to flirt and make new friends (Lenhart & Madden, 2007). In a survey of a diverse sample of urban teens, participants reported similar reasons (keeping in touch with friends and family and making plans with friends) for using social networking sites (see Fig. 5.1) (Reich, Subrahmanyam, & Espinoza, 2009). As with instant messaging, youth, at least those in the USA, use social networking sites as a means of connecting with people who are already in their offline lives.

Some recent research conducted by Subrahmanyam and colleagues confirms the trends revealed by the survey studies. Our goal was to find out "who" exactly youth were interacting with in face-to-face as well as online contexts (SNSs and instant messaging) and to see whether their online and offline networks overlapped (Reich et al., 2009; Subrahmanyam et al., 2008). We wanted to make sure respondents were who they said they were, with regard to age, gender, and other characteristics. But we also wanted to ensure that participants' responses about their online networks were consistent with what they actually did online. Therefore, we used a two-step procedure, in which we first asked participants to complete an in-person survey and then sent them a link to an online survey. Our high school sample comprised 251 youth between 13 and 19 years and our emerging adult sample comprised of 110 college students between 18 and 29 years. Most (88% of the high school and 82% of

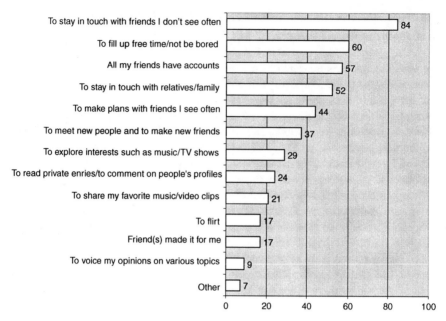

Fig. 5.1 Urban US teens' motives for using SNSs (% participants) (adapted from Reich et al., 2009)

the college students) reported having a social networking site profile, with MySpace being the overwhelming site of choice. For both age groups, social networking site use was reported to be integrated with offline partners and concerns and participants' reasons for using them echoed the findings of the Pew Report (Lenhart & Madden, 2007).

To find out the actual extent of overlap or divergence between young people's offline and online networks, we asked them to list the top 10 people with whom they interacted face-to-face as well as via instant messaging and SNSs. For the most part, respondents interacted online with people they knew offline. However, there was only a low overlap in the friends with whom they were most in contact with online and offline. This means that although online and offline social worlds are connected, they are not mirror images of each other and youth may use different mediums to interact with different partners. Best friends from the online world are not necessarily best friends online and future research should assess whether relationships conducted in different mediums (offline vs. online) offer youth different levels of intimacy and support.

Benefits and Costs of Interacting Online with Peers

An important premise of our developmental framework is that young people use technology in ways that make sense with the issues confronting them at that particular point in their life. This helps to explain the emerging role of online tools for interactions with known peers; however, given some of the features of online communication environments (e.g., disembodied users, anonymity, etc) that we discussed in Chapter 1, we expect that such use may not be without some advantages or disadvantages. In the next sub-sections, we examine the benefits and costs of interacting online with offline friends and peer group members.

Increased access to offline friends and peer groups. First, as we have noted already, opportunities to communicate online with people known offline allow youth to interact and self-disclose to the individuals, who are at that very time becoming important in their lives. According to Boneva et al., two major adolescent needs that are satisfied by their use of instant messaging is maintaining individual friendship and belonging to a peer group (Boneva et al., 2006). In their study, instant messengers were mainly a substitute for in-person talk with local friends and seldom used for communication with strangers; teens also reported gaining the same level of support via instant messengers, phone calls, and face-to-face communication. More importantly, these tools are available 24/7. For instance, Norwegian youth between 10- and 12 years of age, reported that they were able to use whatever medium (Internet, mobile phones) they wished to for interacting with friends and schoolmates; the new technologies facilitates their communication with peers at any time, anywhere, and in an individualized and private way (Kaare, Brandtzaeg, Heim, & Endestad, 2007).

Given this sort of access to peers that technology provides to youth, one would expect that Internet use might occur at the expense of face-to-face interactions. Surprisingly this is not so, according to the WIP data shown in Figs. 5.2 and 5.3. When asked whether face-to-face contact with friends had increased or decreased after gaining access to the Internet, most of the teens from the seven countries reported there had been no change. However, when asked whether their Internet

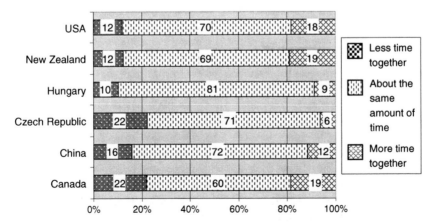

Fig. 5.2 Changes in the time spent interacting face to face with friends after getting access to the Internet (12- to 18-year-olds in the 2007 WIP data)

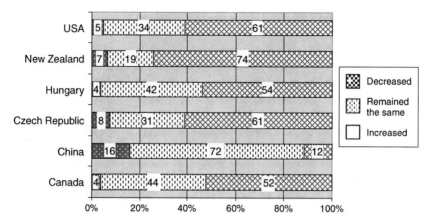

Fig. 5.3 Changes in overall contact with friends after getting access to the Internet (12- to 18-year-olds in the 2007 WIP data)

use had influenced their overall contact with friends, a majority of the teens in six of the seven countries said that it had increased overall contact. Thus, it seems that the Internet is increasing contact with peers, but not necessarily at the expense of face-to-face interactions.

The increased contact with peers also includes a widening or broadening of their peer network. In chat rooms, youth could converse with multiple partners simultaneously in the public space. Using instant messaging, they can talk to several different partners at the same time; moreover, their "buddy list" can have the names of a large number of individuals. Social networking sites take this to another scale altogether – in our study of high school students described earlier, high school students reported between 0 and 793 "friends," with a mean of 176 friends, standard deviation of 166, and a median of 130 "friends." Most (95%) of these "friends" were known offline, and they had frequent interactions with 77% of them (Reich et al., 2009). Every one of these individuals from their offline worlds is now somebody that a youth can potentially interact with either publicly via comments on the profile page, responses to comments on the profile page, or via more privately messages.

Digital tools are clearly increasing young people's access to offline peers, but such access raises several issues that future research must consider. First, the word "friends" itself may be going through a transformation to include not just close, intimate ones, but also those, who previously may have only been considered to be acquaintances. Second, digital tools are widening young people's circle of friends, and allows them to interact with, provide support to, and receive support from peers with whom they might otherwise not have had such interactions. These offline peers are generally outside their intimate circle of friends, and but for the Internet, would very likely not have any significant face-to-face contact with them. Such a "wider circle of friends" might actually be very valuable for adolescents – from an analysis of handwritten messages in high school year books, Giordano has suggested that interactions with more remote peers may help youth learn about themselves and their social world (Giordano, 1995). Third, at least where social networking sites are concerned, many of these interactions are conducted very publicly and for all to see; for example, on Facebook, every one on a teen's network of friends can use the news feed to keep track of the youth's interactions with his/her Facebook friends. We do not know the developmental implications of these rather public peer interactions, in particular their impact on relationship quality, the issue we consider next.

Impact on friendship quality? We saw in the previous section that youth in a number of different countries reported that Internet use had increased and widened contact with their peers. For adolescents, friends are a primary source of support and friendship quality is an important mediator of their well-being. Therefore, it is important to assess whether the increase in contact has an impact on friendship quality and intimacy. In our work on social networking site use among US teens, participants were split on this question – 44% felt that they had made no difference to their relationships with friends, 43% felt that it had made them closer, and 5% even reported that it had created problems (Reich et al., 2009).

There is some evidence that adolescents who interact online more often with their friends also report feeling closer to these friends. Valkenburg and colleagues' survey of 10- to 16-year-old Dutch youth ($n = 794$) revealed that for the 88% who interacted online with face-to-face friends, online communication was positively related to friendship closeness; however, no effects were found for those who mostly communicated with strangers (Valkenburg & Peter, 2007). The positive relationship between online communication and closeness with friends was stable across all developmental stages, as well as for boys and girls. Thirty percent of adolescents stated that they perceived the Internet as more effective than face-to-face communication for self-disclosure of intimate information. These adolescents also reported greater closeness to their existing friends, with whom they communicated online. One should keep in mind that this study was correlational and so we can not separate two potential hypotheses: one, greater communication online led to closer friendships; two, teens with already close relationships communicated online to greater extents. The latter possibility reflects what some researchers have called the "rich get richer hypothesis" (Kraut et al., 2002), an idea that we address in greater detail in Chapter 7.

Even though youth seem to find online interactions very appealing, there may be some hidden costs; in the study by Boneva and colleagues (2006) that we described earlier, teens evaluated instant messaging as less enjoyable than phone and face-to-face conversations and also reported feeling less psychologically close to their instant messaging partners than to their phone or face-to-face partners. Perhaps young people use different settings (face-to-face versus online) and different applications within online contexts for different purposes and to interact with partners of varying relationship levels. Informal discussions with teens suggest that they often use cell phones with more intimate friends and social networking sites with more distant ones. As we noted earlier, more research is necessary to understand the different kinds of support and intimacy that teens receive from these different interactions.

Online Contexts and Relationships with Strangers

According to the Pew Internet Project survey, 32% of online teens were contacted by strangers on the Internet and 21% of them contacted an online stranger to find out more information about that person (Lenhart & Madden, 2007). Among those contacted by a stranger, 23% reported feeling scared or uncomfortable because of that contact. A national survey of social networking site users conducted in 2006 found that 40% of 14- to 22-year olds had been contacted online by a stranger whom they did not know (Annenberg Public Policy Center, 2006); however, this survey was done when social networking sites were just introduced and an unrestricted site, such as MySpace, was dominant. An earlier national survey of US Internet users, found that 25% of children and adolescents aged 10–17 years have established occasional online friendships and 14% had a close virtual friendship (Wolak, Mitchell, & Finkelhor, 2002). Most of these virtual relationships were with same-aged peers (70%) and with members of the opposite sex (71%). Compared to boys, girls established online friendships more often (29% vs. 23%), and reported establishing a close friendship. Of these online friendships, 75% considered them close friendships; 59% were in chat rooms, 30% via instant messaging, 5% in games, and 6% by other means. Most adolescents claimed to share an interest or hobby with their online friends. According to this survey, few adolescents (2%) claimed to have had a negative experience with online friendships. In a different paper based on the same survey, Wolak et al. stated that mainly older adolescents, Caucasians, and those experiencing significant conflict with their parents established online relationships more often (Wolak, Mitchell, & Finkelhor, 2003). According to the authors, the likelihood of an online relationship rises among boys with the absence of communication with their parents and does not increase with the level of conflict with their parents, while it is the opposite in the case of girls.

The potential for meeting strangers and new friends on the Internet is probably closely tied to the particular online context and also the time period under consideration (Subrahmanyam & Greenfield, 2008). For example, because chat rooms brought together people who did not know each other prior to the online contact, one was more likely to interact with strangers online; in contrast, social networking sites assume networks of "friends," so one is typically much more likely to interact with individuals who are already a part of one's social life. Our analyses of adolescents' conversations in chat rooms suggests that the search for partners is as salient an activity while chatting online as it is offline. Almost 11% of 12,258 utterances in chat rooms were requests for partners. There were two partner requests per minute, compared to one sexual request per minute and one obscene utterance every two minutes. The requests were mostly for partners of the opposite sex, but also for communication partners of the same sex. We assume that these requests were made primarily to strangers, since those where who one was more likely to interact in the public chat space. Given that the use of chat rooms itself varied from 31 to 69% across different countries (see Chapter 1), we think it is quite likely that the context may influence teens' attitudes and actual interactions with strangers.

Because a small proportion of adolescents report meeting and forming online friendships with strangers, it is important to know whether such friendships put youth at risk. Wolak et al. investigated this question in a nationally representative sample of US adolescents aged 10–17 years (Wolak, Finkelhor, & Mitchell, 2008). The researchers discovered that many adolescents interact with unknown people with little risk involved. Of youth who communicated with other people online, only 17% were high-risk unrestricted communicators, who engaged in high levels of potentially risky online behaviors. The adolescents most at risk also scored high on a diverse range of problems, such as rule-breaking behavior, depression and social problems. We can therefore hypothesize that adolescents, who are prone to risky behavior offline are also more likely to engage in such behavior online.

Quality of online friendships with strangers. A pervasive concern about purely online interactions is that they are inherently poorer in quality compared to offline face-to-face relationships. The reasoning is that they are impoverished because they occur via machines, and so lack face-to-face cues, such as gesture and gaze and so lead to weaker ties. Thus, it is important to examine the quality of purely online relationships and the factors that mediate it. Researchers in Israel surveyed 987 adolescents (Mean age = 15.5 years) to compare the quality of online and offline relationships (Mesch & Talmud, 2006). Participants reported that compared to their face-to-face friends, they knew their online friends for a shorter time and shared fewer activities with them. They had fewer discussions with their online friends, and the discussions that they did have them were about less personal topics. Youth often shared specific extracurricular hobbies or interests with their online friends, who played more specialized role in the lives. Overall, they perceived their online friendships as being less close than their face-to-face ones. The authors concluded that adolescents' close face-to-face friendships were holistic, and not restricted to particular topics and activities; conversely, their online friendships were not integrated with their everyday life and were restricted to non-personal topics and to activities that did not occur daily.

Mesch and Talmud also analyzed the same data to assess the role of similarity between friends in online and offline relationships (Mesch & Talmud, 2007). Friends made at school were more likely to be similar in age, gender, and place of residence compared to online friends. Participants' perceived their face-to-face friends as being closer to them than their online friends. However, social similarity also mattered for friends who met each other on the Internet: the more similar online friends were in residence and gender, the stronger the relationship.

Self-disclosure may play a role in the perceived quality of online relationships. A cross-cultural study of American, Japanese, and Korean college students revealed that self-disclosure was directly associated with online relationship development (Yum & Hara, 2005). Participants who reported greater self-disclosure online were more likely to report experiencing benefits from their virtual relationships. However, the association between self-disclosure and online relationship quality is not linear and is moderated by factors such as culture and personality. Among US participants, greater self-disclosure was associated with greater trust, for Koreans, higher self-disclosure was inversely associated with trust, and for Japanese, it was not a factor. Similarly personality variables play a role in the way self-disclosure may be connected to online relationship development; extraverted adolescents communicated online more frequently and exhibited more self-disclosure, which facilitated the formation of online friendships (Peter, Valkenburg, & Schouten, 2005). In contrast, introverted adolescents were more strongly motivated to communicate online to compensate for a lack of social skills, which increased their chances of making friends online. This strong motive for social compensation led to more frequent online communication and increased self-disclosure and therefore to more online friendships.

Another variable that plays a role in purely online relationships is duration of the relationship. A study of Hong Kong Internet users between the ages of 16 and 29 years, who were recruited from an online newsgroup revealed that initially, face-to-face relationships were higher in quality, but subsequently there were no differences once both kinds of relationships had lasted more than a year (Chan & Cheng, 2004). The longer the relationship, the more opportunities for exchange of information and the greater the self-disclosure between young Internet users; note that self-disclosure is important in both online and offline relationships. Thus, it appears that purely online relationships are not as high in quality, except if the partners share some offline similarities and if the relationship lasts for a long enough time. In Chapter 7, we will show that despite these limitations, online interactions with strangers may have some benefits for youth.

Adolescents' Romantic Relationships

Theoretical Background

As is widely recognized, romantic relationships are a central part of adolescents' social worlds (Bouchey & Furman, 2004) and according to Erikson, romantic relationships are an integral component in the search for identity (Erikson, 1968). Romantic and sexual relationships have a unique intensity during adolescence (e.g. Miller & Benson, 1999); although adolescents' developing sexuality is an important component of their romantic relationships, romantic and sexual relationships may also be developed by adolescents independently, "one without the other" (Miller & Benson, 1999). Dating and romantic relationships are very dependent on cultural norms and vary as a function of where the teen is living. For instance, the age when youth start to date is related to norms about the age-appropriateness of dating behaviors rather than sexual maturation per se. Research shows that those adolescents who start dating earlier gain sexual experience earlier, and by late adolescence, have more sexual experience with more partners (Thornton, 1990). Thus, the pressure of cultural patterns influences when adolescents become sexually active, irrespective of their actual sexual maturation. Adolescents form romantic relationships for a variety of reasons, including social desirability, seeking safety in a partner (in particular for girls), learning to love and to communicate with a partner, gaining and transferring validation, and the feeling of physical and emotional desire from the partner's side (Miller & Benson, 1999).

Lesbians, gay, bisexual, and transgender (LGBT) adolescents have very similar feelings when searching for validation and the feeling of safety in a relationship. They experience feelings of love and being in love just like their heterosexual counterparts. However, unlike their heterosexual counterparts, LGBT youth may feel less free to express their interest and feelings for potential partners and Chapter 3 examined how the Internet might help them to explore and express their emerging sexual identities.

Online Contexts and Adolescents' Romantic Relationships

As in the case of friendships, we can use the Internet in the service of offline romantic relationships or we can use it to find and establish "purely online" romantic relationships. Most of the existing literature on this topic has focused on the latter kind of online romantic relationships, perhaps because this was more typical in the early days of the Internet. However, we should keep in mind that we can use online technologies to sustain and strengthen offline romantic relationships and where relevant, we point this out.

We saw in the previous chapter that the disembodied nature of online contexts afford opportunities for identity presentation and exploration. We also saw that users adapt to these affordances, sometimes by modifying their behaviors or creating new ones. Online contexts similarly have affordances that are relevant to romantic relationships, and users have adapted to these affordances. For instance, some online contexts do not readily provide information about physical attractiveness, an important ingredient in offline romances, especially at the start. Consequently, beginning a romantic relationship on the Internet becomes more about communication or describing feelings and experiences. Some of the factors of "online attraction" include, proximity, sharing common interests, attitudes and views, sense of humor, self-disclosure, creativity, intelligence, ability to communicate, "virtual charisma" and the spiral of "you like me, I like you, you like me more, I like you more". Factors that decrease online attraction are passivity, inadequate exhibitionism, and aggressiveness (Šmahel & Vesela, 2006; Wallace, 1999). Many online tools are also likely come into play for what are fundamentally offline romantic relationships; in particular online tools such as Google or social networking profiles may be used to find out more about a potential partner as well as to interact with one.

We know surprisingly little about the extent to which young people use different Internet applications in the service of romantic relationships. In a qualitative study of 16 Czech Internet users aged 14–25 years, 13 respondents stated that they used the Internet to look for partners, and, as one girl expressed: *in my opinion, most boys in chat rooms are seeking partners* (Šmahel, 2003). In fact, chat rooms, with their disembodied users and potential for anonymity, showed high rates of sexual exploration and partner selection (e.g., *press 21 if u wanna chat wit a hot and sexy chic*). Our analyses of more than 12,000 utterances in teen chat rooms revealed that on average there were two requests for partners per minute in the public space of the chat room (Šmahel & Subrahmanyam, 2007). Other than expressing identity, the request for a partner was the most frequent content of the chat utterances, even more frequent than greetings.

Although females tended to search for partners more often than males, there was no such difference in sexualized partner requests (Šmahel & Subrahmanyam, 2007). Here we see that the particular features of the virtual context, might moderate the way in which a quintessentially offline behavior is manifested online. We do not know how successful these partner requests were, since the players presumably went into a private space to continue their interaction. We also do not know whether these casual online chat encounters actually led to romantic relationships and if they did, how long they lasted and what they were like.

Partner selection was no doubt so prominent in chat rooms because of their unique communication environment. It was not as dominant in blog entries, perhaps because the audience typically knows the blog author's identity. Although blogs contained romantic content and entries with romantic content had strong emotional tone, topics such as peers, every day life and family were much more frequent. There was also no indication that the blog authors use this forum to connect with potential partners (Subrahmanyam, Garcia, Harsono, Li & Lipana, 2009).

Online dating sites are another Internet context relevant to romantic relationships. To examine teens' online dating behavior, Šmahel and colleagues surveyed a representative Czech sample in September 2008 (unpublished data from the World Internet Project: Czech Republic); of the 2,215 individuals who were surveyed, there were 483 12- to 18-year olds. Approximately 43% of adolescents reported that they *sometimes* visited a dating site and 23% had a profile on that site and had contacted another person to date. There were no gender differences in dating site use. Older adolescents (16- to 18-year-olds) reported visiting dating sites more often (52%) compared to younger adolescents (12- to 15-year-olds) (35%). Thirty percent of adolescents who had profiles on dating sites had called their partners by phone, 9% used web cams, 8% exchanged erotic pictures and 35% had met their online partners face-to-face. Interestingly, only 22% of adolescents who had profiles agreed that they were seeking "serious dating", 64% were seeking noncommittal dating, 46% "pure virtual relationships" and 7% reported that they were looking to have an offline meeting with a sexual contact. Most of the Czech adolescents in this study appear to engage in online dating to explore, to have fun, and to interact with potential partners without actual engagement or commitment. A qualitative study of 16 Czech Internet users between 14 and 25 years adolescents is revealing about young people's reasons for using the Internet for dating and developing online relationships (Šmahel, 2003). Some of their reasons offered were the unlimited source of relationships, ability to form relationships independent of locality, and ease of starting relationships; participants also saw online dating and relationships as being especially valuable for socially handicapped teens who may be overly shy or socially anxious.

From media and press stories, as well as our own observations, we know that teens use instant messaging and social networking sites for romantic relationship development, but given the more private nature of these tools, we do not have the details of such use. As we have already pointed out, the Internet is useful both for romantic relationship formation and for strengthening and maintaining offline romantic connections. The studies on chat room partner selection and online dating sites exemplify the former, whereas the blog study represents the latter category. From casual observation, it is apparent that youth use these technologies to further offline dating and romantic relationships. For instance, they use their Facebook profile to announce the start or break up of a relationship, to declare their feelings for their partner or about the status of their relationship (e.g., 6 months, and so on), and to share publicly what we might consider more private messages. They also use Facebook profiles to find out more about potential partners they meet offline, such as their interests or activities. We do not know how much teens use applications such as Facebook for romantic relationships and whether technology enhances or interferes with their ability to achieve partner intimacy now and in the future.

How "Real" Are Online Romantic Relationships?

Ever since the Internet made it possible for users to interact with total strangers easily and at little cost, concerns have been raised that such interactions are not very rich and lead to "weak ties" (Kraut et al., 1998). Along the same vein, it is important to consider how real online romantic relationships may be to young people. It appears that although adolescents like online dating and on occasion meeting strangers and chatting with them, they mostly view online relationships as "not real", or "not true." A comment from a Czech adolescent exemplifies this nicely: *it is not a real relationship, we just meet and speak* or *we cannot compare real and virtual friendship* (Šmahel, 2003). This is consistent with the finding described previously that online relationships are perceived as being of lower quality (2006; Mesch & Talmud, 2007). Despite the fact that adolescents exchange intimate information with their online romantic partners, they claim that such a relationship is not real and valid. They seem to be ambivalent: it is a relationship yet not "real", intimate details are known about each other, but there is still the feeling of freedom to exit the relationship at any moment. Quite possibly a new kind of relationship is being created on the Internet and a female subject expressed her feelings thus: *the term friendship does not fit, but I do not know what to call it* (Šmahel, 2003).

Youth in this study also seem to believe that online romantic relationships are usually shorter and more superficial than offline relationships. They do not assess pure virtual relationships as being very serious and when they do perceive them as serious, they try to transform their virtual relationship into an offline physical or face-to-face friendship or romantic relationship. As one 19-year-old girl stated (Šmahel, 2003): *Wherever it is nicer and easier on the Internet, you cannot compare it with real life. If you intend only to speak, the Internet is OK. But if you need to feel proximity, embracing, a virtual friend cannot give you these.*

In sum, although adolescents use the Internet to meet new partners, they do not view such relationships in the same light as those with offline partners. They seem to know that online worlds cannot substitute their offline physical relationships. Instead, they appear to use the Internet, particularly the newer tools such as social networking sites and instant messaging, to form and/or extend romantic relationships with people known offline. For example, incoming college freshmen often use Facebook profiles to obtain information and presumably form judgments about roommates. When adolescents' romantic entanglements are exclusively online with people who are not a part of his/her offline life, it should raise a red flag for parents, guardians, and practitioners.

The Role of Culture in Online Romantic Relationships

We saw in the chapter on sexuality and the Internet (Chapter 3) that young people's offline and online sexual behaviors are influenced by the offline cultural contexts within which they are living. Offline dating and romantic relationships are similarly contextually dependent. In most modern Western societies, dating and romantic partners are an important facet of adolescent life; this is not so in more traditional societies such as parts of Asia and the Middle East. In these latter contexts, offline dating is not the norm for adolescents, and some more traditional societies even practice sex segregation (Steinberg, 2008). The role of the Internet for romantic relationship development is likely very different in these more restrictive contexts. This is illustrated in an ethnographic study of the ecology of early adolescents' (12- to 14-year olds) online dating/romance in Mauritius, a relatively conservative country (Rambaree, 2008). The researchers analyzed 136 narrative interviews and conducted eight focus groups; they found that dating and romantic relationships were taboo for early adolescents and parents did not sanction them either. In fact, many young adolescents did not receive any kind of formal sex education. However, the participants revealed that the Internet had become a new and secret environment for them to experience, understand, and fantasize about dating. Rambaree notes that these new and emerging patterns of online dating in Mauritius are similar to behaviors found in face-to-face contexts within Western countries. This study shows nicely that online contexts provide opportunities for users to deal with old concerns, but in new ways. They may provide a new avenue for contact with romantic partners for adolescents living in settings that are more restrictive.

Adolescent's Relationships Within Their Families

Up to this point, we have focused on how technology mediates adolescents' interactions with their peers – friends and romantic partners. Now we turn to the intersection of technology and young people's families. Even though the peer group increases in importance during adolescence, nonetheless the family remains an important context. Technology has become commonplace in the lives of families in the USA, Western Europe, and other parts of the world, and we examine its impact on family dynamics as well teens' relationships with their parents.

According to results of the 2008 Pew Internet Project, both spouses use the Internet in 76% of US households married-with-children, as do 84% of their 7- to 17-year-old children (Kennedy, Smith, Wells, & Wellman, 2008). Eighty-nine percent of such households own multiple cell phones, and 57% of children (7- to 17-year-olds) have their own cell phone in these families. Interestingly, teens (12- to 17-year-olds) and their parents often use similar technologies and with similar frequencies (Macgill, 2007). However, compared to their parents, teens reported more often that technologies made their lives easier. Parents tend to be more concerned about media content than the time that their teens spend using such media and we address parents monitoring of their teens' technology in Chapter 11.

Has Technology Changed Interactions with Family Members?

A key question is whether the pervasive use of technology by both parents and their teens has affected teens' contact with their family members. Implicit here is the concern that teens' use of technology may be coming at the expense of face-to-face interaction with parents and family members. The WIP data depicted in Figs. 5.4 and 5.5 are relevant to this question. Respondents (12- to 18-year-olds) were asked whether interactions with household members and family members had changed since getting home Internet access. Figure 5.4 focuses on household members, defined as individuals living in the same household as the teen and Fig. 5.5

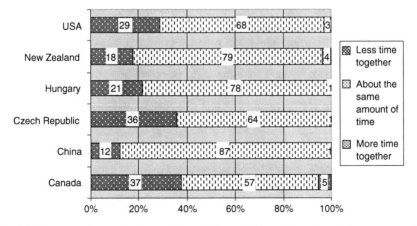

Fig. 5.4 Time spent interacting face to face with household members after getting access to the Internet (12- to 18-year-olds)

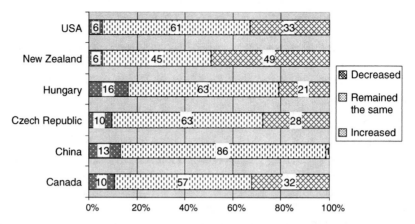

Fig. 5.5 Overall contact with family members after getting access to the Internet (12- to18-year-olds)

shows family members, defined as relatives who do not live together. Across different countries, the majority of youth reported that since getting Internet access, they spent about the same amount of time interacting with household members and that overall contact with family members who lived separately had also remained the same; the only exception was New Zealand, where teens reported that the Internet had increased contact with family members.

Somewhat similar findings were obtained on the Pew Internet project, in which 55% of US Internet users of all ages reported that e-mail has improved their connections to family members (60% women and 51% of men) (Rainie & Kohut, 2000). The charm of technology may lie in the fact that it allows people to interact with family members without some of the costs associated with such contact: in fact, 62% of those who exchange e-mail with relatives opined that they like e-mail as it enables them to stay in touch without having to spend too much time talking to relatives. Furthermore, the results indicated that parents and children who communicated with each other regularly via e-mail also talked often by phone – more than 75% of parents and children who send e-mail to each other communicate this way at least once weekly and call each other with the same frequency. From the survey data, we see that youth feel that new technologies have not changed the amount of time spent interacting with immediate family and more extended family members.

Although youth feel that technology does not affect the extent of their interactions with their family, nonetheless extant research points to a more complex picture. There is no doubt that tools such as cell phones and instant messaging, enable family members to be in much more frequent contact with each other compared to earlier times. According to a majority of the adults on the 2008 Pew Report, technology allowed their family life today to be as close (60%), or closer (25%), than their families were when they were growing up. Respondents also felt that new communication tools allowed them to stay connected with their families, a benefit that could be valuable when teens leave home for college or to live on their own (Kennedy et al., 2008). However, the very tools that enhance contact with family members can also allow teens much more freedom and independence from parents than was possible before. An in-depth interview study of 21 15- to 18-year olds in Israel revealed such a dual role for mobile phones – participants reported that they contributed to both intimacy as well as inter-generational distance (Ribak, 2009).

The issue of mobile phones and generational boundaries is an important one. Parents often get their teens mobile phones for safety reasons, as a means of monitoring them, to coordinate pick up, and for other practical matters. Teens use them primarily to communicate with their peers (Kaare et al., 2007), and sometimes to even shut out their family. A focus group study of Norwegian adolescents, young adults, and parents revealed that teens used the cell phone to establish generational boundaries (for example, screening calls from parents into voice mail) and their frequent mobile phone use often undermined family rituals, such as mealtimes and vacations (Ling & Yttri, 2006). According to Subrahmanyam and Greenfield (2008), the mobile phone might undermine family interaction in favor of peer communication via what they call the individualization of communication: "When peers called one another through a mobile telephone, they knew that they could talk directly with their friends, without any filtering or monitoring from parents or others in the household."

Parents also seem to feel that new technologies are interfering with their family life (Ochs, Graesch, Mittman, Bradburg & Repetti, 2006; Rosen, 2007). From surveying a very diverse sample of parents in Los Angeles, Rosen found that a third of his sample felt that time on MySpace interfered with family life and the proportion increased to half for parents whose teens spent more than 2 h a day on the social networking site (Rosen, 2007). Another study using a completely different approach revealed a similar picture of the role of technology in modern family life (Ochs et al., 2007). In this case, the researchers conducted a detailed 4-year video study of 30 dual-earner families, also in Los Angeles. Children's immersion in their technologies was so complete that parents could not break through it and so frequently retreated. The researchers observed this happening particularly when the working spouse, often the father, came home at the end of the day: generally, the children failed to greet him, did so only a third of the time, and that too with a perfunctory "hi." However, there may be other factors at play as well. In the study by Rosen and colleagues described earlier in the paragraph, adolescents who spent a lot of time on MySpace also reported receiving less support from their parents (Rosen, 2007). Another study found that family interaction was negatively affected only when adolescents used the computer for social purposes, but not when they used it for educational ones (Mesch, 2006b).

Impact on Family Relationships

Just as the relation between technology use and family interaction is a complex one, so is the relation between use and its impact on family relationships. Mesch's work on the impact of the Internet on family relationships has shed some light on this important issue (Mesch, 2003, 2006a, 2006b). In his first study, Mesch studied 1,000 households in Israel with at least one adolescent in the family (Mesch, 2003). The study revealed that there were no differences in the level of closeness between adolescents and parents in families with and without an Internet connection. Parent and adolescent closeness was positively related to parent and adolescent characteristics and the extent to which family members interacted with each other, in particular the amount of time they spent interacting face-to-face. The extent of face-to-face contact was not related to the presence of an Internet connection in the home. Closeness was negatively related to time online, and the more time teens spent online, the less close they were to their parents. Teens' online activities were also relevant: Using the Internet for educational reasons - doing homework, downloading software, and learning Internet skills – was positively related to the quality of adolescent – parent relationships, perhaps because parents value such activities. Mesch concluded that a high frequency of Internet use among adolescents, particularly when it was not used for learning related uses, created intergenerational conflicts.

Indeed research confirms that Internet use is a source of parent-teen conflict and may disrupt the traditional parental position of power. Based on a re-analysis of data from the Pew Internet & American Life Project 2000 (Mesch, 2006a), Mesch reported that adolescent – parent conflict over Internet use was widespread; the data were from interviews of 1,508 individuals from a survey of 754 12- to 17-year old Internet users and one of their parents. Conflicts were reported by 40% of parents in the sample and the extent of conflict was greater if the adolescent was perceived as the family's Internet expert. Teens generally may be more knowledgeable than their parents about using computers and other technologies. In a 2008 survey of Czech Internet users (part of the World Internet Project), 41% of parents with children up to 18 years of age reported that their children were more knowledgeable about computers, whereas only 29% reported the reverse. The older the parent the greater the difference between parents' and children's knowledge. Such adolescent expertise reverses traditional family roles, in which parents typically provide guidance and knowledge to their children. Recall that youth are the digital natives and their parents are the digital immigrants. Thus, the status of youth as the "new experts" could represent a source of power imbalance in the family increasing the potential for conflict.

Parent–adolescent conflict around Internet use may ultimately affect family cohesion. Mesch surveyed 927 13- to 18-year olds to examine the relation between family cohesion and frequency and type of Internet use (Mesch, 2006b). Adolescents who used the Internet for social purposes (online gaming, communication with friends, discussion groups) reported a higher level of family conflict. Internet use for learning or school related purposes was not associated with conflict and reduced family cohesion. More frequent teen Internet use was also associated with lower family cohesion, even when personality characteristics were controlled. The study does not speak to whether there were any positive effects of Internet use.

The foregoing studies by Mesch paint a complicated picture – although the presence of the Internet within the home may not impact closeness within families (Mesch, 2003), it can create intergenerational conflict, especially when the teen is the "Internet expert" (Mesch, 2006a). Family cohesion may also be decreased when the adolescent is a heavy Internet user (Mesch, 2006b). Mobile phones, with their potential for enhancing both communication and distance may similarly have a complex relationship to family relationships and closeness and is deserving of further study. At the same time, we may also see changes in the effect of these new tools as parents become more comfortable with technology, and as technology savvy young adults become parents themselves. It is not clear whether teens will retain their position as the family technology expert or whether parents will assume that mantle restoring the traditional family power balance. As technology becomes more commonplace and as memories of life without technology recede, will technology continue to be such a source of conflict? Only time will tell.

Conclusions

There is no question that digital tools, such as the Internet and cell phones have increased and widened adolescents' contact with the people in their lives – friends, family, romantic partners, and in some cases even with strangers. Their enhanced contact with peers is remarkable, and contrary to fears, teens connect online mostly with people who are already in their offline life and report that their online interactions do not affect the extent of their face-to-face ones. These trends illustrate yet again that developmentally important offline patterns of behavior are emphasized in adolescents' use of digital tools. The Internet allows them to accomplish the dual developmental tasks of autonomy from parents and establishing themselves within their peer groups from the relative comfort and safety of their home. However, several questions remain, particularly with regard to the nature of their online interactions and their impact on friendship quality and family relationships.

As teens' notions about friendship evolve and as some of their peer interactions occur publicly, does it fundamentally alter and transform their peer relationships? Do they accrue different levels of intimacy and support from face-to-face versus digital interactions? Do interactions in different digital contexts (e.g., instant messaging vs. text messaging) offer different levels of support? While digital tools have allowed teens to interact with an expanded network of peers, a valid concern is that they are spreading themselves thin: instead of fewer, more intimate relationships, they may be having more numerous, but less intimate ones. An alternative possibility is that the self-disclosure afforded by the Internet enhances their relationships with close friends while at the same time making it possible for them to interact with a "wider circle of friends" (Giordano, 1995) and the latter interactions may help youth learn about themselves and their social world. More research is necessary to sort through these hypotheses and especially to understand the mechanisms and processes of online self-disclosure that may affect intimacy, relationship quality, and ultimately young people's well-being.

A complicated picture of the effects of technology on family relationships is emerging. Teens report that the Internet has not changed the amount of interactions with their family and tools such as cell phones and social networking sites may even allow them to keep in touch with relatives and family members, with whom they otherwise would not interact. At the same, they may accelerate teens' individuation and autonomy from their family and may even be a source of conflict within the home. When teens, as the digital natives, are more knowledgeable about technology than their digital immigrant parents are, we may see a reversal of traditional roles that may disrupt family relationships.

References

Annenberg Public Policy Center. (2006, September). *Stranger contact in adolescent online social networks*. Philadelphia: Annenberg Public Policy Center, University of Pennsylvania. Retrieved October 19, 2009, from http://www.annenbergpublicpolicycenter.org/Downloads/Releases/Release_HC20060920/Report_HC20060920.pdf

Bee, H. L. (1994). *Lifespan development*. New York, NY: HarperCollins Publishers.

Boneva, S. S., Quinn, A., Kraut, E. R., Kiesler, S., & Shklovski, I. (2006). Teenage communication in the instant messaging era. In R. E. Kraut (Ed.), *Information technology at home* (pp. 612–672). Oxford: Oxford University Press.

Bouchey, H. A., & Furman, W. (2004). Dating and romantic experiences in adolescence. In R. G. Adams & M. D. Berzonsky (Eds.), *Blackwell handbook of adolescence*. Oxford: Blackwell.

Brown, B. B. (2004). Adolescents' relationships with peers. In R. M. Lerner & L. Steinberg (Eds.), *Handbook of adolescent psychology* (2nd ed., pp. 363–394). Hoboken, NJ: Wiley.

Brown, B. B., & Klute, C. (2004). Friendships, cliques, and crowds. In M. R. Lerner & L. Steinberg (Eds.), *Handbook of adolescent psychology* (2nd ed.). Hoboken, NJ: Wiley.

Buhrmester, D., & Prager, K. (1995). Patterns and functions of self-disclosure during childhood and adolescence. In K. J. Rotenberg (Ed.), *Disclosure processes in children and adolescents* (pp. 10–56). New York, NY: Cambridge University Press.

Chan, D. K. S., & Cheng, G. H. L. (2004). A comparison of offline and online friendship qualities at different stages of relationship development. *Journal of Social and Personal Relationships, 21*, 305–320.

Dunphy, D. C. (1963). The social structure of urban adolescent peer groups. *Sociometry, 26*, 230–246.

Erikson, E. H. (1968). *Identity, youth, and crisis* (1st ed.). New York, NY: W. W. Norton.

Furman, W., Brown, B. B., & Feiring, C. (1999). *Contemporary perspectives on adolescent romantic relationships*. New York, NY: Cambridge University Press.

Giordano, P. C. (1995). The wider circle of friends in adolescence. *The American Journal of Sociology, 101*, 661–697.

Gross, E. F. (2004). Adolescent Internet use: What we expect, what teens report. *Journal of Applied Developmental Psychology, 25*, 633–649.

Kaare, B. H., Brandtzaeg, P. B., Heim, J., & Endestad, T. (2007). In the borderland between family orientation and peer culture: The use of communication technologies among Norwegian tweens. *New Media & Society, 9*, 603–624.

Kennedy, T. L. M., Smith, A., Wells, A. T., & Wellman, B. (2008). Networked families. *Pew Internet and American Life Project*. Retrieved September 9, 2009, from http://www.pewinternet.org/~/media/Files/Reports/2008/PIP_Networked_Family.pdf.pdf.

Kraut, R. E., Kiesler, S., Boneva, B., Cummings, J., Helgeson, V., & Crawford, A. (2002). Internet paradox revisited. *Journal of Social Issues, 58*, 49–74.

Kraut, R. E., Patterson, M., Lundmark, V., Kiesler, S., Mukopadhyay, T., & Scherlis, W. (1998). Internet paradox: A social technology that reduces social involvement and psychological well-being? *American Psychologist, 53*, 1017–1031.

Lenhart, A., & Madden, M. (2007). Social networking websites and teens: An overview. *Pew Internet and American Life Project*. Retrieved November 3, from http://www.pewinternet. org/pdfs/PIP_SNS_Data_Memo_Jan_2007.pdf

Ling, R., & Yttri, B. (2006). Control, emancipation, and status: The mobile telephone in teens' parental and peer relationships. In R. E. Kraut, M. Brynin, & S. Kiesler (Eds.), *Computers, phones, and the Internet: Domesticating information technology* (pp. 219–235). New York, NY: Oxford University Press.

Macgill, A. R. (2007). Parent and teenager Internet use. *Pew Internet & American Life Project*. Retrieved November 8, 2008, from http://www.pewinternet.org/pdfs/PIP_Teen_ Parents_data_memo_Oct2007.pdf

Mesch, G. S. (2003). The family and the Internet: The Israeli case. *Social Science Quarterly, 84*, 1039–1050.

Mesch, G. S. (2006a). Family characteristics and intergenerational conflicts over the Internet. *Information, Communication and Society, 9*, 473–495.

Mesch, G. S. (2006b). Family relations and the Internet: Exploring a family boundaries approach. *Journal of Family Communication, 6*, 119–138.

Mesch, G. S., & Talmud, I. (2006). The quality of online and offline relationships: The role of multiplexity and duration of social relationships. *Information Society, 22*, 137–148.

Mesch, G. S., & Talmud, I. (2007). Similarity and the quality of online and offline social relationships among adolescents in Israel. *Journal of Research on Adolescence (Blackwell Publishing Limited), 17*, 455–465.

Miller, B. C., & Benson, B. (1999). Romantic and sexual relationship development during adolescence. In W. Furman, B. B. Brown, & C. Feiring (Eds.), *The development of romantic relationships in adolescence*. Cambridge: Cambridge University Press.

Ochs, E., Graesch, A. P., Mittman, A., Bradbury, T., & Repetti, R. (2006). Video ethnogroaphy and ethnoarcheological tracking. In E. E. Kossek & S. Sweet (Eds.), *The work and family handbook: Multi-disciplinary perspectives and approaches* (pp. 387–409). Mahwah, NJ: Erlbaum.

Peter, J., Valkenburg, P. M., & Schouten, A. P. (2005). Developing a model of adolescent friendship formation on the Internet. *CyberPsychology & Behavior, 8*, 423–430.

Pombeni, M. L., Kirchler, E., & Palmonari, A. (1990). Identification with peers as a strategy to muddle through the troubles of the adolescent years. *Journal of Adolescence, 13*, 351–369.

Rainie, L., & Kohut, A. (2000). Tracking online life: How women use the Internet to cultivate relationships with family and friends. *The Pew Internet & American Life Project*. Retrieved October, 31, 2008 from http://www.pewinternet.org/~/media//Files/Reports/2000/ Report1.pdf.pdf

Rambaree, K. (2008). Internet-mediated dating/romance of mauritian early adolescents: A grounded theory analysis. *International Journal of Emerging Technologies & Society, 6*, 34–59.

Reich, S. M., Subrahmanyam, K., & Espinoza, G. E. (2009, April 3). *Adolescents' use of social networking sites – Should we be concerned?* Paper presented at the Society for Research on Child Development, Denver, CO.

Ribak, R. (2009). Remote control, umbilical cord and beyond: The mobile phone as a transitional object. *British Journal of Developmental Psychology, 27*, 183–196.

Rosen, L. D. (2007). *Me, MySpace and I: Parenting the net generation*. New York, NY: Palgrave Macmillan.

Ryan, A. M. (2001). The peer group as a context for the development of young adolescent motivation and achievement. *Child Development, 72*, 1135–1150.

Šmahel, D. (2003). *Psychologie a Internet: Děti dospělými, dospělí dětmi. [Psychology and Internet: Children being adults, adults being children.]*. Prague: Triton.

Šmahel, D., & Subrahmanyam, K. (2007). "Any girls want to chat press 911": Partner selection in monitored and unmonitored teen chat rooms. *Cyberpsychology & Behavior, 10*, 346–353.

Šmahel, D., & Vesela, M. (2006). Interpersonal attraction in the virtual environment. *Ceskoslovenska Psychologie, 50*, 174–186.

Steinberg, L. (2008). *Adolescence*. New York, NY: McGraw-Hill.

Subrahmanyam, K., Garcia, E. C., Harsono, S. L., Li, J., & Lipana, L. (2009). In their words: Connecting online weblogs to developmental processes. *British Journal of Developmental Psychology, 27*, 219–245.

Subrahmanyam, K., & Greenfield, P. M. (2008). Online communication and adolescent relationships. *The Future of Children, 18*, 119–146.

Subrahmanyam, K., Reich, S. M., Waechter, N., & Espinoza, G. (2008). Online and offline social networks: Use of social networking sites by emerging adults. *Journal of Applied Developmental Psychology, 29*, 420–433.

Thornton, A. (1990). The courtship process and adolescent sexuality. *Journal of Family Issues, 11*, 239–273.

Valkenburg, P. M., & Peter, J. (2007). Preadolescents' and adolescents' online communication and their closeness to friends. *Developmental Psychology, 43*, 267–277.

Valkenburg, P. M., & Peter, J. (2009). Social consequences of the Internet for adolescents. *Current Directions in Psychological Science, 18*, 1–5.

Valkenburg, P. M., Peter, J., & Schouten, A. (2006). Friend networking sites and their relationship to adolescents' well-being and social self-esteem. *CyberPsychology & Behavior, 9*, 584–590.

Wallace, P. M. (1999). *The psychology of the Internet*. New York, NY: Cambridge University Press.

Wolak, J., Finkelhor, D., & Mitchell, K. (2008). Is talking online to unknown people always risky? Distinguishing online Interaction styles in a national sample of youth Internet users. *Cyberpsychology & Behavior, 11*, 340–343.

Wolak, J., Mitchell, K. J., & Finkelhor, D. (2002). Close online relationships in a national sample of adolescents. *Adolescence, 37*, 441.

Wolak, J., Mitchell, K. J., & Finkelhor, D. (2003). Escaping or connecting? Characteristics of youth who form close online relationships. *Journal of Adolescence, 26*, 105–119.

Yum, Y.-O., & Hara, K. (2005). Computer-mediated relationship development: A cross-cultural comparison. *Journal of Computer-Mediated Communication, 11*, 133–152.

Chapter 6
Digital Worlds and Doing the Right Thing: Morality, Ethics, and Civic Engagement

In the previous chapters, we saw that youth bring the core adolescent concerns of sexuality, identity, and intimacy to their online realms. In this chapter, we turn our attention to two equally challenging developmental tasks outlined by Havighurst that are still very relevant in today's world. We examine the role of technology as adolescents construct a moral and ethical set of values and become fully engaged, active members of their social groups, from their local communities to society-at-large. We will show that technology presents both opportunities and challenges to adolescents as they accomplish these tasks.

Consider the Internet: it is both a tool and a social context. As a tool it provides youth with unparalleled and easy access to information (the costs and benefits of such access are discussed in depth in Chapters 8 and 10); but it is also used for plagiarism and to illegally download and share movies, music, and software. As a social context, the Internet allows adolescents to connect and interact with peers and strangers, to participate in online communities, and to engage with their local and more distant communities in ways that would have been unthinkable even a few years ago. Online worlds also come with their own rules, etiquette, and social conventions (Bradley, 2005). Adolescents have to navigate these digital worlds safely and securely and in ways that are at times at odds with offline moral and ethical values. Lying and falsifying of information illustrates this nicely. While online, most people have lied at some point or the other, especially with regard to their identities and their activities. We generally see such online lying and falsification to be prudent, especially with regard to safeguarding privacy. At the same time, online lying can also be dangerous, such as when youth lie about their age to enter a site with mature content. There is no such ambiguity with regard to offline lying, and we teach youth from the beginning that lying is wrong and not sanctioned. Clearly, these are complex issues and in the first part of the chapter, we explore them further in relation to adolescents' developing sense of online morality and ethics; in the second part of the chapter, we focus on young people's use of technology to engage with their local and more distant communities.

K. Subrahmanyam, D. Šmahel, *Digital Youth*, Advancing Responsible
Adolescent Development, DOI 10.1007/978-1-4419-6278-2_6,
© Springer Science+Business Media, LLC 2011

Morality and Ethics Online

Morality and ethics center around standards of right and wrong and offer guide-lines as to how individuals in a society should behave to uphold those standards (Velasquez, Andre, Shanks, & Meyer, 2008). For a society and its institutions to survive and thrive, it is important that people behave in morally correct and eth-ically responsible ways. The collapse of the US sub-prime mortgage market and the 2008 global financial crisis that it triggered are examples of the consequences when individuals in positions of responsibility act unethically. Although a multi-tude of factors led to the debacle, two major contributing factors were the predatory practices of mortgage brokers and the failure of banks to have appropriate lending standards (Klein & Goldfarb, 2008). Young people's ethics have raised concerns as well. According to the Josephson Institute's 2008 Report Card on the Ethics of American Youth ($n = 30,000$ US high school students), within the past year, more than 35% reported that they had stolen from a store, 64% cheated on a test, and 36% used the Internet to plagiarize an assignment (Josephson Institute, 2006). Interestingly their behavior was at odds with their beliefs, as 93% were satisfied with their personal ethics and character and 26% reported that they lied on at least one or two survey questions. While it is very likely that the results were subject to the biases and memory lapses associated with self-report surveys, the results highlight the fact that developing an inner core of values is not an easy task.

The Internet presents special challenges to behaving ethically: Users are dis-embodied and can chose to be as anonymous as they wish. Consequently online contexts decrease the likelihood of being identified and thus allow individuals to remain "faceless" (Freestone & Mitchell, 2004), presumably providing less constraints to behave ethically. Examples of online behaviors that are ethically ques-tionable include: using someone else's e-mail account without permission, hacking into a computer or web site, plagiarizing from online sources, e-mailing assignment and exam answers to their peers, and illegal downloading of music, movies, and more (Jackson et al., 2008). In the next sections, we examine five areas of online behavior where adolescents have to learn to do the right thing (1) maintaining pri-vacy, (2) falsifying information, (3) cheating and stealing, (4) cyber plagiarism, (5) software piracy and illegal downloading of music, movies, and software. Cyber bul-lying and other forms of online harassment are also instances where young people are not doing the right thing, but extant literature has treated them as aggressive behaviors and so they are addressed in Chapter 10.

Maintaining Privacy Online

Youth must come to understand privacy online, their own and that of others, and equally important, learn how to maintain and safeguard it. For instance, they have to learn not to share their electronic passwords with others, understand that another person's e-mail account is private, and that they should not copy and paste and forward an instant message conversation to a third party.

Understanding online privacy. Research on this topic has been motivated by incidents where young people were victimized by predators they had met in online forums (Hinduja & Patchin, 2008). The good news is that most adolescents are careful about not revealing personal information online. Hinduja and Patchin report that only a very small percent of youth MySpace users revealed private details, such as their full name (8.8%), instant messaging name (4.2%), and phone number (0.3%). Similarly, in our own work on blogs, we found that most of the youth bloggers did not reveal personal identifying information. Although self-photos were often used (typically as userpictures and/or uploaded in the blog), most authors were conscious that entries were public and were circumspect about revealing personal and identifying information about themselves (Subrahmanyam, Garcia, Harsono, Li, & Lipana, 2009). There has also been a corresponding decline in reports of unwanted online sexual solicitation and harassment, no doubt due to greater awareness among youth and better enforcement (Mitchell, Wolak, & Finkelhor, 2007) (see Chapter 10).

Safeguarding online privacy. Adolescents actively safeguard their privacy and adopt specific strategies; when faced with web sites that request personal information, they report providing incomplete or inaccurate information about themselves, switching to sites that do not ask for personal information, or leaving the web site. Other strategies that they report using include sending e-mails requesting that their e-mail address be taken off a distribution list, notifying an Internet service provider (ISP) about unwanted mail, and even flaming (angry or abusive e-mail) the senders of spam (Moscardelli & Divine, 2007). Although youth are fairly knowledgeable and proactive about protecting their privacy, not all of their privacy-protection behaviors are smart and effective ones. For instance, it might actually be counterproductive to send requests to be removed from distribution lists, as spammers use such requests to verify e-mail addresses and then sell verified e-mail addresses to third parties (Moscardelli & Divine, 2007). Ironically, this was the second most frequent strategy reported after the providing of inaccurate information. Flaming, too, is a less than effective tactic to deal with spamming, but adolescents seem to prefer it over contacting ISPs about the spammers (Moscardelli & Divine, 2007).

Are adolescents equally careful about safeguarding their privacy when faced with requests from online marketers such as unsolicited e-mail or other offers of free products? Early reports suggested that teens were naive and not very circumspect about protecting their privacy in the face of online marketing (Turow & Nir, 2000). However, as with so many other aspects of the Internet, online behaviors have changed and evolved over time. In recent years, youth have become more well informed about online privacy and more discerning as to the circumstances when they are willing to provide information about themselves. For instance, Youn found that adolescent respondents in her study were more willing to provide generic information about themselves (e.g., age and gender) and their interests and media use, but less willing to provide identifying information (e.g., e-mail address, postal information, parental information, and personal identifiers such as social security number and credit card number). Entertainment (e.g., "listening to music") and communication ("sending instant messages to someone online") benefits were perceived to be more attractive in exchange for information disclosure compared to instrumental benefits such as promotional incentives or product information (Youn, 2005).

Teens' privacy concerns and assessment of risk appear to influence their use of privacy-protection strategies. Adolescents who are more concerned about privacy are also more likely to use privacy protection strategies such as requesting removal of e-mail address and providing inaccurate information (Moscardelli & Divine, 2007). However they appear to be able to balance their concerns about privacy with an appraisal of the risks and benefits of disclosing information; in her study, Youn found that higher levels of risk perception led to lower willingness to disclose personal information and a higher perception of benefits led to a greater willingness to disclose personal information (Youn, 2005).

Concerns about privacy are influenced by variables such as gender and family communication. Boys are less concerned about their online privacy and they also seem to engage in behaviors that may threaten their privacy such as reading unsolicited e-mail, registering on web sites and sending flaming e-mails to spammers (Youn & Hall, 2008). Privacy concerns are also related to family communication styles and are greater among youth who come from families where ideas are presented and discussed, beliefs challenged, and controversies addressed (Youn, 2005). Such parents are referred to as authoritative parents in the developmental psychology literature (Baumrind, 1991). Authoritative parents are warm, use inductive reasoning, exercise control and discipline, and engage in discussions with their children and authoritative parenting is related to positive child and adolescent outcomes. Such parents are also generally more pro-active about monitoring their teens' Internet use such as by setting time limits and using filtering software (Eastin, Greenberg, & Hofschire, 2006). We will see in Chapter 10 that teens who have discussions with their parents about online safety are much less likely to share personal information about themselves to strangers who they meet online. Adolescents who come from homes where intellectual discourse and discussion are encouraged are generally more aware about privacy issues while online.

It is therefore important for parents and even teachers to talk to teens about online privacy and the most appropriate tactics to safeguard it (Moscardelli & Divine, 2007). However, adults themselves have to be knowledgeable about the most appropriate and effective privacy-protection methods. We saw earlier that although teens often write to spammers to request removal of their e-mail address, it might not be the wisest strategy. Even many adults may not be aware of this and so it is important to educate parents and teachers about the most effective strategies so they can pass on these lessons to teens (Moscardelli & Divine, 2007). Boys and girls may also have to be educated differently about privacy concerns (Youn & Hall, 2008). Not only are boys less concerned about online privacy, they are generally more likely to engage in online activities that threaten it. When privacy concerns do increase, boys and girls respond differently; boys do not register on to web sites whereas girls tend to provide inaccurate information. Given the gender differences in levels of concerns and strategies, we should not use a "one size fits all" approach to privacy education.

Falsifying Information Online

Providing incorrect or incomplete information is a technique that youth use not just to safeguard their privacy, but more generally, when they use technology. For instance, Harman and colleagues note that while online, young people may lie about demographic details, such as age, gender, and weight, and their online behavior might be different from their face-to-face behavior (Harman, Hansen, Cochran, & Lindsey, 2005). In teen focus groups that we conducted, participants talked a lot about how their peers often provided inaccurate or embellished accounts of their activities on their MySpace profiles. While there is no firm label for such behavior, they have been variously called "faking" (Harman et al., 2005) or "lying" (Blinka & Šmahel, 2008).

It turns out that lying and faking are not monolithic behaviors that youth engage in whenever they are online, but are more likely in anonymous spaces such as chat rooms (Konečný & Šmahel, 2007), compared to e-mail or instant messaging, which are often used to interact with people from their offline lives. Similarly, what youth lie about also depends on the particular online context within which the lying occurs. Adolescents may lie about their age and appearance in spaces, such as chat rooms, where they are less likely to be discovered, but not in social networking sites, where they interact with offline friends. In the latter context, they may be more apt to inflate their activities for peer approval and engage in what we like to call "creative embellishment." Indeed, adolescents report lying most in chat rooms (in comparison to other applications) and they lie there most about their age; approximately 16% of female and 15% of male chat participants in one study reported that they had done so (Konečný & Šmahel, 2007). Younger adolescents may lie more than older adolescents: with regard to blogs, 52% of 13- to 14-year olds admitted to lying compared to 35% of 15- to 17-year olds (Blinka & Šmahel, 2009). Teens have also become adept at dealing with the lying that they encounter online. In a qualitative study of seven experienced teen chat users, participants acknowledged that lying was commonplace, and that they used deliberate strategies to detect when someone was lying such as their intuition, typographic style, and saving and searching prior communications with a particular nickname (Koubalikova & Šmahel, 2008).

Developmental implications. Given that online lying and faking are common-place and usually do not carry moral sanctions, it is important to consider their developmental implications particularly the relation between online and offline moral behavior. In their correlational study of early adolescents (6–8th grade), Harman et al. concluded that faking was associated with poorer social skills, lower self-esteem, higher levels of social anxiety, and higher levels of aggression (Harman et al., 2005). Jackson and colleagues found that offline moral attitudes and behavior predicted participants' attitudes toward morally questionable online behaviors (e.g., using a friend's Internet account without asking or deleting files or other informa-tion belonging to someone else without asking). Youth who were more willing to accept exceptions to offline moral behavior and who were less moral in their offline behavior were more accepting of morally questionable online behaviors (Jackson et al., 2008).

Although it is too early to conclude that online lying and faking threaten social and psychological well-being, unusually high levels of such behavior should alert parents and teachers to the possibility of other social and psychological problems. We should also consider the potential long-term consequences of online faking and lying behavior for the development of young people's ethics and morality. On the one hand, from early on they are taught that lying is wrong; at the same time, for their safety, they are taught to withhold or even provide false details about themselves while online in order to safeguard their privacy. Youth may also falsify age information to bypass age restrictions (Subrahmanyam & Greenfield, 2008), and most of us have engaged in seemingly harmless online concealment or fabrication at one point or another. Add to that is the difficulty of discriminating faking behavior or embellished accounts from the kind of true identity play (Erikson, 1968) described by Turkle in her early work on the Internet (Turkle, 1995) (online identity play is discussed in greater detail in Chapter 4). More research is necessary to find out when online lying and faking are harmless, when they represent true identity play, and when they might be harmful.

Stealing and Cheating Online

Online stealing and cheating are activities that impinge on moral and ethical development. In 2007, the Dutch police arrested a teenage online thief for stealing furniture from Habbo Hotel, an online Dutch networking site for teens. Apparently, the teen in question had hacked into other users' accounts and stolen online furniture worth 4,000 Euros (Evans & Thomasson, 2007). Less extreme, but more common, are incidents where a user can have the contents of his/her accounts in virtual worlds wiped out; often this happens when a player's password is revealed either accidentally or in exchange for something, such as an avatar makeover (Semuels, 2008). The former happend to the children of the first author when all the points in their Neopets (a virtual world) account was stolen. While the loss had little monetary value, it did sting them – they remember the incident clearly and talk about it several years later. Falling victim to such theft at a young age might ironically be a good lesson for youth and prepare them for increasingly virtual lives, where phishing e-mails are all too common and the theft of one's identity is a real possibility with far-reaching consequences.

More minor forms of cheating have been observed and documented by Fields and Kafai in their ethnographic work in a teen virtual world, Whyville.net (Fields & Kafai, 2007). Whyville is virtual space where members are able to interact with one another as well as play informal science games and activities. Fields and colleagues were interested in the educational value of cheat sites, which they define as "player-generated web sites where players share strategies (or answers if applicable) for solving problems in the virtual games." As part of their ethnographic work in Whyville, they analyzed discussions of cheating that appeared in *The Whyville Times*, the forum's newspaper. Their descriptions of the many creative ways of cheating that Whyvillians devised highlight some of the moral/ethical challenges that come up in virtual worlds. We note a few below, using the original words of the authors to retain the flavor of the incidents.

They note that 10% of the 100 articles on *cheats* contained "explicit warnings against scams, reporting on the many imaginative ways Whyvillians have tried to procure others' passwords with the promise of raising their salaries, giving them makeovers, and even claiming to be site designers." Another devious cheating strategy involved "Smart Car races where instead of going around the track in a traditional race, some players would immediately turn their cars around and cross the finish line, thus triggering a win." About 10% of the articles dealt with "cheating in dating relationships, some of them asking whether it was cheating if one had one boyfriend in the 'real world' and a different one in Whyville." Some articles addressed "issues with ballot stuffing, creating multiple accounts in order to have more votes for oneself in elections for Whyville senator or prom king/queen." Finally Fields and Kafai note of a strategy that they call stealing from Grandma; "Grandma's the place in Whyville where new players can go to receive donated face parts." But "experienced players were going to Grandma's, accepting rather than donating parts, and selling them at the Trading Post for a profit." The latter two are especially worth noting, because they do not break the explicit rules of the virtual world, but nonetheless tested ethical boundaries.

We need research to understand why youth engage in such behavior – Is it because they feel disinhibitied in the online space – that is, do they feel no restraint because they think no can see what they did and so cannot be found out? Alternatively, do they think that offline moral rules do not apply online? Also needed is research on how best to teach youth that moral rules do apply online and that stealing is just as wrong online as it is off. The challenge, of course, is that notions of online property and propriety are very nebulous, as we shall see in the next section, when we discuss cyber plagiarism and the illegal downloading of software, music, and movies.

Cyber Plagiarism

Cyber plagiarism is the unattributed use of information from the web, and ranges from copying and pasting a couple of lines of text to buying whole papers and using digital objects such as images, films, movies, and other online material without crediting the creator. Unlike the cheating, described in the earlier paragraphs, it does not happen online and typically occurs in academic work, which youth turn in at school. In general plagiarism appears to be fairly common among youth, and in a survey conducted at the Center for Academic Integrity, over 60% of high school students admitted to plagiarizing, and half reported that it involved the Internet (McCabe, 2005 cited in Sisti, 2007).

Kinds of cyber plagiarism. The most common way that youth use the Internet to cheat is copying sentences from the Internet without proper citation of the source; less common is buying a paper from a Paper Mill web site (Conradson &

Hernández-Ramos, 2004). In addition to term paper and essay sites, other Internet resources that students use to cheat include, lecture note web sites as well as editorial service sites; see Conradson and Hernández-Ramos for a list of such sites, many of which were active at the time of the writing of this book (Conradson & Hernández-Ramos, 2004). Sometimes the plagiarism may be unintentional such as with cryptomnesia, which Sisti defines as the "unconscious appropriation of another author's work by a plagiarist who thinks the work they are producing is original" (Sisti, 2007). Because of the ease with which one can copy and paste information from the web, some student plagiarism may occur because the writer simply does not have a clear understanding of paraphrasing, use of direct quotes, and citation of sources, particularly digital ones (Conradson & Hernández-Ramos, 2004; Ercegovac, 2005). It is important to distinguish between intentional and unintentional kinds of plagiarism because they are motivated differently.

Intentional plagiarism. Sisti surveyed 160 high school students about their attitudes and justifications for copy-paste plagiarism and term paper purchasing (Sisti, 2007). With regard to copy-paste plagiarism, 54% reported that they always cited sources in their assignments and 35% reported that they had copy and pasted material; roughly 46% of the latter group acknowledged that what they had done was plagiarism. Common justifications were lack of time to do the assignment, feeling unprepared to write the paper, and lack of interest in the subject matter. Only 2% said they had ever bought a paper; two people because they had to make up a grade and did not feel prepared to do the assignment and one person because no one had ever told her not to do it. Other reasons offered by students included fear of failure and parents' high expectations (Ercegovac, 2005). Reasons for not engaging in plagiarism were an awareness that it was cheating, not wanting to spend money for it, feeling they could write a better paper on their own, and fear that they would be caught.

Unintentional plagiarism. Unintentional plagiarism occurs primarily because youth lack a clear understanding of plagiarism. Students must have both a conceptual and procedural understanding of plagiarism; conceptual knowledge entails knowing what plagiarism is (e.g., being able to define it, recognizing when a text has been plagiarized) and procedural knowledge requires one to know how to credit sources obtained online (Ercegovac, 2005). In a case study of 37 junior high school students, Ecegovac found that students had tremendous difficulties with giving credit to authors/creators of non-book sources, such as photographers, choreographers, and cartoon artists. For instance, 40% reported that they would not cite a choreographer for a Romeo and Juliet ballet, 30% thought they did not have to source maps, and only 16% considered that making a DVD album for sale was plagiarism. Students also had difficulty recognizing authorship for digital images such as photographs, computer code on the web, e-mail transcripts, and personal communication. In our own experience as college instructors, we have found that many students think that they have to cite sources only when they are quoted word for word. In Ercegovac's study, 83% of the junior high students similarly said they would credit sources if they had used direct quotes, and only 16% believed that paraphrasing without citing a source was plagiarism. Students' procedural knowledge was similarly mixed – when asked to match one of two citation formats to a source, 84% were able to do so for a book, but only 29% were able to do so for a magazine. Clearly, some instances of cyber plagiarism occur because students do not have a clear understanding of plagiarism, both conceptually and procedurally.

Teachers' role in cyber plagiarism. Research suggests that teachers' perceptions of plagiarism in general are related to student attitudes and behaviors about cheating (Sisti, 2007). Sisti noted that student responses in his study revealed a lack of clarity about plagiarism and suggests that teachers' conflicting instructions could create such confusion among students. Adding to the problem, because students are often technologically more sophisticated than their teachers are, teachers may make errors with regard to clarifying what constitutes plagiarism in the context of Internet sources. Complicating matters, teachers and students are not even in agreement with regard to what academic honesty includes (Ercegovac, 2005).

Several scholars have offered a variety of strategies that can be used to prevent cyber plagiarism among young people (Conradson & Hernández-Ramos, 2004; Ercegovac, 2005; Sisti, 2007). Below is a synthesis of these strategies:

1. Train teachers to teach about cheating (particularly Internet-based plagiarism) and to effectively deal with cheating.
2. Teachers should clearly communicate expectations and standards to students, particularly academic integrity policies.
3. Teach students to get a better understanding of plagiarism – both conceptually as to what it is and when it occurs, and procedurally – how to properly cite sources and avoid plagiarism. Students may need special training to learn that sources have to be cited regardless of format (e.g., text versus audio or digital images) and to deal with electronic sources and digital objects that are easily available online.
4. Developing new and innovative assignments instead of traditional essays and research papers and requiring evidence of content synthesis from students.
5. Using technological solutions such as Turnitin to detect plagiarized content – educational institutions, especially high schools and colleges, are increasingly using such tools to deter plagiarism. It is too early to know how effective they are at curbing plagiarism; more important, they are deterrents, but do not get to the heart of the problem, which is the lack of a clear moral or ethical understanding of the issue.

Software Piracy and Illegal Downloading of Digital Content

Perhaps the most vexing of all is online piracy, which is the unauthorized copying and sharing of digital products, such as music, software, and other digital content (Yar, 2007). Online piracy came to the fore with peer-to-peer (P2P) file sharing networks, which are networks of computers that allow users to directly search for and download files (such as audio and video files) from other computers in the network.

After *Napster* was famously shut down, P2P software such as *Kazaa*, *LimeWire*, and *Direct Connect* allowed users to connect to each other directly without a central entity routing transactions between computers. Such networks are used to illegally download software, music, music videos, and movies and can result in criminal prosecution. Since 2003, the Recording Industry Association of America (RIAA) has aggressively pursued copyright infringement lawsuits against individual file sharers, including teenagers and college students (Yar, 2007). E-mail attachments, online auction sites, file transfer protocol (FTP) are other ways that people use the Internet for digital piracy. In the USA, digital piracy also includes copying and burning of music CD, games, and DVDs from one's collection for others as well as purchasing of pirated copies of music, software, movies, etc.

Across the world, digital piracy is reported to be most frequent among young people (Freestone & Mitchell, 2004; Kini, Ramakrishna, & Vijayaraman, 2003). Although there is not much scholarly research on this topic, there have been several surveys conducted by business organizations that have a vital stake in this issue. At least within the USA, the incidence of illegal downloading of copyrighted digital materials may be decreasing. For instance in a 2004 survey of 1,100 US 8- to 18-year olds, conducted for the Business Software Alliance, 53% admitted to downloading music files without paying, 22% downloaded software, and 17% downloaded movies (Harris Interactive, 2004). In a similar survey conducted in 2007, 30% downloaded music, 11% software, and 8% movies (Harris Interactive, 2007). No doubt, some of this decrease may be due to the RIAA's aggressive litigation in the USA and the accompanying media publicity. We may also be witnessing a change in users' online behaviors, as they understand the issues and nuances involved, and as the marketplace itself changes (it is now possible to legally and inexpensively download music from sites such as iTunes). We also do not know whether declines in illegal downloading are occurring more broadly in other parts of the world or whether they are specific to the USA, where there has been greater enforcement.

Reasons for online piracy. As with cyber plagiarism, one of the main reasons that young people engage in online piracy is that they do not know the laws governing downloading and sharing online content. In a 2008 survey conducted by KRC Research for Microsoft, 7th–10th graders reported that they were less likely to download and share online content when they were aware of the laws surrounding such behavior (KRC Research, 2008). They also reported that they would not continue to download or share content online, after hearing about the laws surrounding such activities. Those who knew the laws about downloading were also more likely to state that violators should be punished. Parents were an important source of such rules and adolescents whose parents had specific rules about illegal downloading were less likely engage in such behavior (Harris Interactive, 2007; KRC Research, 2008).

Knowledge of intellectual copyright rights alone is not enough to stop illegal downloading as financial reasons are also at work (KRC Research, 2008). In the 2004 Harris Interactive survey, although a majority of the respondents reported knowing that books, movies, music, software, and games were copyrighted, they nonetheless downloaded such materials at relatively high rates. Not having the money was their main reason for doing so, even when the same item was available for sale either in a store or online, and more youth were concerned about accidentally downloading a virus than with violating the law.

The third and perhaps most interesting reason for illegal downloading, is that adolescents do not view violations of copyright law as seriously as other offenses, suggesting that forces of moral reasoning may be at play here. Teston examined the moral developmental dimensions of piracy among seventh grade students (approximately 12–13-year olds) and concluded that adolescents hold different moral orientations toward computer-based property compared to tangible property (Teston, 2001). Whereas about 60% found it acceptable to pirate software via the Internet, and 85% found it acceptable to illegally download music files in MP3 format, only 10% thought the same for a bike theft. Participants viewed software as "public property," and a majority believed that the property rights of the owner/developer were terminated at the time of purchase. Almost 7 years later, the KRC Microsoft study obtained similar results; survey respondents did not view illegal downloading of online content as seriously as the theft of other objects such as mobile phones and a bike and only about 7 in 10 teens felt that it should be punished. Crowell and colleagues suggest that "to the extent that digital objects or materials are perceived as being less private than their more tangible counterparts, a greater moral permissiveness is likely to be attached to behavior involving those objects or materials" (Crowell, Narvaez, & Gomberg, 2005, p. 29). Thus we see that adolescent users seem to separate digital representations of intellectual property, such as software and music, from the creators/owners of such intellectual property. We do not know if these morally permissive views toward digital property are more pervasive in younger people (e.g., teens and young adults) than in older adults. We also do not know if today's youth will continue to hold such views even as they themselves get older – in other words, will these digital natives, who are perhaps the first generation to have grown up with technology their entire lives, retain such qualitatively different views about digital objects as they become older?

Political and Civic Engagement Online

In this section, we examine the intersection between technology and civic engagement, which is the process by young people become engaged with their communities. Traditionally, we define civics as the rights and duties of citizens. In democracies, one very important civic duty is that of participating in politics and government, primarily by voting in elections. Over time, participation in politics and government has been declining, not just in the USA, but also in other democratic countries such as Germany, Sweden, and the United Kingdom (Bennett, 2007a; Carpini & Michael, 2000). Compared to older people, young people are much less likely to vote and their seeming lack of participation in the political process has been viewed as a serious problem for the future of effective democracies (Bennett, 2007c). However, as noted below in greater detail, the 2008 US elections saw a surge in voter turnout among 18–29-year olds (CIRCLE, 2008); only time will tell whether this trend was a reflection of the historic nature of this particular election or whether it was a harbinger of a true shift in voting behavior among youth.

Bennett notes that young people's apparent declining participation in politics and government is paralleled by their seeming "civic engagement in nongovernmental areas, including increases in community volunteer work, high levels of consumer activism, and strong involvement in social causes from the environment to economic injustice in local and global areas" (pp. 1–2). In fact, he argues that there are in reality two paradigms of youth engagement – first, the just described traditional view of youth as largely disengaged and passive, and a second, perspective of youth as active and engaged (Bennett, 2007b). In this latter view, peer networks and online communities are important and civic participation in public online forums such as MySpace and Facebook counts as civic engagement. Civic action no longer only includes voting but includes "more personally defined acts such as consumerism, community volunteering, or transnational activism" (Bennett, 2007b) that are sustained through loosely defined online friendship networks. Bennett points out that some scholars have suggested that we should broaden our notions of civic engagement to include public, shared activity (e.g., protests, petitions, etc.) in online forums such as blogs, games, as well as fan and entertainment sites. Digital worlds, with their easy access to public spaces, make it easy for people to engage with their peers and their communities.

Although adolescents can and do vote in elections involving organizations in their school (e.g., student government), they generally cannot vote in state, local, and national elections. Thus even though their participation in the political process is important for their future participation in the democratic process as adults, we focus primarily on their use of technology to engage with their communities, including local, national, and even global ones (Bennett, 2007a; Montgomery, 2007). Such civic engagement is no less important than voting and participating in government. It can contribute positively to the development of a sense of civic identity and social responsibility among youth (McGuire & Gamble, 2006; Metz, McLellan, & Youniss, 2003), as well as can provide psychological benefits to adolescents' self-esteem and mental health and may even help to discourage problem behavior (Steinberg, 2008). Next, we briefly consider how technology may mediate traditional forms of civic engagement such as voting and political participation and then consider how adolescents use the Internet and other tools to engage with their peers and communities.

The Internet, Youth, and Politics

The Internet has become an integral part of the political process. Within the USA, the 2004 and 2008 elections were the first to make widespread and innovative use of various forms of technology including e-mail, text messages, blogs, and social networking sites (Montgomery, 2007; Sanson, 2008). Such use has the potential to boost voter turnout, a key factor in elections. In fact, one study estimated that during the 2008 US primaries, reminders sent via text messaging on Super Tuesday (February 5, 2008) boosted turnout in the targeted sample by 4.6% compared to 2.1% for messages sent the day before election day (New Voters Project, 2008). In fact, technology likely played a role in boosting youth voter turnout in the 2008 US elections – early estimates provided by the Center for Information and Research on Civic Learning and Engagement indicate that voter turnout among 18–29-year olds was up by 2.2 million compared to 2004 levels (CIRCLE, 2008). Clearly, technology is helping to draw young adults to the voting booth. Youth also seem to believe that Internet use can help individuals to increase their political power; see Fig. 6.1, which presents the WIP data showing respondents' views about the relation between Internet use and political power. We hope that these beliefs will lead youth to be active in politics and governments during their adult years.

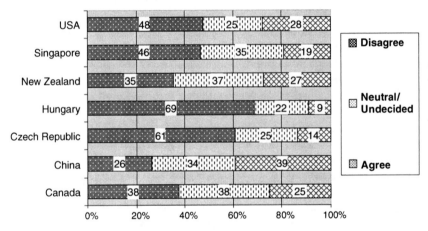

Fig. 6.1 Responses (in percentages) to the question, 'By using the Internet one can have more political power' among 12- to 18-year olds (Data from WIP 2007)

The Internet, Adolescents, and Civic Engagement

We begin by describing some of the ways – some typical and some entirely new and creative – that young people use technology for civic engagement. Since we wanted to give readers a flavor of what real teens are doing in their lives, we use both anecdotal examples as well as ones drawn from published research. By no means are we implying that our examples are common or even typical of teens. Instead, these were ones that illustrate how youth take advantage of the Internet's opportunities to connect with their peers and their larger communities.

As one of us is a parent of a teen in high school and of an emerging adult in college, many instances came to mind where teens have used tools such as Facebook to engage with their fellow students, sometimes in positive ways, other times less so. Two years ago, this author's son was wrongly placed in an "art concentration" prior to his freshman year in high school. It was his fourth choice and he as well as we, were very disappointed. It was summer and we had no immediate way of finding out whether it would be as poor a fit as we thought it would be. This author's older daughter, who had just graduated from the same high school, posted a note on Facebook asking for more information, the difficulty level, requirements and so forth. Literally, in a matter of hours, she received more than 10 responses from students who had taken the art course, all of which convinced us that the assignment was indeed as bad a choice for him as he had feared. The incident had a good ending for us, in large part, because the information he gleaned from the Facebook posts convinced him to get his concentration changed. We have also observed instances when teens have used Facebook to inform their peers about community service projects, impending student rallies, and other kinds of student actions. But most poignant were our observations of how they used Facebook to create RIP (Rest in Peace) groups, and posted very touching notes about their peers, who had met untimely deaths. In addition to these more positive uses, teens also figure out ways of using the Internet for less than ideal reasons. While driving carpool, the author learnt of an instance where an enterprising student used a cell phone to take a picture of the exam which the teacher had left on the desk and stepped out of the room; the student reportedly then uploaded the picture on Facebook for all to see.

There is now systematic research that has documented how adolescents are putting the Internet to use for civic purposes (Bers & Chau, 2006; Cassell, Huffaker, Tversky, & Ferriman, 2006; Ito et al., 2007; Montgomery, 2007). From this body of work, we describe three studies as they demonstrate nicely the Internet's potential for youth civic engagement. The first study shows how one very basic online tool, a web site, can be put to use for civic and political causes. In a 2004 study, a team of researchers at American University surveyed more than 300 web sites created for and by young people (Montgomery, 2007). The web sites were diverse in terms of their goals (exposure to public art in St. Paul, Minnesota, fighting hate, gay and lesbian issues, and environmental concerns), target audience (broad audience versus specific groups such as urban or rural teens), and how innovatively they used the interactive potential of the web (Montgomery, 2007).[1] Montgomery noted that the sites offered youth a variety of online tools to express themselves and communicate with others (e.g., polls, discussion boards, and means of expressing oneself via artwork, essays etc); she speculated that they could foster a sense of belonging, and help youth to engage with peers, consolidate their identities, and help refine their civic skills such as fundraising, volunteering, and even contacting political leaders (Montgomery, 2007).

In addition to the vast resources of the web, the Internet provides access to closed virtual spaces that can also be valuable for youth civic engagement. We describe two diametrically different studies that have done just that – one is a case study of 12 users in a three-dimensional multi-user environment (Bers & Chau, 2006) and the other involved an online global community of over 3,000 adolescents

---

[1] For the full report of the sites surveyed, see Montgomery, Gottlieb-Robles, & Larson, 2004.

(Cassell, 2002; Cassell et al., 2006). The study by Bers and Chau utilized Zora, a virtual world which allowed users to "hold conversations with each other, to express ideas easily and safely in both synchronous and asynchronous ways, to tell stories, and to create virtual objects that are personally meaningful to them" (Bers & Chau, 2006). It allowed youth users to "design and inhabit a virtual city" 750 and offered them the opportunity for civic actions and civic discourse. Civic actions were defined as online behaviors such as creating virtual objects (e.g., Hero objects such as Tim Duncan or Einstein or Villain objects such as Backstreet Boys or Saddam Hussein), associating descriptions or stories with them, as well as creating definitions for common values and ethics (e.g., equality, charity, etc) shared by all the members. Civic discourse included *dialogues*, where participants shared ideas and perspectives and *deliberation*, where they engaged in to reach some sort of consensus. Bers and Chau reported that when given the opportunity to explore this virtual environment without adult direction or supervision, the 11- to 17-year-old participants wrote about civic issues such as equality and wealth on their own volition. They also engaged in discourse centered on topics related to civic engagement such as participants' religious and ethnic backgrounds, current affairs, and solution for racism and discrimination. Such civic discourse was surprisingly frequent and made up approximately 44% of the total conversation during the study period. Interestingly, civic dialogue occurred more often but was relatively brief, whereas civic deliberation occurred less frequently, but when it did occur, such discourse was more extensive and at a deeper level.

On an entirely different scale, the JUNIOR SUMMIT online community hosted at the Massachusetts Institute of Technology (MIT) in Cambridge, MA, consisted of 3,062 adolescents from 139 countries and brought together young people of varying backgrounds (e.g., socio-economic status, urban versus rural, and computer experience) from around the world. Participants ranged in age from 9 to 16 years and were selected from over 8,000 applications; some participated individually, others as part of a group with their friends or as part of their school class. The focus of the online community was to find ways for using technology to make the world a better place. The youth members first engaged in conversation and discussion on this topic, then elected 100 leaders from amongst themselves; these leaders represented the online youth community at a meeting at MIT where they met with political and business leaders from around the world to discuss how technology could be harnessed positively (Cassell et al., 2006). Cassell reported that without any sort of adult direction, the youth "debated the role that technology could play in improving the world for children, came up with action plans, voted for delegates to represent them at the in-person summit, and began to implement their plans" (Cassell, 2002). The Junior Summit officially ended in 1998, but between 1998 and 2002, the youth participants exchanged 50,000 messages (Cassell et al., 2006). Cassell (Cassell, 2002; Cassell et al., 2006) has noted that 3 years later, participants remained active, communicating online in the forum and pursuing their Junior Summit work offline. For example, in 2001, some participants received funding to continue their work in the online country of *Nation 1*. As of 2005, online participation had even continued for 7 years (Cassell et al., 2006). By all accounts, the effort was quite successful in engaging a diverse group of youth on a topic of common interest for the collective good, and seemed to translate into offline action, which persisted long after their participation in the project.

Developmental implications. The foregoing examples, anecdotal and research-based, attest that young people are using technology in new and sometimes unexpected ways to engage with their peers and communities. As developmental psychologists, our interests go beyond merely describing how youth use technology for civic purposes. We are interested in understanding the relation between civic engagement and the more informal uses of online peer forums. Research suggests that among youth, media use does facilitate civic engagement and political awareness (Pasek, Kenski, Romer, & Jamieson, 2006). In their survey of a large national sample of 14–22-year olds, Pasek et al. found that using the Internet for information purposes, reading books, and watching national television shows were associated with enhanced civic actions and political awareness; civic actions were assessed by asking participants about extracurricular voluntary activities as well as community service activities. The authors speculate that informal media use might help young people develop shared interests and contribute to community building and social capital. From the studies and anecdotal examples described earlier, it is apparent that online spaces, even informal ones such as social networking sites, may help young people build social capital and contribute to civic and political engagement. Future research should examine whether informal peer engagement in online contexts can similarly help build civic engagement and participation.

In addition to using technology to create new and alternative pathways to engage with their communities (Bennett, 2007b), youth are developing their own unique modes of civic engagement and leadership in online contexts (Cassell et al., 2006). When Cassell et al. analyzed the discourse within the online Junior Summit community, they found that youth leaders adopted a very different leadership style compared to that observed in adult leaders, who offer many ideas, are task-oriented, and use powerful language. Youth leaders also contributed more than their peers did, but tended to be more group-oriented – they kept group goals central, referred to the group rather than to themselves, and often synthesized posts in an effort to help the group arrive at a consensus.

There are preliminary indications that civic actions in online contexts may have some limited effects. Cassell reported that children who filled out a questionnaire of self-worth after participating in the online Junior Summit forum for 1 month reported greater levels of self-worth than those completed prior to the online forum. Participation in the online forum was also associated with greater "meaningful instrumental activity;" those activities that require skills and resulted in desired goals were associated with greater self-worth and well-being. All told, participation in the online youth program appeared to have short-term benefits; unknown at this time is whether these effects are cumulative and longer lasting (Cassell, 2002). Other potential areas of influence include adolescents' attitudes and beliefs about civic engagement as well their civic actions in the present and in the future as adults. Of singular relevance is whether adolescents' online engagement with peers and communities will translate into adult participation in civic institutions such as politics and government, the cornerstone of all democracies.

Conclusions

As teens navigate digital contexts, they have to learn to deal with moral and ethical issues just as they have to do so in their offline lives. While they often do the right thing when it comes to safeguarding their own privacy, we cannot say the same for cyber plagiarism and digital piracy. Some reasons for their difficulties in these areas include a poor understanding of the ethical issues, lack of knowledge about the laws, and financial constraints. We are confident that we can address these gaps in their understanding through systematic education by parents, teachers, and law enforcement. More challenging may be the fact that youth have different moral orientations toward different kinds of property. They do not treat the theft of digital property as seriously as that of a tangible one such as a bike, even though the latter may have much lower value. One reason for this may be the psychological distance that is present when computer screens and digital objects are involved. Lying and falsifying information online may similarly hinge on the distance between an individual and his/her actions. As the physical increasingly becomes virtual, it will be important for youth to overcome this psychological distance and recognize that morality and ethics must be adhered to even when interacting via a screen. Less challenging, but perhaps more promising for adolescent development are the numerous opportunities for political and civic engagement that technology offers. It is our hope that by allowing individuals to engage with their communities during their formative years, technology can help to transform them into healthy and politically active adults.

References

Baumrind, D. (1991). The influence of parenting style on adolescent competence and substance use. *The Journal of Early Adolescence, 11,* 56–95.

Bennett, W. L. (2007a). Changing citizenship in the digital age. *The John D. and Catherine T. MacArthur Foundation Series on digital media and learning,* 1–24. Retrieved February 20, 2009, from http://www.mitpressjournals.org/doi/abs/10.1162/dmal.9780262524827.001

Bennett, W. L. (2007b). *Changing citizenship in the digital age.* Paper presented at the OECD/INDIRE Conference on Millennial Learners, Florence, Italy. Retrieved February 20, 2009, from http://www.oecd.org/dataoecd/0/8/38360794.pdf

Bennett, W. L. (2007c). Civic learning in changing democracies: Challenges for citizenship and civic education. *Young citizens and new media: Learning for democracy.* New York, NY: Routledge. Retrieved September 20, 2009, from http://depts.washington.edu/ccce/assets/documents/bennet_civic_learning_in_changing_democracies.pdf

Bers, M. U., & Chau, C. (2006). Fostering civic engagement by building a virtual city. *Journal of Computer-Mediated Communication, 11,* 748–770.

Blinka, L., & Šmahel, D. (2008). Matching reality and virtuality: Are adolescents lying on their weblogs. In F. Sudweeks, H. Hrachovec, & Ch. Ess (Eds.), *Cultural attitudes towards technology and communication* (pp. 457–561). Australia: School of Information Technology, Murdoch University.

Blinka, L., & Šmahel, D. (2009). Fourteen is fourteen and a girl is a girl: Validating the identity of adolescent bloggers. *CyberPsychology & Behavior, 12,* 735–739.

Bradley, K. (2005). Internet lives: Social context and moral domain in adolescent development. *New Directions for Youth Development, 108*, 57–76.

Carpini, M. X. D., & Michael, X. (2000). Gen.com: Youth, civic engagement, and the new information environment. *Political Communication, 17*, 341–349.

Cassell, J. (2002). "We have these rules inside": The effects of exercising voice in a children's online forum. In S. Calvert, R. Cocking, & A. Jordan (Eds.), *Children in the digital age: Influences of electronic media on development* (pp. 123–144). New York, NY: Praeger Press.

Cassell, J., Huffaker, D., Tversky, D., & Ferriman, K. (2006). The language of online leadership: Gender and youth engagement on the Internet. *Developmental Psychology, 42*, 436.

CIRCLE. (2008). *Preliminary circle projection: Youth voter turnout up.* Retrieved February 23, 2009, from http://www.civicyouth.org/?p=322

Conradson, S., & Hernández-Ramos, P. (2004). Computers, the Internet, and cheating among secondary school students: Some implications for educators. *Practical Assessment, Research and Evaluation, 9.* Retrieved October 26, 2009, from http://pareonline.net/getvn.asp?v=9&n=9

Crowell, C. R., Narvaez, D., & Gomberg, A. (2005). Moral psychology and information ethics: Psychological distance and the components of moral behavior in a digital world. In L. A. Freeman & A. G. Peace (Eds.), *Information ethics: Privacy and intellectual property* (pp. 19–37). Hershey, PA: Information Science Publishing.

Eastin, M. S., Greenberg, B. S., & Hofschire, L. (2006). Parenting the Internet. *Journal of Communication, 56*, 486–504.

Ercegovac, Z. (2005). *What students say they know, feel, and do about cyber-plagiarism and academic dishonesty: A case study.* Retrieved June 10, 2009, from http://www.asis.org/Conferences/AM05/abstracts/42.html

Erikson, E. H. (1968). *Identity: Youth and crisis.* New York, NY: WW Norton & Company.

Evans, D., & Thomasson, E. (2007). *Dutch police arrest teenage online furniture thief.* Retrieved February 24, 2009, from http://uk.reuters.com/article/oddlyEnoughNews/idUKL1453844620071114

Fields, D. A., & Kafai, Y. B. (2007). *Stealing from grandma or generating cultural knowledge? Contestations and effects of cheats in a tween virtual world.* Paper presented at the Situated Play, Proceedings of Digital Games Research Association 2007 Conference, Tokyo, Japan.

Freestone, O., & Mitchell, V. (2004). Generation y attitudes towards e-ethics and Internet-related misbehaviours. *Journal of Business Ethics, 54*, 121–128.

Harman, J. P., Hansen, C. E., Cochran, M. E., & Lindsey, C. R. (2005). Liar, liar: Internet faking but not frequency of use affects social skills, self-esteem, social anxiety, and aggression. *CyberPsychology & Behavior, 8*, 1–6.

Harris Interactive. (2004). Tweens' and teens' Internet behavior and attitudes about copyrighted materials. Retrieved November 20, 2008, from http://www.bsa.org/country/Research%20and%20Statistics/Research%20Papers.aspx

Harris Interactive. (2007). BSA and Harris youth and interactive study – Youth downloading statistics and chart. Retrieved November 20, 2008, from http://www.bsa.org/country/Research%20and%20Statistics/Research%20Papers.aspx

Hinduja, S., & Patchin, J. W. (2008). Personal information of adolescents on the Internet: A quantitative content analysis of MySpace. *Journal of Adolescence, 31*, 125–146.

Ito, M., Davidson, C., Jenkins, H., Lee, C., Eisenberg, M., & Weiss, J. (2007). Civic life online: Learning how digital media can engage youth. *The John D. and Catherine T. MacArthur Foundation Series on Digital media and learning.* Cambridge, MA: MIT Press. Retrieved February 24, 2009, from http://www.mitpressjournals.org/toc/dmal/-/1

Jackson, L. A., Zhao, Y., Qiu, W., Kolenic, A., Fitzgerald, H. E., Harold, R., et al. (2008). Cultural differences in morality in the real and virtual worlds: A comparison of Chinese and US youth. *CyberPsychology & Behavior, 11*, 279–286.

Josephson Institute. (2006). *The ethics of American youth: 2006.* Retrieved November 11, 2008, from http://charactercounts.org/programs/reportcard/2006/index.html

Kini, R. B., Ramakrishna, H. V., & Vijayaraman, B. S. (2003). An exploratory study of moral intensity regarding software piracy of students in Thailand. *Behaviour & Information Technology*, *22*, 63–70.

Klein, A., & Goldfarb, Z. (2008, June 15). Anatomy of a meltdown: The credit crisis. *Washington Post*. From http://www.washingtonpost.com/wp-srv/business/creditcrisis/

Konečný, Š., & Šmahel, D. (2007). *Virtual communities and lying: Perspective of Czech adolescents and young adults*. Paper presented at Internet Research 8.0: Let's Play (Association of Internet Researchers), Vancouver, Canada.

Koubalikova, S., & Šmahel, D. (2008). Fenomen lhani v prostredi internetu. [Phenomenon of lying on the Internet.]. *Ceskoslovenska Psychologie*, *52*, 289–301.

KRC Research. (2008). *Topline results of Microsoft survey of teen attitudes on illeagal downloading*. Retrieved November 22, 2008, from http://www.microsoft.com/presspass/download/press/2008/02-13KRCStudy.pdf

McGuire, J. K., & Gamble, W. C. (2006). Community service for youth: The value of psychological engagement over number of hours spent. *Journal of Adolescence*, *29*, 289–298.

Metz, E., McLellan, J., & Youniss, J. (2003). Types of voluntary service and adolescents' civic development. *Journal of Adolescent Research*, *18*, 188–203.

Mitchell, K. J., Wolak, J., & Finkelhor, D. (2007). Trends in youth reports of sexual solicitations, harassment and unwanted exposure to pornography on the Internet. *Journal of Adolescent Health*, *40*, 116–126.

Montgomery, K. C. (2007). Youth and digital democracy: Intersections of practice, policy, and the marketplace. In W. Bennett (Ed.), *The John D. and Catherine T. MacArthur Foundation Series on Digital media and learning* (pp. 25–49). Cambridge, MA: The MIT Press.

Montgomery, K. C., Gottlieb-Robles, B., & Larson, G. O. (2004). *Youth as e-citizens: Engaging the digital generation*. Washington, DC: American University. Retrieved February 23, 2009, from http://www.centerforsocialmedia.org/ecitizens/youthreport.pdf

Moscardelli, D. M., & Divine, R. (2007). Adolescents' concern for privacy when using the Internet: An empirical analysis of predictors and relationships with privacy-protecting behaviors. *Family and Consumer Sciences Research Journal*, *35*, 232–252.

New Voters Project. (2008). *Text reminders increase primary youth turnout*. Retrieved February 24, 2009, from http://www.newvotersproject.org/uploads/Mv/wt/MvwtSTcFqKDlkNloOS0Onw/2008_texting_fact_sheet.pdf

Pasek, J., Kenski, K., Romer, D., & Jamieson, K. H. (2006). America's youth and community engagement: How use of mass media is related to civic activity and political awareness in 14-to 22-year-olds. *Communication Research*, *33*, 115–135.

Sanson, A. (2008). Facebook and youth mobilization in the 2008 presidential election. *gnovis Journal*. Retrieved March 3, 2009 from http://www.gnovisjournal.org/files/Facebook-Youth-Mobilization.pdf

Semuels, A. (2008, July 2). In virtual worlds, child avatars need protecting – from each other. *Los Angeles Times*. Retrieved from http://articles.latimes.com/2008/jul/02/business/fi-kidssafe2

Sisti, D. A. (2007). How do high school students justify Internet plagiarism? *Ethics & Behavior*, *17*, 215–231.

Steinberg, L. (2008). *Adolescence*. New York, NY: McGraw-Hill.

Subrahmanyam, K., Garcia, E. C., Harsono, S. L., Li, J., & Lipana, L. (2009). In their words: Connecting online weblogs to developmental processes. *British Journal of Developmental Psychology*, *27*, 219–245.

Subrahmanyam, K., & Greenfield, P. M. (2008). Online communication and adolescent relationships. *Future of Children*, *18*, 119–146.

Teston, G. (2001). *A developmental perspective of computer and information technology ethics: Piracy of software and digital music by young adolescents*. Minneapolis, MN: Walden University.

Turkle, S. (1995). *Life on the screen: Identity in the age of the Internet*. New York, NY: Simon & Schuster.

Turow, J., & Nir, L. (2000). *The Internet and the family 2000: The view from parents, the view from kids*. Philadelphia, PA: Annenberg Public Policy Center of the University of Pennsylvania.

Velasquez, M., Andre, C., Shanks, T. S. J., & Meyer, M. J. (2008). *What is ethics*. Retrieved November 11, 2008, from http://www.scu.edu/ethics/practicing/decision/whatisethics.html

Yar, M. (2007). Teenage kicks or virtual villainy? Internet piracy, moral entrepreneurship, and the social construction of a crime problem. In Y. Jewkes (Ed.), *Crime online: Committing, policing and regulating cybercrime* (pp. 95–108). Oxfordshire: Willan Publishing.

Youn, S. (2005). Teenagers' perceptions of online privacy and coping behaviors: A risk-benefit appraisal approach. *Journal of Broadcasting & Electronic Media, 49*, 86–110.

Youn, S., & Hall, K. (2008). Gender and online privacy among teens: Risk perception, privacy concerns, and protection behaviors. *CyberPsychology & Behavior, 11*, 763–765.

Chapter 7
Internet Use and Well-Being: Physical and Psychological Effects

In the foregoing chapters, we explored the intersection between technology and development as young people confront and deal with the challenges and issues that are present in their lives. In the next few chapters, we shift gears and look at the practical implications of their interactions with technology. This chapter takes an in-depth look into how adolescents' online activities influence their well-being. Does spending time on the Internet make youth obese? Are teens becoming sleep-deprived because they stay up late talking with their friends? Is machine-based communication impoverished and does it result in weaker relationships? Does the Internet make young people depressed and lonely? Does talking online to strangers hurt adolescents' well-being? In this chapter, we tackle some of these questions with regard to adolescent physical and psychological well-being.

Understanding the Influence of the Internet

Concerns about how media may influence young people have been around ever since the advent of media itself. Research on this question has drawn from the media effects model (discussed earlier in Chapter 2), which suggests that media influences users' attitudes and behaviors. Extrapolating to the Internet, the expectation is that online use, like the use of television and video games, will have effects on the user. One mechanism of influence centers on online time use. The idea is that online activities represent not only time spent on the Internet but also time away from other activities. This idea is reflected in the displacement hypothesis, which argues that since time is a finite quantity, time spent on the Internet comes at the expense of other activities (Nie & Hillygus, 2002). With regard to young people, activities that may be displaced because of Internet use include sleep, participation in physical activities (e.g., organized sports), and social interactions with "real people" in face-to-face contexts as well as over the phone. A second mechanism of influence involves the nature of online interactions and communication. As described in Chapter 1, such interactions typically occur via a screen, involve text, and may lack important face-to-face cues, such as gesture, gaze, and body language (Greenfield & Subrahmanyam, 2003). Thus online interactions may be

K. Subrahmanyam, D. Šmahel, *Digital Youth*, Advancing Responsible
Adolescent Development, DOI 10.1007/978-1-4419-6278-2_7,
© Springer Science+Business Media, LLC 2011

"artificial" or "poor" or "impoverished" and result in what sociologists call "weaker ties" (Granovetter, 1973; Subrahmanyam, Kraut, Greenfield, & Gross, 2000). It is speculated that such Internet-engineered weaker ties may ultimately lead to lowered psychological well-being (Kraut et al., 1998; Subrahmanyam & Lin, 2007).

A third pathway of influence stems from the vast and virtually unlimited content of the Internet that we can access at any time with little effort. Some of this content can be used for considerable benefit such as for school work, to answer questions about wellness and illness (see Chapter 8), and general information needs (e.g., jobs, internships, careers, community events, etc). Unfortunately, the Internet also includes content that can be potentially harmful for young people, for instance, aggressive and hateful sites as well as pornographic material. For the remainder of this chapter, we pursue the implications of the first two mechanisms of influence; because Internet activities may not only displace physical and social activities, but also potentially replace "higher quality" face-to-face activities with "lower quality online social activities," we consider the influence of the Internet on both physical and psychological well-being. We examine content effects separately; Chapter 3 covered pornography, Chapter 8 deals with young people's use of the Internet for health, wellness, and illness, and Chapter 10 focuses on violent, hateful, and other problematic content.

Effects on Physical Well-Being

To understand the physical effects of young people's online behavior, it is important to consider some of the changes that occur during adolescence and how technology might affect these changes. The biological changes of puberty include rapid growth in height and weight as well as the appearance of secondary sex characteristics (e.g., breast development, facial and body hair, etc.) leading to sexual maturation (Tanner, 1978) and eventually to a dramatically changed and more adult-like physical appearance. Aspects of adolescents' lives that could mediate the inevitable weight gain of adolescence includes increasing or decreasing levels of physical activities (e.g., because of their involvement in or dropping out of organized sports) or increasing levels of sedentary activities, such as watching television and using the Internet.

The biological changes that occur at puberty are also related to changes in adolescent sleep patterns, called the delayed phase preference, and result in older adolescents going to bed later at night and also getting up later in the morning (Carskadon, Vieira, & Acebo, 1993). Because many high schools within the USA start early in the morning, this results in reduced sleep quantity on school days; typically, adolescents sleep later on weekend nights and get up even later on weekend mornings in order to catch up with the chronic shortage of sleep that occurs during the week (Tarokh & Carskadon, 2008). Environmental factors such as lighting and mass media may also have a role in the later bedtimes of young people and we will examine the relation between technology use and adolescent sleep patterns. Next we show that like television, computers, and electronic games, the Internet also has both direct and indirect effects on users' physical well-being (Subrahmanyam, 2010; Subrahmanyam et al., 2000).

Direct Effects

Extrapolating from findings that use of computer and video games are associated with injuries and changes in physiological arousal, such as heart rate (Subrahmanyam et al., 2000), we expect that Internet use has the potential for injuries and may affect arousal and consider these possibilities next.

Physical injuries. One documented injury as a result of excessive computer game playing is a form of tendinitis, called Nintendinitis (Brasington, 1990), which is characterized by severe pain in the extensor tendon of the right thumb as a result of the repeated pressing of buttons during game play. Excessive computer use, while online, might similarly impact young people's eyes, back, and wrists, just as adults have reported such injuries as a result of prolonged computer use (Mendels, 1999). With laptops becoming the norm, and young people using them at younger and younger ages, it is probably a good idea to educate them about safe computer use, including precautions, such as taking frequent breaks and positioning equipment properly. Excessive texting has been reported to lead to a new condition called texting tenosynovitis or text-messenger's thumb, in which repetitive use leads to pain and tenderness of the thumb (Storr, de Vere Beavis, & Stringer, 2007). Virgin mobile even has a web site with "textercises" to promote safe texting (http://www.practisesafetext.com) (see Fig. 7.1). There have also been reports of teens texting during driving and getting involved in accidents, some even fatal.

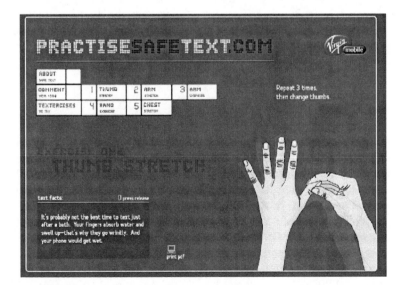

Fig. 7.1   Screenshot of a "textercise" to promote safe texting (from www.practisesafetext.com)

Physiological arousal. Generalized physiological arousal is a bodily response manifested by changes in breathing, heart rate, and blood pressure. According to arousal theory, media-induced arousal lingers after exposure, and may have an energizing effect leading to agitation and restlessness in children's behavior (e.g., while playing or interaction with peers) (Valkenburg, 2004); features of media that may trigger arousal include violent content, lots of action, fast pace, and loud music. Meta analyses have confirmed that exposure to violent video increases physiological arousal (Anderson & Bushman, 2001; Anderson, 2004), generally measured by systolic blood pressure, diastolic blood pressure, and heart rate. Although systematic research on the effects of teen Internet use on arousal is lacking, there are indications that the two are related. In one study, the researchers experimentally manipulated mood such that college students were over simulated/stressed (they had to complete a GRE-type test under time pressure) or bored (they had to thread metal washers on a shoelace). Bored participants surfed online at high levels compared to the over stimulated ones, who went to much fewer Internet sites (Mastro, Eastin, & Tamborini, 2002).

Another experiment found that download speed affected arousal as measured by skin conductance; the direction of the effect varied with the content of the image being downloaded (Sundar & Wagner, 2002). For a high-arousal image (an erotic image of a couple), slower download led to greater arousal, presumably because of the anticipation. In contrast, for a low-arousal image (a flower), faster download speed led to higher arousal. Worth noting is that download speed, a non-message feature of new media, is able to induce physiological changes in the viewer. Although participants in both studies were college students, we have no reason not to expect similar effects on adolescents' physiological arousal. Technology-induced arousal may contribute to teens' delayed bedtime and reduced sleep patterns, a topic we will address later. Research is needed to understand the short-term (e.g., sleep) and long-term (e.g., sustained effects of high arousal) effects of such Internet-related arousal on young people.

Indirect Effects

According to the displacement hypothesis described earlier, time online can displace other important activities, thereby indirectly affecting well-being. Here we consider two potential indirect effects on physical well-being, obesity, and decreased sleep.

Internet use and obesity. Relevant to this concern are trends about the prevalence of obesity among youth. In the USA, between 2003 and 2006, 31.9% of children and adolescents between 2 and 19 years were at or above the 85th percentile of the body mass index (BMI) for their age, with 16.3% considered obese as they were at or above the 95th percentile for their age (Ogden, Carroll, & Flegal, 2008). These prevalence estimates of overweight children and adolescents are from the 2003–2004 and 2005–2006 National Health and Nutritional Examination Survey (NHANES), a nationally representative sample. According to the CDC, although the rates of obesity have not increased in recent years, the current rates of obesity among adolescents is triple of what it was in the late 1970s (about 5%) (Centers for Disease Control and Prevention, 2004). As obesity increases the risk for a variety of health conditions ranging from hypertension and osteoarthritis to Type 2 diabetes, stroke, and gall bladder disease, current prevalence rates among young people are a public health issue.

In the search for reasons to account for the rates of obesity among young people, media have been implicated along with other factors such as sedentary lifestyles, increased consumption of fast food and portion sizes, and decreased physical activity (e.g., reduction in physical education classes in secondary schools) (Kaiser Family Foundation, 2004). Although the limited research on this question does suggest that media may play a role, most of this research was on television and only a handful of studies have looked at computers, video games, and the Internet. First, we review what we know about television's role in obesity and then we turn to research on computers and the Internet.

In one of the most comprehensive reviews of research on this topic, involving more than 40 studies, the 2004 Kaiser report found that youth who used more media were more obese; keep in mind that the report did not distinguish between different kinds of media and only studies focusing on television were included in their write-up. Of interest is that television displaced other equally sedentary activities, but not physical activities. Thus, children who watched less television were also involved in other similarly less active behaviors, such as talking on the phone, playing board games, and reading books, suggesting that television may not directly contribute to obesity by displacing physically more challenging activities. However, the report also examined studies that analyzed the content of the television watched by children, in particular, food advertising. Incidentally, content analyses reveals that children are exposed to significant amounts of television advertising, and may watch more than 40,000 television ads in 1 year alone (Kunkel, 2001). Most of these ads are for fast foods, sodas, cookies, and other not very healthy foods. The Kaiser Report concluded that such advertisements influence children's food choices and may even cause them to be confused about the relative merits of different kinds of food. Media content, particularly food advertising on television, could have a role in the increases in obesity rates. Of course, this also raises the intriguing possibility that television could successfully promote anti-obesity messages (e.g., information about exercising and healthy eating) to youth.

Evidence regarding the relation between youth, obesity, and interactive technologies, such as video games and the Internet is even sparser. From epidemiologic data, we know that over the course of adolescence, there are the dual trends of decreasing amounts of vigorous physical activity and increasing amounts of leisure-time computer use (Nelson, Neumark-Stzainer, Hannan, Sirard, & Story, 2006). One study has found a more direct link between interactive media use and obesity. Using a large sample of 922 Swiss elementary school children, researchers (Stettler, Singer, & Sutter, 2004) examined the role of environmental factors and obesity as measured by overweight (BMI) and overfat (skinfold thickness). In addition to information about the time spent playing electronic games and watching television, a variety of other potential environmental variables were assessed including, physical activity, number of siblings, smoking status of parents, job status of parents, etc. Relative to the other variables, time spent watching television and playing electronic games were much more strongly related to obesity.

The sedentary nature of young people's online behavior does seem to be associated with the prevalence of obesity in them. Less clear are the reasons for this association. Schneider, Dunton, and Cooper (2007) point out that obesity among youth can be attributed to either energy intake or energy expenditure. The displacement hypothesis is relevant to the energy expenditure part of the equation – if Internet use is displacing physical activities then it is indirectly contributing to a decrease in energy expenditure and eventually to obesity. To assess the role of energy expenditure in obesity, the researchers assessed the relation between physical activity, television, and interactive media use and percentage body fat and BMI among 194 adolescent females between 14 and 17 years of age. They found that use of interactive media, such as video games and Internet surfing, was associated with obesity indicators of percentage body fat and BMI. The relationship held even after controlling for the extent of physical activity and cardiovascular fitness indicating that reduced physical activity engendered by Internet use might not be the mediating mechanism.

What about energy intake? The Kaiser report speculated that television might play a role in the energy intake side of the energy balance equation. However, unlike television, we generally need both hands while using interactive media and so increased energy intake might not have a role in the relation between interactive media use and body fat. Instead Schneider et al. speculate that non-exercise activity thermogenesis or NEAT might play a role – specifically "increased time spent engaged in interactive media could result in decreased NEAT throughout the day and, therefore, bring about increased body fat" (p. 2334). Thus, interventions to reduce the risk of obesity should not only seek to increase physical activity but should also seek to reduce interactive media use. There are some indications that NEAT may have a genetic basis – thus interactive media use might have different effects on obesity based on individual differences in NEAT (Schneider et al., 2007).

We should also keep in mind that youth multitask when using interactive media and we have to disentangle the effects of different media used when studying their relation to obesity. The Schneider et al. study actually compared the relative relation between obesity and television and interactive media use but found no effect of television use. They even took care to address the issue of multi-tasking, but because their study was limited to girls, it is too early to say whether interactive media has a stronger relationship to obesity than television. The little research we have suggests that interactive media use does relate to physical being, not because it displaces other physical activities, but because it may change other underlying processes. This is an important point to keep in mind when we look at the Internet's effect on psychological and social well-being.

Technology and sleep patterns. Earlier in this chapter, we saw that because of their changing circadian rhythms, older adolescents start sleeping later. Furthermore, between 1974 and 1993, adolescents' bedtime has been getting later and the time of awakening has remained unchanged, leading to a decrease in the total time spent sleeping (Iglowstein, Jenni, Molinari, & Largo, 2003). The greater availability of television, video games, and the Internet late in the night and in young people's bedrooms is undoubtedly responsible to some extent. For instance, a 2004 Belgian study of 2,546 adolescents found that those with televisions in their bedrooms went to bed later on weekdays and weekends and got up later on weekends. Teens who spent more time online slept later on weekdays, and during the weekend got up later on the weekend, slept less overall, and also reported feeling more tired (Van den Bulck, 2004). At the time of the study, only a small proportion of the sample had Internet access in their rooms; the increasingly wired nature of young people's bedrooms since then leads us to expect effects on sleep similar to those of having a television in the bedroom.

Also part of young people's wired lives are cell phones and other mobile devices. Youth seemed glued to these devices, including while in the shower and in bed, adding further impediments to good quality sleep (Van den Bulck, 2003). A recent online survey by Teenage Research Unlimited found that nearly a quarter of teens in a romantic relationship have communicated with a boyfriend or girlfriend hourly between midnight and 5 a.m. using a cell phone or text messaging. Incredibly, one in six communicated ten or more times an hour through the night (Teenage Research Unlimited, 2007). Mobile phone use late at night after lights out was associated with tiredness, and these associations were likely to hold up to a year later; less than 40% of adolescents in this study reported that they did not use their mobile phone after they turned the lights off in preparation for going to bed (Van Den Bulck, 2007). In addition to keeping adolescents up late at night, Internet and mobile phone use may also lead to arousal and we discussed earlier some of the issues surrounding arousal.

The aforementioned studies suggest that the use of Internet and other mobile technologies by adolescents may be extending their already delayed bedtime leading to sleep deprivation and excessive sleepiness during the day. Such chronic lack of sleep is not without its costs, some relatively minor and others more serious and even fatal. Chronic lack of sleep among adolescents is associated with mood regulation problems, learning and memory problems, poorer school performance including school tardiness and absenteeism, impulsivity and risk taking as well as substance abuse (Fredriksen, Reddy, Way, & Rhodes, 2004; Tarokh & Carskadon, 2008). Among youth between 16 and 24 years of age, fatigue and falling asleep at the wheel are one of the risk factors for fatal motor vehicle crashes (Zhang, Fraser, Lindsay, Clarke, & Mao, 1998). Tarokh and Carskadon note that more than 50% of car crashes caused by the driver falling asleep involved drivers between 16 and 25 years of age (Tarokh & Carskadon, 2008). Educating adolescents about these risks, encouraging them to turn off their phones at night, charging their phones outside their bedroom, and parental monitoring of teen cell phone records are some ways of limiting technology use late at night.

Effects on Psychological Well-Being

In addition to the changing nature of their bodies, adolescents have to deal with many social changes, especially in their relationships with their peers and parents, as well as in their increased autonomy (see Chapter 5). One casualty of all these changes is loneliness, which is common and quite intense during adolescence (Brennan, 1982; Woodward & Frank, 1988). Research suggests that adolescents' loneliness is related to their peer relations (Degirmencioglu, 1995; Storch, Brassard, & Masia-Warner, 2003; Valas, 1999) as well as to self-esteem, family strengths, and mother-adolescent communication (Brage, Meredith, & Woodward, 1993). Peer relationships become increasingly important during adolescence and are related to well-being. Adolescents with strong friendship networks, that is, those who are well connected and have cohesive, highly interconnected friendships report being less lonely, less depressed, and receiving more support from their friends (Degirmencioglu, 1995). Another indicator of well-being, self-esteem, particularly barometric self-esteem appears to fluctuate during adolescence (Rosenberg, 1986) and is also related to problems in peer relationships (Bukowski, Newcomb, & Hartup, 1996; Hartup, 1996) as well as perceived regard or support from others (Harter, 1985). Self-esteem and loneliness are related and adolescents with lower self-esteem report greater loneliness (Brage et al., 1993). Social support from significant others is important for psychological well-being (Raja, McGee, & Stanton, 1992; Sarason, Sarason, & Pierce, 1990), especially at a time such as adolescence, when there are so many changes occurring seemingly at the same time (Kef & Dekovic, 2004).

As the foregoing attest, there are several threats to well-being during adolescence. Although not every adolescent is necessarily at risk, it is nonetheless important to consider how technology might further add to or detract from adolescent well-being. Per the two mechanisms of influence we described earlier, Internet use entails interactions via machines that may displace "real interactions" and as a result substitute adolescents' strong ties with peers and family with weak ties; research suggests that weak ties typically provide less consequential social support than more intimate ties (Krackhardt, 1994). Thus, persistent Internet use may be associated with weaker social ties, which over time could lead to lowered well-being, such as greater depression and loneliness.

This was precisely the reasoning that motivated the landmark Home Net study. Conducted by Kraut and colleagues at Carnegie Mellon University, the study was published in the American Psychologist (Kraut et al., 1998), and triggered a firestorm of publicity, academic and non-academic. Even though, the study did not focus on adolescents, given its seminal role in the debate concerning Internet use and well-being, we describe it in some detail.

From 1995 to 1998, the researchers had conducted a field trial involving 93 families (208 adults and 110 children and teens) in the Pittsburg area, who received home computers and access to the Internet. They obtained data from the families via in-home interviews, periodic questionnaires, and software programs automatically recorded whenever family members went online. The results indicated that more heavy users of the Internet showed a decline in social involvement (communication within the family and size of people's social networks) and increases in loneliness and depression. Among the teens in the sample, greater use of the Internet was tied to declines in social support.

The results were controversial and the study was widely criticized for not having a control group (a comparable group of participants without Internet access), using an opportunity sample, as well as for the particular measures that were used to assess social and psychological well-being. A subsequent follow-up study designed to address these criticisms clarified the original findings (Kraut et al., 2002). First, a follow-up of the original 208 participants revealed that generally positive effects of the Internet replaced the earlier negative ones. Second, a comparison of 406 new television and computer purchasers revealed that Internet use had generally positive effects on both social and psychological well-being as well as communication and social involvement. Most important, they found that the positive benefits of using the Internet were greater for those with greater social resources, such as extroverts and those reporting greater social support. Thus compared to introverts, the extroverts had greater increases in community involvement and self-esteem, as well as larger declines in loneliness, negative effect, and feelings of time pressure. Similarly, among people who reported having more social support, computer use was associated with greater family communication and increases in computer skill. Kraut et al. have called this the "rich-get-richer" model, in which users with more offline resources, in this case greater social resources, also accrued more benefits from their online activities. When gains from greater Internet use occurred, adults and teens benefited differently. For adults, more Internet use increased their face-to-face communication with others and their emotional closeness to distant friends, whereas teens gained more social support and increased their family communication as their Internet use increased (Subrahmanyam, Greenfield, Kraut, & Gross, 2001).

Since the landmark HomeNet studies, the Internet has become extremely diffuse and online applications have changed dramatically. The relation between Internet use and well-being has continued to be the focus of several research studies. Despite the approximately 10 years of research on this question, we only have a murky picture of the relationship between Internet use and well-being among adolescents. What they have shown is that the relationships between adolescent Internet use and well-being is a complex one, based not just on the time spent online, but also mediated by other factors, some surprising, others less so.

It is Not All About Time

Perhaps the most vexing question of all is the extent to which time spent online relates to well-being. In the HomeNet study, greater use of the Internet was associated with declines in adolescents' well-being and with weaker social ties (Kraut et al., 1998); but in the follow-up study, time spent online was not related to aspects of social networks, such as size of local and distant social circles and amount of face-to-face communication (Kraut et al., 2002). In contrast, Mesch has found that frequent Internet users in Israel were more likely to report lower levels of attachment to close friends (Mesch, 2001, 2003). Frequency of Internet use was also found to be negatively related to adolescents' perception about the quality of family relationships (Mesch, 2003). Still other studies have not found a link between adolescents' time online and their dispositional or daily well-being (Gross, Juvonen, & Gable, 2002) as well as their loneliness (Subrahmanyam & Lin, 2007).

One reason for this conflicting picture is that early studies simply used time online to measure use. The HomeNet study used software to automatically record time use; but such a procedure raises privacy concerns and is also expensive to carry out. Few studies since have used this method to measure time. Instead, most have asked subjects to estimate the average amount of time they spend online per day. Such measures are at best approximations and are subject to the usual biases of estimation, subjectivity, and memory. Indeed, in one of our own studies (Subrahmanyam & Lin, 2007), some subjects gave answers that were improbable and at times mathematically impossible, given the amount of time teens typically spend in school on a week day as well as the number of hours in a day. A partial solution to the time measurement problem is the one that Gross et al. (2002) adopted, which required subjects to keep daily logs of their Internet use for 3 days. When time online was measured using such daily dairies, no relation was found between Internet use and well-being. Another challenge for participants is estimating their time online when such use occurs in a multitasking environment. Even when researchers use software to track every key stroke, it is still difficult to estimate the actual attention directed to the different applications running at the same time. Indeed, we have to re-conceptualize how we measure Internet use and develop paradigms that do not focus entirely on the amount of time spent online.

Do Online Activities Matter?

Complicating matters, the early studies compounded the problem by not distinguishing between different kinds of Internet use. For instance, among adolescents, emailing and chatting with school friends might contribute to well-being, surfing the web for information about sports, music, or movies might have no impact on well-being, and accessing pornographic materials could even threaten well-being. While the latter is admittedly an extreme example, it nonetheless drives home the point that what one does online might be equally, if not more important, than how much time one spends online.

In fact, a study of 161 youth between 18 and 25 years found that more time spent in chat rooms, online browsing, and games was related to higher levels of social anxiety among older adolescent and young adult males, but not females (Mazalin & Moore, 2004). A similar relation between depression and chat room use was found in a study with a large sample of adolescents ($N = 2{,}373$) between 11 and 16 years of age ($M = 12.8$ years) (Sun et al., 2005). However, muddying the picture are the results of a longitudinal study of Dutch adolescents in which 663 students between 12 and 15 years of age were tested in two waves (Eijnden, Meerkerk, Vermulst, Spijkerman, & Engels, 2008). Compared to non-communication uses such as information seeking and surfing, some communication uses were related to certain aspects of well-being. Thus, there was a positive relationship between instant message use and feelings of depression, but not loneliness. Emailing and chatting in chat rooms were not related to either depression or loneliness. Instant messaging use during the first wave of data collection was positively related to levels of depression reported during the second wave of testing, 6 months later.

One reason for this contradictory pattern of results is that the findings are from different countries, where different applications were popular at different points in time. People in different contexts might use different applications in very different ways. For instance, within the USA, Internet users are more likely to interact with strangers in chat rooms compared to other online forums, such as instant messaging. None of the studies asked participants whom they were interacting with using the different communication tools. Thus, the key variable might not be the particular application used, but what users do and whom they interact with within a particular digital context. This was borne out in the findings of the Youth Internet Safety Survey, which was a nationally representative telephone survey of 1,501 online youth between 10 and 17 years of age. The data were collected between Fall 1999 and Spring 2000 (Ybarra, Alexander, & Mitchell, 2005). Adolescents who reported symptoms of depression were much more likely to talk with strangers online compared to those who did not report such symptoms. In fact, 80% of teens with major symptoms of depression and 62% with minor symptoms reported talking online with a stranger; in contrast, only 53% of youth with mild or no symptoms of depression reported talking to a stranger. Of course, we cannot tell whether participants became more depressed because of their interactions with strangers or whether they interacted with strangers in the first place because they were depressed and were looking for support, which they may have been lacking in their offline lives. However, the previously described Dutch longitudinal study, which tested alternative causal models, found no relationship between depression and online communication 6 months later. Together the studies seem to indicate that young people's online communication partners might determine whether their online activities relate to their well-being or not.

Given that communication is usually a two-way street, the quality and nature of young people's online interactions may to influence what young people derive from their online communications. This is the finding that emerged from another large study of Dutch adolescents by Valkenburg and her colleagues on the newer social networking sites that allow users to meet and interact with both strangers as well as known others. They surveyed 881 Dutch adolescents to assess the impact of using a friend networking site (CU2) on their self-esteem and well-being (Valkenburg, Peter, & Schouten, 2006). Using structural equation modeling (complex statistical techniques that seeks to confirm causal relationships among measured and latent/underlying variables), the researchers concluded that participants' self-esteem was affected only by the tone of the feedback that they received on the social networking profiles; positive feedback was associated with higher self-esteem and negative feedback with lowered self-esteem. Two other variables tested in the model, frequency of reactions to profiles, and the number of relationships formed on the site, were not associated with self-esteem.

Only a very small percentage of adolescents (7%) reported receiving negative feedback always or predominantly often, but for these adolescents, use of social networking sites was associated with reduced self-esteem. The authors did not test alternative models, so we have no way of knowing whether negative feedback per se reduced self-esteem or participants with lower self-esteem typically perceived the feedback they received as more negative, which in turn caused a further dip in their self-esteem. Regardless, the study provides the first indication that quality of one's online interactions might mediate the effect of such experiences on well-being.

Do User Characteristics Matter?

An implicit assumption in the early research on Internet use and well-being is that Internet use has similar effects regardless of user characteristics. This is also a basic premise of the media effects model described in Chapter 2. However, the co-construction model, also discussed in Chapter 2, suggests that users chose what to do online and so they bring their respective nature and histories to what they do. There is mounting evidence that user characteristics might in fact mediate the relation between adolescents' online behavior and their well-being. Recall that in the 2002 follow-up of the initial HomeNet study, Internet use was associated with declines in loneliness among extroverted teens, but not introverted teens (Kraut et al., 2002). This finding indicates that individuals with greater offline social resources, such as extroverts, were able to leverage their offline strengths in online contexts to enhance their well-being. Perceived resources, particularly online ones, may also play a role in well-being. In our study of urban teens in Los Angeles, loneliness was not related to the total time spent online, nor to the time spent on email, but was predicted by participants' gender (male adolescents were more lonely) and their perceptions regarding their online relationships (Subrahmanyam & Lin, 2007). Adolescents who felt that their relationships with online partners were ones that they could turn to in times of need were lonelier. Although one possible reason for this finding was that these teens had less offline support, this does not seem very likely as we found no evidence that there was a relation between Internet use and perceived support from offline sources (e.g., parents and offline close friends). Keep in mind that we conducted the study at a time when chat rooms were very popular and instant messaging was new. Thus, many of these subjects were also likely interacting with people who were not part of their offline lives. Because this was a correlational study, we cannot say which came first, loneliness or online relationships. In other words, we cannot rule out the possibility that lonely subjects were more actively seeking online relationships, and hence felt that they could depend on them at times of need.

Two longitudinal studies are relevant to questions of directionality regarding Internet use and well-being. Although neither focused exclusively on adolescents, we discuss them as they shed some light on this question. Bessière, Kiesler, Kraut, and Boneva (2008) followed 1,222 adults over a 6–8 month period, and 15% were younger than 19 years of age. Although overall time online was not related to changes in well-being, using the Internet to meet new people and using it for entertainment did lead to reduced depressive effect, but only for people with better social resources. For people with poor resources, using the Internet to meet people was actually associated with reduced depressive effect. Social resources in this study was measured via a variety of measures including interpersonal activity, group memberships, social network size, community involvement, perceived social support, extraversion, and shyness. The second study by Steinfield, Ellison, and Lampe tracked students at Michigan State University for a 2-year period and looked at the relation between Facebook use, social capital, and self-esteem. Social capital refers to the resources accrued from one's social relationships and the researchers were looking at bridging social capital, which are the resources that stem from one's weaker ties. Because of the longitudinal nature of the data, these researches were able to conclude that Facebook use led to gains in bridging social capital. But more importantly, participants with lower self-esteem reported more gains in their social capital from their Facebook use (Steinfield, Ellison, & Lampe, 2008). Although social capital is not strictly a measure of psychological well-being, it is related to measures of well-being, such as self-esteem and life satisfaction (Bargh, McKenna, & Fitzsimons, 2002; Helliwell & Putnam, 2004).

At first glance, the results of the two studies are contradictory but we should keep two points in mind about the study by Bessiere and colleagues. First, they collected their data in 2001 and 2002, before social networking sites were available; also, only using the Internet for meeting new people affected depression. The power of sites such as Facebook, which was the focus of the Michigan State study, is that they allow users to create a vast and layered network of people from various offline spheres, such as their college community, high school, or family and relatives. Second, the participants spanned a wider age range, and younger users might have well used the Internet very differently and benefited very differently as well. Regardless of these differences, two conclusions that we can draw from these studies are as follows: (1) The Internet provides unique opportunities to expand one's social networks and relationships and consequently one's well-being; (2) not all users benefit equally from these opportunities; gains can vary based on variables, such as an individual user's resources (e.g., self-esteem) or the particular kinds of relationships sought (meeting anyone on the Internet versus meeting people from offline sphere's such as one's college community).

Short-Term Effects on Well-Being

Much of the research on Internet use and well-being are based on two assumptions. First, online communication entails weaker ties because it occurs via a computer, lacks face-to-face cues, and may involve strangers. Second, a cumulative effect is presumed, that is over time, the weaker ties encouraged by the Internet lead to reduced well-being. There is very limited research as to whether online communication might bestow more immediate benefits to young people. Researcher Elisheva Gross suspected that this might be the case when she found that time online was not related to dispositional well-being (Gross et al., 2002). Adolescents who reported feeling lonely or socially anxious on a given day were more likely to communicate that day via instant messaging with people whom they did not know well. She speculated that online interactions with unknown peers may help adolescents to recover from the sting of social rejection. In one of the few experimental studies on this topic, Gross used a cyberball task (the computer equivalent of playing catch) to simulate social inclusion or exclusion among adolescent participants; subsequently they were asked to either participate in an instant message conversation with an unknown opposite-sex peer or to play a computer game (Gross, 2009).

Adolescents who experienced social exclusion reported greater negative affect (for example, lower self-esteem, shame, and anger) than those who were included. Among the participants who were excluded, online communication with an unknown peer facilitated recovery from negative affect better than solitary computer game play. Gross concluded that interactions with unknown peers in forums, such as chat rooms and social networking sites, may help adolescents cope with threats to "belonging" in their offline lives; she has suggested that "policies are needed to promote the creation and maintenance of safe spaces for youth to interact online." Creating such safe online spaces is akin to the practice of setting aside outdoor parks and others similar open areas, a tradition of cities and communities in many parts of the world.

The idea that interactions with strangers could help teens is contrary to much of the conventional wisdom that has prevailed since the communication applications of the Internet became as popular as they have among youth. A widely held assumption is that online communication will have deleterious effects on well-being because they occur via machines and especially in the early years of the Internet, with people who were strangers or acquaintances rather than close friends. Gross's finding raises the intriguing possibility that weaker ties, of the kind involved in communication with strangers and even acquaintances from offline settings, such as school might help young people deal with some of the anxiety and heartache that is part and parcel of this challenging period in their lives. Indeed that may explain the popularity of instant messaging and social networking sites. In Chapter 5, we had noted that digital tools allow teens to widen their networks and interact, however fleetingly, with peers with whom they might not otherwise do so. Gross's study points to the potentially beneficial role of such interactions.

For some teens, such online spaces might represent the only sources of social support in their lives, offline or on (Tynes, 2007a). Tynes description of her experience conducting a research study with instant messaging highlights this so well that we reproduce it here in its entirety:

In my research on ethnic identity and online interaction among youths, I collected data from teens via instant messaging (IM). Teens participating in the study would continually contact me and my research assistant via IM to ask questions that ranged from the mundane to the serious. In one instance, a participant contacted my research assistant and told her that she had been cutting herself and that she was going to do it again. My research assistant got in touch with me and I began to talk to the teen, still through IM. We talked for more than an hour about her problems in school, her feelings of social isolation, and the teasing she endured because she was a cutter. We began on a very grim note, but over the course of the conversation, there was a dramatic shift in her mood. By the end, she was in good spirits and agreed to talk to her family about the cutting. Several days later, she messaged me again and said that she had seen a therapist and was feeling better. It is not clear that my research assistant and I were her only form of social support – we were just two of a number of online friends on her "buddy list" that she could have contacted. But contacting someone outside of her family and peers at school was crucial, and the online setting provided that opportunity.

Thus, parents, teachers, and others who work with teens should recognize that young people might draw benefits from online interaction and communication with strangers and acquaintances, particularly those from other spheres of their offline lives, such as their school, church, or other community organizations. Quite possibly such interactions may serve as a buffer against some of the stress that adolescents surely experience from their interactions with close friends and even parents and other family members. At the same time, it is legitimate, and even important, to continue to be concerned when young people interact and get intimate with total strangers online, especially when such interactions form the bulk of their social interactions or when their partners are older adults. We discuss the issue of youth victimization by predatory adults in Chapter 10.

Effect of Negative Interactions on Well-Being

Although the Internet's potential for disembodied and anonymous interactions can be potentially liberating and empowering to users, it has its disadvantages. These very same features of the Internet may also disinhibit users leading to negative online interactions, such as very public displays of racism (Tynes, 2005) (*Note*: The issue of hateful content and racist sites is tackled in Chapter 10). Chat rooms, bulletin boards, e-mails, blogs, and social networking sites are all venues where such negative interactions may occur. Tynes and colleagues provide the following example of a negative interaction that they recorded in an unmonitored online teen chat room (Tynes, Reynolds, & Greenfield, 2004):

21. bigbootygirl: where'd the racist fucker go
23. gaanas 49: no where
24. chulischick: SORRY EKE NO ME GUSTAN LOS RASISTAS
27. gaanas 49: right here u f u c king mexican
29. cinsea: RIGHT HERE DUMB MEXICan
429. bigbootygirl: why does everyone hate me cuase i'm mexican?
439. gaanas 49: cause your mexican
440. gaanas 49: duh

According to the researchers, this was an excerpt from an approximately 30-min interaction. They deconstructed the interaction as representing a strong attack on the user *bigbootygirl*, where other users addressed her with racial epithets (lines 27 and 29) and the stereotype of an uneducated Mexican (line 29). Tynes et al. note that some of the online negative stereotypes and racial hostility were similar to those seen in offline contexts.

In their study of monitored and unmonitored chat rooms, Tynes and colleagues (2004) found that racial slurs and comments were much more common, for example, in unmonitored chat rooms for older adolescents compared to monitored chat rooms frequented by younger adolescents. Chat participants openly identified their racial/ethnic group membership and mentioned race and ethnicity often in the chat conversations: 37 out of 38 half-hour transcripts had at least one reference to race or ethnicity. The authors observed: "While most references had a neutral or positive valence in both monitored and unmonitored chat rooms, chat participants nonetheless had a 19% chance of being exposed to negative remarks about a racial or ethnic group (potentially their own) in a session of monitored chat and a 59% chance in unmonitored chat" (p. 667). These findings indicate that in the absence of social controls, such as a monitor or peer pressure, youth in online contexts may be more likely to express racist attitudes that may otherwise be lurking under the surface. A frequency of one in five online sessions is a relatively high rate for racist remarks; although we have no firm data on the extent of negative, racially tinged interactions in adolescents' offline peer interactions, it would be surprising indeed to see such a high rate offline, and to actually hear such remarks in face-to-face settings. This is an instance where a behavior is more intense online compared to offline contexts. Of course, it is possible that the incidence of online racism is higher because the unit of analysis in this case was the chat room rather than that of an individual user. However, validation of the findings of online racism come from another study by Tynes in which she interviewed adolescents recruited by instant messaging from a teen chat room. Participants in her study reported that while online, they had been exposed to negative stereotypes and racial prejudice against their own and other ethnic groups (Tynes, 2007b). We do not know the actual extent to which youth may experience or witness prejudice in online contexts. But, even if it were relatively infrequent, it would be very difficult "to imagine the extent of the psychological damage that such remarks do" (Subrahmanyam & Greenfield, 2008).

Conclusions

When Kraut and colleagues first released the findings of the HomeNet study in the late 1990s, there was a plethora of headlines in the press such as "Is the Internet a sad, depressing world?" "Researchers Find Sad, Lonely World in Cyberspace" "Net use causes depression." Since then, the Internet itself has changed and evolved, as have online users and the way they use various applications. Research on the effects of Internet use on youth well-being has revealed a very different and complex picture than initially feared. Simply spending a lot of time online does not automatically lead to lowered well-being. Instead, what users do with that time and in particular, whom they interact with, moderates effects on well-being. Teen users' psychological and social resources are also relevant, but we need more research to clarify how they mediate the Internet's effect on psychological well-being.

One important message to take away is the need for more education. Youth must be educated to use the Internet and mobile devices moderately and safely, and in ways that will not cause them physical harm. When adolescents, particularly younger ones, are not able to self-regulate their technology use, parents must step in and be more proactive. Although it is crucial for us to be aware of the possible adverse effects from Internet use, we must also be willing to see its benefits where we least expect them, such as when teens interact with strangers. The bottom line is that the Internet is fundamentally a tool, and so the particular ways that teens use it will ultimately determine its effects on their well-being.

References

Anderson, C. A. (2004). An update on the effects of playing violent video games. *Journal of Adolescence, 27*, 113–122.

Anderson, C. A., & Bushman, B. J. (2001). Effects of violent video games on aggressive behavior, aggressive cognition, aggressive affect, physiological arousal, and prosocial behavior: A meta-analytic review of the scientific literature. *Psychological Science, 12*, 353–359.

Bargh, J. A., McKenna, K. Y. A., & Fitzsimons, G. M. (2002). Can you see the real me? "Activation and expression of the true self" on the Internet. *Journal of Social Issues, 58*, 33–48.

Bessière, K., Kiesler, S., Kraut, R. E., & Boneva, B. (2008). Effects of Internet use and social resources on changes in depression. *Information Community and Society, 11*, 47–70.

Brage, D., Meredith, W., & Woodward, J. (1993). Correlates of loneliness among midwestern adolescents. *Adolescence, 28*, 685–693.

Brasington, R. (1990). Nintendinitis. *New England Journal of Medicine, 322*, 1473–1474.

Brennan, T. (1982). Loneliness at adolescence. In L. A. Peplau & D. Perlman (Eds.), *Loneliness: A sourcebook of current theory, research and therapy* (pp. 269–290). New York, NY: Wiley.

Bukowski, W. M., Newcomb, A. F., & Hartup, W. W. (1996). *The company they keep: Friendships in childhood and adolescence*. Cambridge: Cambridge University Press.

Carskadon, M. A., Vieira, C., & Acebo, C. (1993). Association between puberty and delayed phase preference. *Sleep, 16*, 258–262.

Centers for Disease Control and Prevention. (2004). *Overweight among U.S. children and adolescents*. National Health and Nutrition Examination Survey. http://www.cdc.gov/nchs/data/nhanes/databriefs/overwght.pdf

Degirmencioglu, S. M. (1995). *Changes in adolescents' friendship networks: Do they matter?* Detroit, MI: Wayne State University.

Eijnden, R., Meerkerk, G. J., Vermulst, A. A., Spijkerman, R., & Engels, R. (2008). Online communication, compulsive Internet use, and psychosocial well-being among adolescents: A longitudinal study. *Developmental Psychology, 44*, 655–665.

Fredriksen, K., Reddy, R., Way, N., & Rhodes, J. (2004). Sleepless in Chicago: Tracking the effects of sleep loss over the middle school years. *Child Development, 74*, 84–95.

Granovetter, M. S. (1973). The strength of weak ties. *American Journal of Sociology, 78*, 1360.

Greenfield, P. M., & Subrahmanyam, K. (2003). Online discourse in a teen chatroom: New codes and new modes of coherence in a visual medium. *Journal of Applied Developmental Psychology, 24*, 713–738.

Gross, E. F. (2009). Logging on, bouncing back: An experimental investigation of online communication following social exclusion. *Developmental Psychology, 45*, 1787–1793.

Gross, E. F., Juvonen, J., & Gable, S. L. (2002). Internet use and well-being in adolescence. *Journal of Social Issues, 58*, 75–90.

Harter, S. (1985). *Manual for the self-perception profile for children*. Unpublished manuscript, University of Denver, Denver, CO.

Hartup, W. W. (1996). The company they keep: Friendships and their developmental significance. *Child Development, 67*, 1–13.

Helliwell, J. F., & Putnam, R. D. (2004). The social context of well-being. *Philosophical Transactions of the Royal Society B: Biological Sciences, 359*, 1435–1446.

Iglowstein, I., Jenni, O. G., Molinari, L., & Largo, R. H. (2003). Sleep duration from infancy to adolescence: Reference values and generational trends. *Pediatrics, 111*, 302–307.

Kaiser Family Foundation. (2004). *The role of media in childhood obesity*. Retrieved [Date] from http://www.kff.org/entmedia/entmedia022404pkg.cfm

Kef, S., & Dekovic, M. (2004). The role of parental and peer support in adolescents well-being: A comparison of adolescents with and without a visual impairment. *Journal of Adolescence, 27*, 453–466.

Krackhardt, D. (1994). The strength of strong ties: The importance of philos in organizations. In N. Nohria & R. Eccles (Eds.), *Networks and organizations: Structure, form, and action* (pp. 216–239). Boston, MA: Harvard Business School Press.

Kraut, R. E., Kiesler, S., Boneva, B., Cummings, J., Helgeson, V., & Crawford, A. (2002). Internet paradox revisited. *Journal of Social Issues, 58*, 49–74.

Kraut, R. E., Patterson, M., Lundmark, V., Kiesler, S., Mukopadhyay, T., & Scherlis, W. (1998). Internet paradox: A social technology that reduces social involvement and psychological well-being? *American Psychologist, 53*, 1017–1031.

Kunkel, D. (2001). Children and television advertising. In D. Singer & J. Singer (Eds.), *Handbook of children and the media* (pp. 375–393). Thousand Oaks, CA: Sage Publications.

Mastro, D. E., Eastin, M. S., & Tamborini, R. (2002). Internet search behaviors and mood alterations: A selective exposure. *Media Psychology, 4*, 157–172.

Mazalin, D., & Moore, S. (2004). Internet use, identity development and social anxiety among young adults. *Behavior Change, 21*, 90–102.

Mendels, P. (1999). A warning on class computers. *New York Times*, p. 16.

Mesch, G. S. (2001). Social relationships and Internet use among adolescents in Israel. *Social Science Quarterly, 82*, 329–339.

Mesch, G. S. (2003). The family and the Internet: The Israeli case. *Social Science Quarterly, 84*, 1039–1050.

Nelson, M. C., Neumark-Stzainer, D., Hannan, P. J., Sirard, J. R., & Story, M. (2006). Longitudinal and secular trends in physical activity and sedentary behavior during adolescence. *Pediatrics, 118*, e1627–e1634.

Nie, N. H., & Hillygus, D. S. (2002). Where does Internet time come from? A reconnaissance. *IT & Society, 1*, 1–20.

Ogden, C. L., Carroll, M. D., & Flegal, K. M. (2008). High body mass index for age among us children and adolescents, 2003–2006. *The Journal of the American Medical Association, 299*, 2401–2405.

Raja, S. N., McGee, R., & Stanton, W. R. (1992). Perceived attachments to parents and peers and psychological well-being in adolescence. *Journal of Youth and Adolescence, 21*, 471–485.

Rosenberg, M. (1986). Self-concept from middle childhood through adolescence. In J. Suls & A. Greenwald (Eds.), *Psychological perspectives on the self* (Vol. 3, pp. 107–136). Hillsdale, NJ: Erlbaum.

Sarason, B. R., Sarason, I. G., & Pierce, G. R. (1990). *Social support: An interactional view*. Hoboken, NJ: Wiley.

Schneider, M., Dunton, G. F., & Cooper, D. M. (2007). Media use and obesity in adolescent females. *Obesity, 15*, 2328–2335.

Steinfield, C., Ellison, N. B., & Lampe, C. A. C. (2008). Social capital, self-esteem, and use of online social network sites: A longitudinal analysis. *Journal of Applied Developmental Psychology, 29*, 434–445.

Stettler, N., Singer, T., & Sutter, P. (2004). Electronic games and environmental factors associated with childhood obesity in Switzerland. *Obesity Research, 12*, 896–903.

Storch, E. A., Brassard, M. R., & Masia-Warner, C. L. (2003). The relationship of peer victimization to social anxiety and loneliness in adolescence. *Child Study Journal, 33*, 1–18.

Storr, E. F., de Vere Beavis, F. O., & Stringer, M. D. (2007). Case notes: Texting tenosynovitis. *New Zealand Medical Journal, 120*, 107–108.

Subrahmanyam, K. (2010). Technology and physical and social health. In P. Peterson, E. Baker, & B. McGaw (Eds.), *International encyclopedia of education* (Vol. 8, pp. 112–118). Oxford: Elsevier.

Subrahmanyam, K., & Greenfield, P. M. (2008). Online communication and adolescent relationships. *Future of Children, 18*, 119–146.

Subrahmanyam, K., Greenfield, P. M., Kraut, R. E., & Gross, E. F. (2001). The impact of computer use on children's and adolescents' development. *Journal of Applied Developmental Psychology, 22*, 7–30.

Subrahmanyam, K., Kraut, R. E., Greenfield, P. M., & Gross, E. F. (2000). The impact of home computer use on children's activities and development. *The Future of Children, 10*, 123–144.

Subrahmanyam, K., & Lin, G. (2007). Adolescents on the net: Internet use and well-being. *Adolescence, 42*, 659–677.

Sun, P., Unger, J. B., Palmer, P. H., Gallaher, P., Chou, C. P., Baexconde-Garbanati, L., et al. (2005). Internet accessibility and usage among urban adolescents in Southern California: Implications for web-based heath research. *CyberPsychology & Behavior, 8*, 441–453.

Sundar, S. S., & Wagner, C. B. (2002). The world wide wait: Exploring physiological and behavioral effects of download speed. *Media Psychology, 4*, 173–206.

Tanner, J. M. (1978). *Growth at adolescence* (2nd ed.). Oxford: Blackwell.

Tarokh, L., & Carskadon, M. A. (2008). Sleep in adolescents. In L. R. Squire (Ed.), *Encyclopedia of neuroscience* (pp. 1015–1022). Oxford: Academic Press.

Teenage Research Unlimited. (2007). *Tech abuse in teen relationships study*. Retrieved September 25, 2009, from http://www.loveisrespect.org/wp-content/uploads/2009/03/liz-claiborne-2007-tech-relationship-abuse.pdf

Tynes, B. M. (2005). Children, adolescents and the culture of online hate. In N. E. Dodd, D. E. Singer, & R. F. Wilson (Eds.), *Handbook of children, culture and violence* (pp. 267–289). Thousand Oaks, CA: Sage.

Tynes, B. M. (2007a). Internet safety gone wild? Sacrificing the educational and psychosocial benefits of online social environments. *Journal of Adolescent Research, 22*, 575–584.

Tynes, B.M. (2007b). Role taking in online "classrooms": What adolescents are learning about race and ethnicity. *Developmental Psychology, 43*, 1312–1320.

Tynes, B. M., Reynolds, L., & Greenfield, P. M. (2004). Adolescence, race, and ethnicity on the Internet: A comparison of discourse in monitored vs. unmonitored chat rooms. *Journal of Applied Developmental Psychology, 25*, 667–684.

Valas, H. (1999). Students with learning disabilities and low-achieving students: Peer acceptance, loneliness, self-esteem, and depression. *Social Psychology of Education, 3*, 173–192.

Valkenburg, P. M. (2004). *Children's responses to the screen: A media psychological approach.* Mahwah, NJ: Lawrence Erlbaum Associates.

Valkenburg, P. M., Peter, J., & Schouten, A. P. (2006). Friend networking sites and their relationship to adolescents' well-being and social self-esteem. *CyberPsychology & Behavior, 9*, 584–590.

Van den Bulck, J. (2003). Text messaging as a cause of sleep interruption in adolescents, evidence from a cross-sectional study. *Journal of Sleep Research, 12*, 263.

Van den Bulck, J. (2004). Television viewing, computer game playing, and Internet use and self-reported time to bed and time out of bed in secondary-school children. *Sleep, 27*, 101–104.

Van Den Bulck, J. (2007). Adolescent use of mobile phones for calling and for sending text messages after lights out: Results from a prospective cohort study with a one-year follow-up. *Sleep*, *30*, 1220–1223.

Woodward, J., & Frank, B. (1988). Rural adolescent loneliness and adolescent coping strategies. *Adolescence*, *23*, 559–565.

Ybarra, M. L., Alexander, C., & Mitchell, K. J. (2005). Depressive symptomatology, youth Internet use, and online interactions: A national survey. *Journal of Adolescent Health*, *36*, 9–18.

Zhang, J., Fraser, S., Lindsay, J., Clarke, K., & Mao, Y. (1998). Age-specific patterns of factors related to fatal motor vehicle traffic crashes focus on young and elderly drivers. *Public Health*, *112*, 289–295.

Chapter 8
Technology and Health: Using the Internet for Wellness and Illness

In the previous chapter, we saw the relation between adolescents' Internet use and their well-being; in this chapter, we examine how they use the Internet in the service and on occasion, disservice, of their health and well-being. We will show that adolescents take advantage of the Internet's communication and information capabilities of the Internet to enhance wellness and deal with illness. We have discussed the communication applications in the preceding chapters and so they need no further discussion. Next, we briefly consider the information capabilities afforded by the Internet. The world wide web on the Internet has become an information behemoth not witnessed before in the course of human history.

In July 2008, Google search engineers estimated that there were one trillion unique URLs on the web (Alpert & Hajaj, 2008). Combined with the power of search engines such as Google, and now Bing, the web can instantly deliver answers to most of our questions. We turn to it whenever we need information on just about any topic, be it politics, popular culture, movie listings, directions, or health, wellness, and illness, the focus of this chapter. After a visit to the doctor, many of us have gone straight to Google or Wikipedia to obtain more information about our diagnosis and recommendations. In addition to providing free and unfettered access to vast amounts of publicly available information, the Internet also allows individuals to store and access personal medical information via online accounts or briefcases. For instance, there are free web sites, where users can create profiles that allow them to track their weight loss or smoking cessation progress. Thus, the Internet provides access to both publicly available and privately stored information resources to improve and enhance health and well-being.

In this chapter, we first focus on adolescents' use of online health-related information resources. After we describe the nature and extent of this use, we examine the opportunities and challenges that ready access to such information may present for youth. Next, we turn to the Internet as a tool for treatment delivery, with particular attention to the factors that may limit the efficacy of such interventions with this age group.

K. Subrahmanyam, D. Šmahel, *Digital Youth*, Advancing Responsible
Adolescent Development, DOI 10.1007/978-1-4419-6278-2_8,
© Springer Science+Business Media, LLC 2011

Adolescents' Use of Online Health Resources

On the web, a variety of health-related resources are available such as web sites, bulletin and discussion boards, physician blogs, and sites that allow users to ask physicians a medical question (e.g., www.MDAdvice.com). Web sites range from those hosted by government entities (e.g., www.cdc.gov) and universities to independent organizations focused on a particular health issue (e.g., American Cancer Society), corporations, as well as individuals suffering from a particular health condition (e.g., diabetes or cancer). The topics of the sites are just as varied, and include those relevant to youth such as general adolescent concerns about puberty and sexual health and more specific topics such as sexually transmitted diseases (STDs), smoking cessation, suicide, mental health, and pro-anorexia sites.

How Much Do Adolescents' Use Online Health Resources?

Like adults, young people report using the Internet to access health information and by all accounts this use has been increasing since these trends have been tracked (Borzekowski & Rickert, 2001; Rideout, 2001; Roberts, Foehr, & Rideout, 2005). In a 2005 national survey of 8- to 18-year-olds in the USA, half of all those surveyed reported looking for health information online (Roberts et al., 2005). A qualitative study of 210 Canadian adolescents found even greater use of technology for health-related questions. Although the participants used the Internet more often to look for information related to school, peers, and social concerns, health-related issues were very popular as well and 67% reported looking for information on specific medical conditions, 63% for information on body image and nutrition, and 56% for information about sexual health (Skinner, Biscope, Poland, & Goldberg, 2003). Use of online resources for health information is also found among youth in other parts of the world, (Cole et al., 2008) and has even been documented in Ghana, a third-world developing country (Borzekowski, Fobil, & Asante, 2006).

Frequency data from the WIP show that although adolescents do use the Internet for health-related searches, it is not something they report doing very often (See Fig. 8.1). That is, the frequency with which they search online is at acceptable levels and, for the moment, we do not have to worry about information overload. In general, searching data from search engines reveal that health information searches make up only 5% of all daily online searches, indicating that for most people searching for health information, although common, is not the most frequent online activity (Eysenbach, 2008).

Health Topics That Adolescents Seek Information About

A content analysis of a health-related online bulletin board for adolescents revealed that the most frequent health-related concerns/questions were on the following topics: sexual health, pregnancy/birth control, body image, and grooming of genital areas (Suzuki & Calzo, 2004). Along similar lines, on the 2001 Kaiser Report,

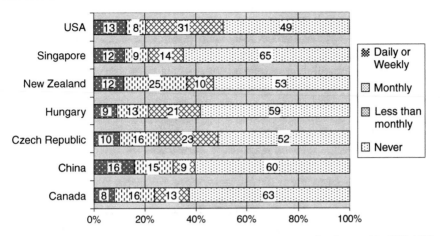

Fig. 8.1 Frequency of looking for health related information among 12- 18-year olds (WIP 2007 data)

sexual health, sexual health issues such as pregnancy, AIDS, and other STDs, were the second most frequently searched topic after diseases like cancer and diabetes (Rideout, 2001).

The particular focus of teens' online inquiries is related to offline demographics such as gender, age, and even ethnicity in some cases (Gilbert, Temby, & Rogers, 2005; Rideout, 2001). The Kaiser report described earlier found that compared to adolescent males, adolescent females were more likely to have reported looking for information online about a sexual health topic (e.g., pregnancy and birth control) as well as about depression, eating disorders, and weight control. Similarly, greater proportions of adolescent males reported looking for information about puberty and teen sexuality, whereas female adolescents reported looking for information about contraception, relationships/dating, general and specific STD information such as prevention, symptoms, testing, transmission, treatment, teen pregnancy, and virginity (Gilbert et al., 2005).

With regard to age, older adolescents are more likely to use the Internet to search for information about health, fitness, and dieting (Lenhart, Rainie, & Lewis, 2001). An online survey of a teen STD prevention web site found that younger teens, who were between 13- and 14-years old, reported looking for information about puberty, whereas older teens between 15- and 17 years reported looking for specific information about sexuality such as contraception, general STD information, STD symptoms, transmission, and teen pregnancy. Such age- and gender-based trends in online health information seeking reveal that developmental trends in online searching parallel trends in adolescents' offline concerns.

Adolescents' Health Information Seeking Behaviors

Search engines have become the gateways for seeking out health information. When looking for health information online, young users report going to multiple sites and averaged five sites in their most recent online search (Rideout, 2001). The Internet is a tool kit, as Greenfield and Yan point out (Greenfield & Yan, 2006), and different online applications such as web pages, bulletin boards, and even chat rooms can be used to access health-related information. Each of these applications affords different opportunities and has different constraints – web pages allow users to get information easily from trusted sources such as the Center for Disease Control (CDC) or the American Heart Association, whereas bulletin boards have a more interactive format where users can get answers both from experts and from their peers. When looking for health information, adolescents and emerging adults report that confidentiality is an important consideration, along with ease of finding information, knowing the source of the information and being able to ask questions, and to hear different sides of an issue (Rideout, 2001). In addition, females and younger women report that they want to hear about the real experiences from other people near in age to them. Given the foregoing, not only are different applications likely to differ in how well they disseminate different kinds of information, but they are also likely to differ in their appeal to different groups of youth.

Self-report data about online searching suggest that youth are turning to the Internet to find out more about specific adolescent concerns, especially sensitive ones, which they may not be comfortable discussing with parents, teachers, or physicians. Their developing autonomy might also be driving them to turn to the Internet and away from the adult sources on which they relied when they were younger (Eysenbach, 2008). The information they obtain from the Internet may even lead them to talk about this information with their peers and parents. However, it does not consistently lead to long lasting behavior changes and only a very small minority reports going to the doctor because of information they saw online (Rideout, 2001).

Less evident at the moment is whether online resources are their first choice or whether they turn to them when they have exhausted all other options (Eysenbach, 2008; Gray, Klein, Cantrill, & Noyce, 2002). Adult trends provide some clues regarding this question. The Internet may be a "source of first resort" for younger adults. Compared to older adults (65 and older), younger adults (18- to 34-year olds) report greater trust and preference for getting health information (e.g., information about cancer) from the Internet; further, when they have sought information, they report using the Internet rather than seeing a health care provider (Hesse et al., 2005). Extrapolating from their tendency to be early adopters of technology in general, we suspect that adolescents would also use the Internet as their first stop when looking for health information. The following quote from a participant in one of the focus groups conducted by Gray and colleagues illustrates a sense of empowerment and independence from health care providers that young people may get from finding health information online (Gray, Klein, Noyce, Sesselberg, & Cantrill, 2005):

> I think that patients – they just want to be more clued up nowadays, and know what's going on for themselves instead of like just going to a doctor and him telling them that 'This is wrong with you, and you're going to have to do this.' They want to be able to do things for themselves, help themselves, and not be totally reliant on seeing doctors and things, and not making out that they're just completely stupid. (UK female, 17–18 years)

Despite this reliance on online sources for information and empowerment, we think it is unlikely that adolescents will self-treat themselves in the event of serious illnesses, but instead may use online sources to inform themselves both prior to and after a meeting with their doctor (Eysenbach, 2008; Gray et al., 2005). In fact, there have been very few documented cases of harm from health-related Internet information (Eysenbach, 2008). Eysenbach points out that the Internet provides access both to low-quality information with potential to harm as well as large amounts of high-quality information from trusted organizations that could greatly enhance public health. Because of these contradictions as well as the many changes occurring in adolescents' body, mind, and social lives, we consider both the opportunities and challenges that online health information presents for adolescent well-being.

Online Health Resources: Opportunities for Adolescents

The potential for anonymity on the Internet makes it appealing as a source of health-related information for young people who may not be comfortable asking adults (e.g., parent or physician) sensitive health-related questions in person (Gray et al., 2005; Suzuki & Calzo, 2004). Other advantages include the Internet's 24/7 availability, the option to passively obtain information (e.g., by looking at other people's questions and the responses they received), and the ability to get advice and suggestions from more individuals than would be possible from one's circle of face-to-face friends (Suzuki & Calzo, 2004). The latter two benefits are very significant and we consider each of them next.

Within digital contexts, we call the passive exposure to online content as lurking. Adolescents may be able to obtain health-related information through lurking, such as via advertisements and passive participation in online groups (e.g., bulletin or discussion boards). Gray and colleagues provide the example of a young woman who reported that she saw a condom advertisement when working on a biology topic. They also describe advertisements for other more questionable products including Viagra and weight-loss medications. At this time, we really do not know whether adolescents are influenced by such messages, and if they are, we suspect that it could be a positive or a negative depending on the message content. Lurking in online health-related forums such as bulletin boards can occur both at the time when the interchange occurs and later on, since many sites retain conversation threads for a long time, some indefinitely. Thus, adolescents who may be hesitant or too shy to post questions themselves, or who may not be concerned about a particular issue at that time can still benefit from the ongoing public exchange of information. Being able to expand the circle of people whom one can tap into can be very beneficial, especially for youth, who otherwise might not have access to such offline resources, because of location (e.g., rural areas, areas steeped in poverty), social isolation, or illness (e.g., teens with cancer). We describe research on some of these groups of young people to show how the Internet can empower them and provide access to resources which otherwise might not be available to them.

One such group consists of young adolescents living in impoverished third-world conditions. Borzekowski and colleagues found that approximately 53% of 15- to 18-year-olds living in Accra, Ghana, used the Internet to search for health information; the Internet was a more important source for youth who were out of school (Borzekowski et al., 2006). Some of the topics that the youth in this study searched for most frequently were sexually transmitted diseases, sexual abuse, sexual activities, as well as diet/nutrition, fitness, and exercise. The results indicate that the Internet has tremendous potential to reach poor, disadvantaged youth in the area of health education.

Another group consists of adolescents who suffer from physical and psychological illnesses such as cancer, eating disorders, and self-injury. Not only can they use the Internet to obtain general health information, but they can also use it to obtain and disseminate information about specific diseases and illnesses as well as to receive support from others who have experienced or are experiencing the same illness. Researchers have studied two online applications that illustrate these uses, web pages and bulletin boards devoted to specific illnesses. For adolescents and young adults (between 16 and 22 years) suffering from a chronic illness such as cancer, searching for information on the Internet has been found to be a good coping strategy (Kyngas et al., 2001). Suzuki and Beale (2006) studied the personal web pages created by teens with cancer and found three potentially beneficial functions: self-presentation (e.g., essays and poetry), information dissemination (e.g., lists, charts, and hyperlinks), and interpersonal connection (e.g., guestbook entries). They concluded that adolescent cancer sufferers were using such web pages for "self-expression, information access, and contact with peers." The access to information that technology affords is particularly important given the finding that exposure to cancer information in young patients is related to lowered anxiety and depression as well as to less anxiety about treatments (Suzuki & Beale, 2006).

The interpersonal connections with peers that technology makes possible may also be particularly valuable for isolated youth (e.g., those living in small towns or rural areas), youth suffering from relatively rare illnesses, as well as youth suffering from illnesses that they may not be comfortable talking about with their offline peers (e.g., AIDS, eating disorders, self-injury behavior). Online bulletin boards and chat rooms are Internet venues that allow youth to form such connections. Whitlock, Powers, and Eckenrode studied a large number of online message boards targeting self-injurious behaviors (e.g., cutting) and found that they were most popular among young females between 14 and 20 years of age, the group also most at risk for such behavior (Whitlock, Powers, & Eckenrode, 2006). This is also the case of bulletin boards focusing on eating disorders, which are also much more common among adolescent females (Winzelberg, 1997). In an eating disorder electronic support group, the most common message themes were self-disclosure, requests for information, and direct provision of emotional support, and most of the messages were posted between 7 p.m. and 7 a.m (Winzelberg, 1997). The value of such interactive online channels lies in their ability to connect teens with their peers, who may be battling similar issues to exchange and share information, especially at times during the day when other more traditional face-to-face sources of support are not usually available. Of course, such connections may not always be a good thing, especially if incorrect or even dangerous information is exchanged and this is addressed in the next section.

Online Health Resources: Challenges for Adolescents

Information challenges. The vast amounts of health-related information that adolescents can access online, some of them of questionable quality, present challenges and raise concerns. A simple Google query with the search terms "cancer teens" conducted in September 2008 yielded 15,400,000 results in 0.12 s. How good are teens at searching for health-related information to find the answers that they are looking for? In addition, how good are they at sifting through all the results, 15 million in the above instance that do pop up? Not very good it turns out: in the Kaiser survey, only 4 out of 10 respondents indicated that the health information that they found was very useful. Finding personally relevant, high-quality information online is a barrier for adolescents looking to find answers to their health questions (Skinner et al., 2003). A female participant in Gray and colleagues' focus group study (Gray, Klein, Noyce, Sesselberg, & Cantrill, 2005) was frustrated that, at times, search engines yield information that is not specific and not very relevant to the queries and complained thus:

> Like on search engines. . .If you're looking up. . .sports or something. . .sometimes it never gives that sport. . ..It could have like millions of different things. It's annoying. (US female, 16–18 years)

Further challenges come from adolescents' search behavior and an observational study provides a contradictory picture. Approximately 69% of the 68 observed searches yielded a correct and useful answer to a health-related question. A little less than a quarter of the searches used incorrect spellings of search terms. However, participants often used a trial and error approach to form search strings, randomly scanned pages, and failed to consider the source of the content (e.g., site hosted by an individual versus a government entity) they had found (Hansen, Derry, Resnick, & Richardson, 2003).

Another issue concerns the quality of information that is available online. Not all information on the web is of equal quality and generally web sites hosted by universities or government organizations are the most accurate and trustworthy. With regard to youth, some of the credibility concerns for online information are as follows (Eysenbach, 2008):

(1) Lack of quality controls such as via editorial boards or peer review and a low-cost publishing process has lowered publishing standards compared to the more conventional format of print (e.g., peer-reviewed journals or books).
(2) Youth may not be able to distinguish material that has gone through a rigorous peer-review from material that has not undergone such a review.
(3) There is often a deficit of context, which is a lack of information about who produced or sponsored a web site, and why and how they did so. For instance,

lay and unqualified individuals can create very professional looking web sites that may be inherently deceptive in nature.

(4) There may be a blurring of the lines between different information genres such as advertising versus informational content. For instance, companies with a stake in a product can create very convincing sites about the benefits of that product.

Research is scarce on the question of whether adolescents take into account credibility considerations when looking online for health-related information. In the 2001 Kaiser Report, only 17% of the 18- to 24-year-old respondents said that they trusted online health information. Although respondents reported a healthy level of skepticism about health information from the Internet, they still reported relying on online sources. They also do not consistently check source credentials when doing online searches, even though they say that this information is important to them when looking for health information (Rideout, 2001). Although some experimental research suggests that college students take into account both the source and the content when evaluating the credibility of online information, we do not know how adolescents process information online. Even though remarkable cognitive advances occur during adolescence, it is hard to say if these advances actually translate to more informed behavior while online (Eastin, 2001).

Lack of sustained attention to the credibility of a site is an important concern given the wide variability in the quality of information that is available online. Another review similarly concluded that adolescents' use of the Internet for information about health and sexuality was often limited by their health/online literacy skills (Gray & Klein, 2006). Borzekowski has also pointed out that although it is generally assumed that adolescents are technologically sophisticated, we do not yet know how young people incorporate the information they find online into their lives (Borzekowski, 2006). It is very likely that adolescents are not equally effective in terms of accessing and benefiting from the health-related resources that are available online. Until there is systematic research on these issues, it would be premature to conclude that the Internet's health-related information access is of benefit to all adolescent users.

Dangerous and harmful content online. Although teens can benefit from high-quality health-related information on the web, it is also possible for them to access sites with harmful and potentially dangerous content. Two such sites relevant to adolescents that we consider here are (1) sites that endorse eating disorders and (2) those that sell prescription drugs.

The Internet has become an important source of information about eating disorders, known to be much more prevalent among young adolescent girls compared to all other demographic categories. Of concern to us are sites developed by youth, which promote anorexia and bulimia (Wilson, Peebles, Hardy, & Litt, 2006) and are called pro-eating disorder (ED) sites or pro-ED sites or pro-ana (standing for pro-anorexia) sites. According to Wilson and colleagues, such sites create online communities for disordered eaters and either promoted EDs as a life style choice or as an illness. Regardless of which approach they take, they include 'thinspiration' (mages of thin and cachectic women), poetry, weight-loss advice, methods for avoiding detection by family and health care providers, forums, merchandise, and links to other, related sites (Wilson et al., 2006). Sites which adopt a recovery perspective are called pro-recovery sites and are much less common; in a 2003 study, the results of an online search revealed 500 pro-ED sites, 100 pro-recovery sites, and 30 professional sites (Chesley, Alberts, Klein, & Kreipe, 2003). Adolescents with eating disorders may be at risk for learning new and dangerous behaviors from online forums with a pro-eating disorder tilt.

One survey study of patients (10- to 22-year olds evaluated for eating disorders) and their families (76 patients and 106 parents) indicates that although a majority (49%) of the youth with ED had not visited either kind of site, 41% reported that they had visited pro-recovery sites, 36% had visited pro-ED sites, and 25% reported using both kinds of sites. Chance searching led many of the patients to pro-ED and pro-recovery sites. Worryingly, those who knew of pro-ED sites reported that they learnt new techniques of purging and weight loss, as well as learned about diet pills, laxatives, and supplements. Contrary to what one might expect, the youth also reported learning high-risk eating behaviors (e.g., new methods of weight loss or purging, new diet aids, and how to obtain them) from pro-recovery sites (Wilson et al., 2006). As has become par for the course, parents had incomplete knowledge – a majority did not know about pro-recovery sites, and more than half were aware of pro-ED sites. Parents who knew of pro-ED sites did not know whether their child visited them or not, and only 10% reported knowing that their teen visited them. In recent years, there has been a significant increase in the number of pro-anorexia sites, many of which contain both text and graphic pictures (Davis, 2008) that seem intent on shocking their viewers. Notwithstanding its many potential benefits in the area of illness and disorders, the Internet may serve to normalize a potentially dangerous behavior such as anorexia and bulimia.

It is doubtful that such sites in and of themselves could cause individuals to have an eating disorder, but the easy availability of such online images may nonetheless have negative consequences. In an experimental study, female undergraduate students ($M = 18.7$ years) saw one of three kinds of web sites – a pro-anorexic web site, a web site of female fashion showing average-sized models, or a home décor site. Pre- and post-treatment questionnaires suggested that among participants who viewed the pro-anorexic web site, there was a decrease in self-esteem, appearance self-efficacy, and perceived attractiveness, and an increase in negative affect and perceptions of being overweight (Bardone-Cone & Cass, 2006). While we cannot pinpoint the direction of influence, it is clear that viewing pro-ana or pro-ED content online is associated with negative effects about the body. Based on the finding that self-injurious behavior follows epidemic-like patterns in hospitals and other institutions, Whitlock and colleagues (2006) have speculated that such problem behaviors might even be socially contagious through the Internet. This is an important concern considering that the Internet is now home to innumerable sites that provide detailed information and instructions about several dangerous behaviors that are gaining popularity among some adolescents (e.g., sniffing glue, choking oneself, etc).

Another example of the potentially harmful information that is available on the Internet is the online availability and portrayal of prescription stimulants, particularly those which adolescents tend to abuse. Schepis and colleagues analyzed the results of Google searches involving the names of controlled stimulants (e.g., Amphetamine, Ritalin, etc.) (Schepis, Marlowe, & Forman, 2008). They found that the majority of the substances were easily available online without a prescription; although one stimulant, methamphetamine was not available online, instructions to manufacture it were easy to find. The portrayal of the stimulants varied and seemed to depend on the drug – some were mostly associated with anti-use sites, whereas others were associated with neutral or even pro-use sites. The authors speculated that negative portrayals might not be enough to dissuade adolescents from misusing stimulants. As of now, we do not know the extent to which adolescents actually utilize such sites to obtain illegal prescription drugs, but their easy availability points to the need for more research on this question. Although the Internet may empower many adolescents by providing them with easy access to health-related information, the two examples discussed in this section indicate that parents, physicians, and clinicians need to be aware of the very real dangers that specific kinds of online health-related content may present for some adolescents.

The Internet as a Tool for Treatment Delivery

Given its interactive nature as well as its 24/7 availability, the Internet can be used to deliver interventions/treatments and to disseminate prevention programs (Borzekowski, 2006). There are many home-based Internet delivery programs for health-related issues such as overweight and eating disorder symptoms (Doyle et al., 2008; Williamson et al., 2005), smoking cessation (Buller et al., 2006; Patten et al., 2006), and conflict training (Carpenter, Frankel, Marina, Duan, & Smalley, 2004). Research on the effectiveness of these programs is mixed. Therefore, instead of providing an exhaustive description and review of all of them, we focus here on the factors that may limit or enhance the Internet's potential to deliver treatment and interventions.

One study compared two Internet-based programs for weight management in overweight African-American adolescent girls, who also had one obese biological parent (Williamson et al., 2005). Participants were randomly assigned to either a more passive online health-education program or a more interactive behavioral intervention program, which included Internet counseling. Face-to-face sessions were included for all participants. Although only 50% of the participants completed the 6-month trial, measurements taken at baseline and 6 months later showed that adolescents in the interactive behavioral program lost more body fat and their parents lost more body weight and both parents and adolescents showed lowered dietary fat intake. This study indicated that passive Internet health education programs might not be as effective as interactive ones.

Another study compared overweight adolescents who either took part in a 16-week cognitive behavioral program online or were in the usual care program (Doyle et al., 2008). The Internet-delivered program resulted in a modest reduction in weight status; initially there were differences between the two groups in weight status, but 4 months later participants in both groups showed similar improvements. The program also did not lead to any change in eating disorders attitudes and behaviors. One reason for the modest effects was that participants who received the intervention via the Internet actually had very limited exposure to treatment materials; one third of participants accessed less than 10% of the content suggesting that there was low adherence to the program. Because program satisfaction was high among participants in the online intervention, the authors suggest that treatment providers might need to use innovative means to improve program adherence, for example sending reminders via cell phone or text messages or even providing incentives to enhance adherence.

Efforts at enhancing adolescents' log on rates to online interventions have yielded somewhat mixed results. For instance, researchers examined the factors that may influence the efficacy of the Food, Fun and Fitness Internet program, an obesity prevention program at Baylor University (Thompson, Baranowski, Cullen, & Watson, 2007; Thompson, Baranowski, Cullen, & Watson, 2008). They found that the schedule of incentives influenced log on rates – adolescent girls who received weekly incentives had a slightly higher, though not statistically significant, log on rate. Similarly, participants who were recruited via media also had higher log on rates, but they reported a drop between the 4th and 5th week of the program. Disappointing results have also been found in studies that examined the efficacy of smoking-prevention programs targeting adolescents (Buller et al., 2006; Patten et al., 2006). However, the study by Buller et al. suggested that there was a reduction in smoking when participants adhered to the program. Thus, it appears that the Internet may have potential to deliver treatment for important adolescent concerns such as overweight and smoking, but we can harness its potential only if we are able to devise better ways of getting adolescents to actually log on and adhere to the intervention program. Of course, this is also the same challenge involved in getting adolescents to use condoms to prevent STDs and pregnancy, not drink and drive, and not text and drive, so it may unfortunately be a considerably more difficult problem than we realize.

Conclusions

For youth, the Internet has become both an important social context and a tool, and in this chapter we focused on how adolescents use it in the service of their health, wellness, and illness. Like adults, adolescents use the health-related resources that the Internet provides access to and do so mostly about topics relating to their general health and sexuality. However, if youth are to take advantage of these resources, they will need health literacy training to search more effectively and evaluate the credibility of online information. At the same time, the Internet also provides youth with easy access to potentially harmful content (e.g., pro-eating disorder sites) and parents for the most part are in the dark about such sites. A first step is to educate parents so they can more effectively monitor their teen's use of such sites. We also need to understand how we can most effectively combat the potentially harmful and normalizing effects that such content can have on youth. Finally, the Internet can help to deliver low-cost interventions targeting youth for health-related goals such as weight modification or smoking cessation, but we need more research to identify the particular program features that will ensure long-term changes in behavior.

References

Alpert, J., & Hajaj, N. (2008). *We knew the web was big. . .* [web log]. Retrieved November 2009 from http://googleblog.blogspot.com/2008/07/we-knew-web-was-big.html

Bardone-Cone, A. M., & Cass, K. M. (2006). Investigating the impact of pro-anorexia websites: A pilot study. *European Eating Disorders Review, 14,* 256–262.

Borzekowski, D. L. G. (2006). Adolescents' use of the Internet: A controversial, coming-of-age resource. *Adolescent Medicine Clinics, 17,* 205–216.

Borzekowski, D. L. G., Fobil, J. N., & Asante, K. O. (2006). Online access by adolescents in Accra: Ghanaian teens' use of the Internet for health information. *Developmental Psychology, 42,* 450–458.

Borzekowski, D. L. G., & Rickert, V. I. (2001). Adolescents, the Internet, and health: Issues of access and content. *Journal of Applied Developmental Psychology, 22,* 49–59.

Buller, D. B., Borland, R., Woodall, W. G., Hall, J. R., Hines, J. M., Burris-Woodall, P., et al. (2006). Randomized trials on consider this, a tailored, Internet-delivered smoking prevention program for adolescents. *Health Education Behavior, 35,* 260–281.

Carpenter, E. M., Frankel, F., Marina, M., Duan, N., & Smalley, S. L. (2004). Internet treatment delivery of parent-adolescent conflict training for families with an ADHD teen: A feasibility study. *Child and Family Behavior Therapy, 26,* 1–20.

Chesley, E. B., Alberts, J. D., Klein, J. D., & Kreipe, R. E. (2003). Pro or con? Anorexia nervosa and the Internet. *Journal of Adolescent Health, 32,* 123–124.

Cole, J. I., Suman, M., Schramm, P., Zhou, L., Salvador, A., Chung, J. E., et al. (2008). *World Internet project: International report 2009.* Los Angeles, CA: Center for the Digital Future, USC Annenberg.

Davis, J. (2008). Pro-anorexia sites – A patient's perspective. *Child and Adolescent Mental Health, 13,* 97–97.

Doyle, A. C., Goldschmidt, A., Huang, C., Winzelberg, A. J., Taylor, C. B., & Wilfley, D. E. (2008). Reduction of overweight and eating disorder symptoms via the Internet in adolescents: A randomized controlled trial. *Journal of Adolescent Health, 43,* 172–179.

Eastin, M. S. (2001). Credibility assessments of online health information: The effects of source expertise and knowledge of content. *Journal of Computer-Mediated Communication, 6,* 0–0. From http://dx.doi.org/10.1111/j.1083-6101.2001.tb00126.x

Eysenbach, G. (2008). Credibility of health information and digital media: New perspectives and implications for youth. In M. J. Metzger & A. J. Flanagin (Eds.), *Digital media, youth, and credibility* (pp. 123–154). Cambridge, MA: MIT Press.

Gilbert, L. K., Temby, J. R. E., & Rogers, S. E. (2005). Evaluating a teen STD prevention web site. *Journal of Adolescent Health, 37,* 236–242.

Gray, N. J., & Klein, J. D. (2006). Adolescents and the Internet: Health and sexuality information. *Current Opinion in Obstetrics and Gynecology, 18,* 519–524.

Gray, N. J., Klein, J. D., Cantrill, J. A., & Noyce, P. R. (2002). Adolescent girls' use of the Internet for health information: Issues beyond access. *Journal of Medical Systems, 26,* 545–553.

Gray, N. J., Klein, J. D., Noyce, P. R., Sesselberg, T. S., & Cantrill, J. A. (2005). Health information-seeking behaviour in adolescence: The place of the Internet. *Social Science & Medicine, 60,* 1467–1478.

Greenfield, P. M., & Yan, Z. (2006). Children, adolescents, and the Internet: A new field of inquiry in developmental psychology. *Developmental Psychology, 42*, 391–394.

Hansen, D. L., Derry, H. A., Resnick, P. J., & Richardson, C. R. (2003). Adolescents searching for health information on the Internet: An observational study. *Journal of Medical Internet Research, 5*, e25.

Hesse, B. W., Nelson, D. E., Kreps, G. L., Croyle, R. T., Arora, N. K., Rimer, B. K., et al. (2005). Trust and sources of health information the impact of the Internet and its implications for health care providers: Findings from the first health information national trends survey. *Archives of Internal Medicine, 165*, 2618–2624.

Kyngas, H., Mikkonen, R., Nousiainen, E. M., Rytilahti, M., Seppanen, P., Vaattovaara, R., et al. (2001). Coping with the onset of cancer: Coping strategies and resources of young people with cancer. *European Journal of Cancer Care, 10*, 6–11.

Lenhart, A., Rainie, L., & Lewis, O. (2001). *Teenage life online: The rise of the instant-message generation and the Internet's impact on friendships and family relationships.* Washington, DC: Pew Internet & American Life Project.

Patten, C. A., Croghan, I. T., Meis, T. M., Decker, P. A., Pingree, S., Colligan, R. C., et al. (2006). Randomized clinical trial of an Internet-based versus brief office intervention for adolescent smoking cessation. *Patient Education and Counseling, 64*, 249–258.

Rideout, V. (2001). *Generation rx.Com: How young people use the Internet for health information.* Retrieved December 18, 2008, from http://www.kff.org/entmedia/upload/Toplines.pdf

Roberts, D. F., Foehr, U. G., & Rideout, V. (2005). *Generation m: Media in the lives of 8–18 year-olds – Report.* Retrieved December 16, 2008, from http://www.kff.org/entmedia/7251.cfm

Schepis, T. S., Marlowe, D. B., & Forman, R. F. (2008). The availability and portrayal of stimulants over the Internet. *The Journal of Adolescent Health, 42*, 458–465.

Skinner, H., Biscope, S., Poland, B., & Goldberg, E. (2003). How adolescents use technology for health information: Implications for health professionals from focus group studies. *Journal of Medical Internet Research, 5*, e32.

Suzuki, L. K., & Beale, I. L. (2006). Personal web home pages of adolescents with cancer: Self-presentation, information dissemination, and interpersonal connection. *Journal of Pediatric Oncology Nursing, 23*, 152–161.

Suzuki, L. K., & Calzo, J. P. (2004). The search for peer advice in cyberspace: An examination of online teen bulletin boards about health and sexuality. *Journal of Applied Developmental Psychology, 25*, 685–698.

Thompson, D., Baranowski, T., Cullen, K., & Watson, K. (2007). Food, fun and fitness Internet program for girls: Influencing log-on rate. *Health Education Research, 23*, 228–237.

Thompson, D. I., Baranowski, T., Cullen, K. W., & Watson, K. (2008). Food, fun and fitness internet program for girls: Influencing log-on rate. *Health Education Research, 23*, 228–237.

Whitlock, J. L., Powers, J. L., & Eckenrode, J. (2006). The virtual cutting edge: The Internet and adolescent-self-injury. *Developmental Psychology, 42*, 407–417.

Williamson, D. A., Martin, P. D., White, M. A., Newton, R. W., Walden, H., York-Crowe, E., et al. (2005). Efficacy of an Internet-based behavioral weight loss program for overweight adolescent African-American girls. *Eating and Weight Disorders, 10*, 193–203.

Wilson, J. L., Peebles, R., Hardy, K. K., & Litt, I. F. (2006). Surfing for thinness: A pilot study of pro-eating disorder web site usage in adolescents with eating disorders. *Pediatrics, 118*, e1635–e1643.

Winzelberg, A. (1997). The analysis of an electronic support group for individuals with eating disorders. *Computers in Human Behavior, 13*, 393–407.

Chapter 9
When Is It Too Much? Excessive Internet Use and Addictive Behavior

As young people are living enmeshed in technology, the issue of extreme use and dependence on these newer tools is one that we must address. Consider the case of "Jamie," a 16-year British college student described by Griffiths, who interviewed him face-to-face as well as online (Griffiths, 2000a). Jamie's parents were divorced and he was an only child, living with his mother. According to Griffiths, Jamie spent about 70 h/week on the computer, including two 12-h sessions on weekends. Jamie described himself as "sci-fi mad" and reported spending hours in Usenet discussions on the TV program "Star Trek." Preoccupied with the Internet, Jamie stated that it was the most important activity in his life and that it was on his mind even when he was offline. He reported that the Internet seemed to influence his mood, either exciting him or calming him down and described having withdrawal symptoms when he could not go online. He had difficulty controlling the time he spent online and his efforts to cut back on his Internet activities were futile as he found "the lure of cyberspace too strong to resist" (p. 213). He also could not limit the time he spent offline in front of the computer (he used a non-permanent modem connection in 2000), and upgraded his computer 11 times in 2 years. He described his computer use in this way: "I log on literally until I am physically unplugged by someone else ... I can't work or live without it – my social and intellectual life are linked directly to it" (p. 213).

Because of such intense Internet use, Jamie's sleeping patterns suffered and he even missed his college classes at times when he overslept. Once when he attempted to stop his Internet use, he was able to resist going online for only 3 days. Jamie reported that he had no friends outside his online life and used the Internet to socialize and meet people. Interestingly, he denied having a problem with his Internet use and did not consider himself addicted to the Internet. Although we find such excessive Internet use among all age groups, it is especially prevalent among adolescents and emerging adults (Šmahel, Sevcikova, Blinka, & Vesela, 2009b; Tsai & Lin, 2003).

We begin the chapter by examining whether we can use the term "addiction" in the context of Internet users and describing what addictive behavior on the Internet entails. Then we discuss the prevalence of addictive behavior among adolescents, highlighting that as a group they are the most at risk for online addictions. Next,

K. Subrahmanyam, D. Šmahel, *Digital Youth*, Advancing Responsible
Adolescent Development, DOI 10.1007/978-1-4419-6278-2_9,
© Springer Science+Business Media, LLC 2011

we discuss the symptoms considered to be red flags for Internet-related addictive behavior and describe the personal and social context of addictive behavior on the Internet. A separate section describes the four areas of online addictions, which have been the topic of the most research: online gaming, online relationships (communication), virtual sexual behavior, and online gambling. Finally, we describe the therapeutic approaches used to treat addictive behavior on the Internet.

Is the Term "Addiction" Applicable to Internet Use?

A casual examination of Jamie's case suggests that his Internet use was excessive, as it seemed to be affecting other aspects of his life. In fact, some of his symptoms, such as his withdrawal difficulties, are reminiscent of those experienced by individuals addicted to nicotine, alcohol, and other substances. Even though we see the term "Internet addiction" used to describe such excessive online activities, mental health experts disagree as to whether "addiction to the Internet" exists, even calling to question the use of the term "addiction" in the context of Internet use. In June 2007, the American Medical Association discouraged the American Psychiatric Association from including "Internet Addiction Disorder" as a formal diagnosis in the next edition of the DSM (Diagnostic and Statistical Manual of Mental Disorders) and did not recommend categorizing "video game addiction" as a serious mental disorder (Grohol, 2007). According to Grohol (2005), it is not clear whether Internet addiction results from/or is a cause of certain life issues, and whether it is a problem in itself or a manifestation of other illnesses; most people who consider themselves "addicted to the Internet" likely have difficulty solving conflicts and problems in their lives. He warns that much of the early research on addictive behavior on the Internet was explorative and did not address causal relationships and so is speculative at best. Others, such as British psychologist, Mark Griffiths (Griffiths, 2000a, 2000b, 2000c, 2001a, 2001b), use the term "addiction" to describe the overuse of the Internet as such use displays the characteristic properties of other addictions, including substance addictions. Griffiths argues that Jamie, the male teenager described earlier, showed symptoms characteristic of other addictions such as salience, mood modification, tolerance, withdrawal symptoms, conflict, and relapse.

Young, who has done seminal work on this topic, has described Internet addiction "as any online-related, compulsive behavior which interferes with normal living and causes severe stress on family, friends, loved ones, and one's work environment." Internet addiction has been called Internet dependence and Internet compulsivity (Young, 1998a, 1998b). The key element is that the excessive Internet use completely dominates the addict's life. Researchers who disagree with the characterization of such excessive behavior as "Internet addiction" have instead used other terms such as "addictive behavior," "dependence," "high engagement," "compulsive behavior," "excessive use," and "problematic use" (Beard & Wolf, 2001; Beard, 2005; Charlton & Danforth, 2004; Goldsmith & Shapira 2006; Morahan-Martin & Schumacher, 2003; Morahan-Martin, 2005; Shapira, Goldsmith, Keck, Khosla, & McElroy, 2000).

There is also the question of whether we should distinguish between "addiction on the Internet" and "addiction to the Internet" (Griffiths, 2000c; Widyanto & Griffiths, 2007). "Addiction on the Internet" implies that the Internet is merely an environment within which a deeper and original problems play out. In the absence of the Internet, it is likely that the problem will manifest itself in other ways. In this case, the Internet might even be considered a relatively safe environment for the problem to emerge in, as opposed to it taking the form of more risky symptoms or behaviors, such as drug use, self harm, or anorexia (Šmahel, 2003). In contrast, "addiction to the Internet" implies that the behavior of concern would not have shown up in any other context (Griffiths, 2000b; Widyanto & Griffiths, 2007). That is, the Internet and its various forums create environments that allow people to do things, they would not do elsewhere (e.g., cybersex, cyber stalking) (Griffiths, 2000b).

Clearly, there is the need for further research to determine whether the extremes of Internet use represent the characteristic symptoms of a "real addiction." In light of these issues, we use the term "addictive behavior on the Internet," to characterize excessive Internet use, without presuming that the Internet itself is the originator of this addictive behavior. Given the current state of research, we concur that the term "Internet addiction" does not apply to Internet users. However, for the sake of consistency, we adopt the particular terms used by the authors when describing their research, including the term "Internet addiction."

Prevalence of Addictive Behavior on the Internet

To get a handle on the problem of addictive behavior among youth in online contexts, we examine how prevalent it actually is among adolescents and emerging adults. We will also discuss if and why youth may be the most at-risk in terms of addictive behavior. Here we only provide general prevalence statistics on online addiction; statistics concerning specific applications (e.g., online games) can be found in the sections that address addiction to those applications.

Because rates of addictive behavior on the Internet are very variable across contexts, we present prevalence rates separately by country. In the USA, Morahan-Martin and Schumacher surveyed 277 US undergraduate Internet users and identified 8.1% of the sample as pathological users, who showed at least four of six symptoms of pathological Internet use (Morahan-Martin & Schumacher, 2000). Pathological Internet users spent an average of 8.5 h on the Internet weekly. While the average hours spent on the Internet seem low, in fact, the authors argued that it was indicative of problems surfacing during short periods of being on the Internet. Pathological users accessed the Internet more to play interactive games, meet new people for emotional support, and behaved in a more uninhibited way. Troublingly, there is a dearth of information about prevalence rates among US adolescents and at the time of writing, we could not find more recent estimates as well as estimates of addiction among adolescents in the USA. In contrast, as we will see next, there has been more research on this topic in Asian countries such as China and Taiwan, perhaps reflecting the urgency created by news stories about Internet cafes in these countries, filled with mostly young males, eyes glued to the screen, immersed in online games (Macartney, 2008).

Among Chinese adolescents, Cao and Su (2007) found 2.4% of their sample ($n = 2,620$) 12- to 18-year olds of adolescent Internet users to be addicted. Addicted Internet users spent an average of 11 h/week compared to 3 h/week spent by the non-addicted group. Interestingly, addicted users were much more likely to be male (83%) than female (17%). This is different from studies in the USA and Europe, where no gender differences have typically been found (e.g., Johansson & Gotestam, 2004; Šmahel et al., 2009b).

Within the European context, Johansson and Götestam (2004) surveyed 3,237 Norwegian youth, between 12- and 18 years of age. They used Young's Diagnostic Questionnaire (1998c) and found that 2% of the youth had "Internet addiction," and 8.7% were at-risk for excessive Internet use. Forward regression analyses with Internet addiction as the dependent variable showed significant values for extent of Internet use and type of online activities. Individuals in the addictive behavior group reported greater frequency and time online; these individuals also reported greater use of discussion groups, reading/sending e-mail, playing games, buying and ordering goods and services, and reading newspapers and magazines. The researchers did not find a relation between demographic variables (age, gender, geography and social background variables such as schooling, work, and domicile type) and addictive behavior on the Internet.

There is a general perception that young people are at greater risk for addictive behavior on the Internet compared to adults and so it is important to actually compare addiction prevalence or addiction scores between adolescents, emerging adults, and adults. We did such a comparison using the data from questions on online addictive behavior that were a part of the World Internet Project in the Czech Republic (Šmahel et al., 2009b). We collected the data in September 2008 from 2,215 respondents ages 12 and up using face-to-face interviews. The data set had two parts; the original sample was representative of the Czech population and consisted of 1,520 respondents, who were 12 and older and the second sample consisted of 695 respondents aged 12–30 years. The questions on online addictive behavior measured five dimensions based on Griffiths (2000a, 2000c), Beard and Wolf (2001) and Beard (2005): (1) cognitive and behavioral salience, (2) tolerance, (3) positive and negative mood change, (4) conflict aspects, (5) time aspects – unsuccessful attempts to cut down time on Internet use. Two groups were created according to the following criteria: Group A (addictive behavior on the Internet) – all five dimensions had to be present and Group B (at risk for addictive behavior on the Internet) – conflict and at least three other factors had to be present.

Four percent of Czech Internet users demonstrated all symptoms of addictive behavior on the Internet (Group A) and 8.6% of Internet users were at risk for online addictive behavior (Šmahel et al., 2009b). Figure 9.1 shows the age trends in prevalence of addictive behavior on the Internet among Internet users. Addictive behavior on the Internet was most prevalent among 12- to 15-year-olds (8% showed all symptoms of addictive behavior), followed by 20- to 26-year olds (5.3%). The groups with addictive behavior symptoms decrease sharply with age and among Internet

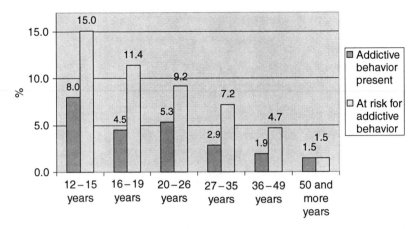

Fig. 9.1 Prevalence rate (in percentage) of addictive behavior on the Internet as a function of age (2008 Czech WIP data)

users 36 years old and up, less than 2% exhibit all addictive symptoms. Furthermore, the slope of the line for the group at risk for addictive behavior was steep and the number of at-risk adolescents and emerging adults was very high. Keeping in mind that Fig. 9.1 includes only data from Internet users and Internet usage decreases with age, the actual risk for younger individuals relative to the rest of the population, particularly adults, is probably even greater. Interestingly, there were no gender differences in the rate of addictive behavior on the Internet. For youth (12- to 19-year olds), time online was associated with increased risk: those who exhibited all symptoms of addictive behavior (Group A) reported using the Internet at home for an average of 15.1 h/week compared to 9.8 h reported by adolescents who were not at risk.

One reason for the higher prevalence rates of addictive behavior among youth may be the presence of conflict more generally in their lives. Figure 9.2 suggests that adolescents in three countries (Chile, Sweden and the Czech Republic) (Šmahel, Vondrackova, Blinka, & Godoy-Etcheverry, 2009c) were more likely to report having conflict over their Internet use compared to emerging and older adults. According to some researchers, conflict concerning Internet use may be the most important dimension of addictive behavior (Beard & Wolf, 2001). Thus, its increased presence during adolescence may be responsible for the greater likelihood of addictive behavior in this age group.

Identifying Youth Who May Be Addicted to the Internet

An important step to understanding addictive online behavior is identifying youth whose online activities might be excessive and pathological. To assess addictive behavior on the Internet, Young designed a brief questionnaire (Young, 1995, 1998b, 1998c) based on the criteria for pathological gambling in offline contexts, which was

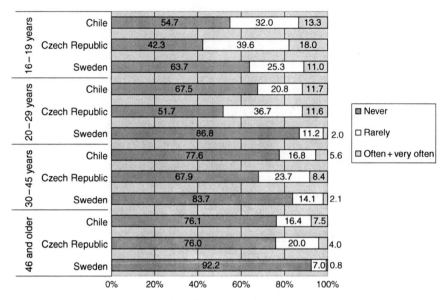

Fig. 9.2 Percent of respondents who reported on the conflict over Internet use with family, friends, and partners as a function of age in Chile, Czech Republic and Sweden (2008 WIP data)

classified as an impulse control disorder in the DSM-IV. Findings from this short questionnaire were then used to develop the 20-item Internet Addiction Test (IAT), which is available at the web site for the Center for Internet Addiction Recovery directed by Young (1998a).

Based on the general criteria of the DSM-IV, Griffiths (2000a, 2000b, 2000c) and Widyanto & Griffiths, (2007) have proposed the following six basic components of addictive behavior on the Internet (Griffiths, 2000a), which have informed questionnaires used with adolescents (i.e. Ko, Yen, Chen, Chen, & Yen, 2005; Lemmens, Valkenburg, & Peter, 2009; Šmahel et al., 2009b):

(1) Salience: When an online activity becomes the most importan in an individual's life and dominates cognitive and emotional processes and behavior
(2) Mood modification: When the online activity influences the Internet user's subjective experiences
(3) Tolerance: An ongoing process, wherein larger and larger "doses" of the online activity are required to experience the original mood
(4) Withdrawal symptoms: Negative feelings and emotions follow the termination of or inability to conduct an online activity
(5) Conflict: Interpersonal (mostly with family and friends) or intrapersonal conflict is caused by the online activities
(6) Relapse: A tendency to relapse and go back to addicted behavior even after periods of relative control.

Griffiths suggests that an individual is addicted only if all components are present. For instance, in five case studies, Griffiths (2000a) showed that when individuals exhibit only a few of the dimensions, excessive use was purely symptomatic and that the Internet may have been used to counteract other problem areas, such as problems in relationships, concerns about physical appearance, disability, and so on. For this reason, a high score in some questionnaires (without all components present) may not really indicate that an Internet user is "addicted," but rather that their excessive use is symptomatic of other underlying issues. Psychologists and counselors should be careful when using questionnaires such as Young's, which do not distinguish between "addiction" and "excessive use."

The above criteria for diagnosing addictive behavior on the Internets are general, and are common to adults, emerging adults and adolescents. But for diagnosing addictive behavior on the Internets among adolescents, we believe that the criteria should be modified since many of the current criteria are based on negative family dynamics such as conflicts surrounding Internet use, complaints made by close family members, (such as parents), lying to family members, etc. As Fig. 9.2 showed, conflict between adolescents and their parents is relatively common during adolescence and is often present in some form or the other, regardless of the extent to which a teen may use the Internet. Thus, current questionnaires may overestimate the addiction scores of adolescents and we should use them with caution.

In an attempt to create special diagnostic criteria for adolescents, researchers in Taiwan (Ko et al., 2005) surveyed 468 adolescents between 12- and 19 years of age. Respondents completed the questionnaire on Internet addiction (CIAS) and seven psychiatrists used a diagnostic interview to assess for addictive behavior on the Internet. The results revealed 13 diagnostic criteria, divided into three groups (Ko et al., 2005):

(A) *Maladaptive pattern of Internet use*: Leads to clinically significant impairment or distress, and occurring at any time within the same 3-month period. Six (or more) of the following symptoms have to be present:

1. Preoccupation with Internet activities
2. Recurrent failure to resist the impulse to use the Internet
3. Tolerance: a marked increase in the duration of Internet use needed to achieve satisfaction
4. Withdrawal, as manifested by either of the following:

    i. Symptoms of dysphoric mood, anxiety, irritability, and boredom after several days without Internet activity
    ii. Use of the Internet to relieve or avoid withdrawal symptoms

5. Use of the Internet for longer than intended
6. Persistent desire and/or unsuccessful attempts to cut down or reduce Internet use
7. Excessive time spent on Internet activities
8. Excessive effort spent on activities necessary to obtain access to the Internet

9. Continued heavy Internet use despite knowledge of having a persistent or recurrent physical or psychological problem likely to have been caused or exacerbated by Internet use

(B) *Functional impairment*: One (or more) of the following symptoms have to be present:

1. Recurrent Internet use resulting in a failure to fulfill major role-related obligations at school and home
2. Internet use results in impairment of social relationships
3. Internet use leads to behavior that violates school rules or laws

(C) *Not explained by any other psychiatric condition*: The addictive behavior on the Internet cannot be accounted for by a psychotic disorder or bipolar I disorder.

Given the complexity entailed in diagnosing addictive behavior on the Internet, Beard and Wolf (2001) recommend that "diagnosis should be based on the extensive clinical interview and the results of any testing that was completed. The clinician should be able to see whether the information obtained fits the suggested criteria to diagnose Internet addiction" (p. 379). We echo their sentiments with regard to the need for caution when evaluating addiction among adolescents, and stress the importance of using a clinical interview to diagnose addictive behavior on the Internet.

Correlates of Addictive Behavior on the Internet

Research suggests that adolescents with addictive behavior on the Internet also have problems in other aspects of their lives such as in their academics (a drop in grades, avoiding school), family relations (conflicts and having to hide their excessive Internet use from parents), physical health (sleep deprivation) mental health (depression), and finances (Internet expenses), substance abuse, and cyber bullying (Chou, Condron, & Belland, 2005; Griffiths, 2000a; Ko et al., 2006; Kraut et al., 1998; Kubey, Lavin, & Barrows, 2001; Tsai & Lin, 2003; Young, 1998a). In one survey of 576 college students (mean age = 20.25 years), about 9% of participants reported that they may be psychologically dependent on the Internet; although there were no age effects, males were more likely to be "dependent" and 14% of the students reported that their schoolwork had been hurt due to Internet use (Kubey et al., 2001). Heavier Internet use was highly correlated with impaired academic performance. Self-reported Internet dependence and impaired academic performance were both associated with greater use of all Internet applications, but was strongest among those who used chat rooms and MUDs (textual virtual worlds).

Substance use is another problem behavior that has been associated with addictive behavior on the Internet. Ko and colleagues surveyed 3,662 Taiwanese junior and senior high school students, who ranged in the age from 11- to 21 years (Ko et al., 2006). Participants completed the Tridimensional Personality Questionnaire

(TPQ), the Chen Addiction Scale, and the Questionnaires for Experience in Substance Use. Adolescents with higher Internet addiction scores were more likely to report substance use. Addictive behavior was associated with high novelty seeking, high harm avoidance and low reward dependence; high novelty seeking, low harm avoidance and low reward dependence predicted greater levels of substance use. The authors concluded that adolescents with high novelty seeking scores and low reward dependence scores should be provided with strategies for preventing Internet addiction and substance use.

The association between Internet addiction and substance use is similar to that of cyber bullying and substance use (i.e. Hinduja & Patchin, 2007), which we address in the next chapter. Czech data from the World Internet Project reveals a similar moderate correlation between cyber bullying and two components of addictive behavior, conflict, and salience (Šmahel, Blinka, & Sevcikova, 2009a). Cao and Su's study (2007) of Chinese 12- to 18-year olds revealed that participants who displayed symptoms of addictive behavior on the Internet scored higher on subscales of neuroticism, psychosis, lying, emotional symptoms, conduct problems, hyperactivity, and overall difficulties. The Internet addiction group also scored lower on the subscales of sense of control over time, sense of value of time, sense of time efficacy and pro-social behavior. Together, these results provide further evidence that problems in young people's offline and online lives may be related to each other. Indeed, it appears that offline and online problem behaviors among teens such as substance abuse and excessive Internet use may be interconnected and may even be indicative of deeper psychological and emotional difficulties.

Not surprisingly, family variables such as satisfaction, economic status, parents' marital status, and household alcohol use, are also related to online addiction (Yen, Yen, Chen, Chen, & Ko, 2007). Yen and colleagues report that higher parent-adolescent conflict, habitual alcohol use by siblings, perceived positive parental attitude to adolescent substance use, and lower family functioning were related to Internet addiction. Internet addiction and substance abuse share similar family factors indicating that both may be subsumed under problem behavioral syndromes.

Common Areas of Online Addictive Behavior

In the next sections, we discuss four common areas of online addictive behavior that may be the most problematic aspects of excessive Internet use among youth: (1) online gaming, (2) online relationships (communication), (3) virtual sexual behavior, and (4) online gambling.

Online Games and Addictive Behavior

According to the results of the Pew Internet Project, 97% of US teens play computer, web, hand-held, or console games, 50% played games yesterday, and 80% played five or more different game genres (Lenhart et al., 2008). Playing computer games seems to be a generally widespread activity among adolescents in developed countries. In the WIP data, online games were played by 59–87% of 12- to 18-year-old Internet users (see Fig. 1.6 in Chapter 1). Online gaming thus has a central place in young people's online lives and is also prominent in the context of excessive Internet use; the issue of violence and online gaming is examined separately in Chapter 10.

Here we focus on one kind of online games, Massively Multiplayer Online Role-Playing Games, described earlier in Chapter 1, as research on addiction has mostly focused on this gaming environment. Research indicates that MMORPG and MMO games have substantial potential to create game "addictive behavior" among many of their players (e.g., Rau, Peng, & Yang, 2006; Wan & Chiou, 2006a, 2006b). We start with a case study illustrating addictive behavior in the context of online games; then we discuss player characteristics and game features that are relevant to excessive online gaming.

Consider the case of a 11-year-old British male, Martin, who had problems with playing MMORPGs (Wood, 2008, p. 173):

> Martin is an only child who did not have many friends, at least not in the "real" world and he spent most of his spare time playing the massively multiplayer online role playing game (MMORPG) World of Warcraft. Martin enjoyed playing his game and explained how he enjoyed the various adventures that he was involved in with his gaming friends. Martin was concerned that his parents were trying to stop him from playing as they thought he was "addicted" to the game. He admitted that he did play as much as he could and was happiest when he was playing. However, Martin confided that he was being bullied at school and hated going there. His game playing was his way of coping with the experience, and it allowed him to socialize without going outside and possibly being bullied again. He had not told anyone else about the bullying. His parents noticed his reluctance to go to school, that his teachers were concerned about his performance, and that he was spending so much time on his own in his room playing his game. They believed that the game was the cause of his problems and were threatening to take it away from him. Martin was distraught, not only was he getting bullied, his only escape from the reality of his existence was being threatened. If Martin could not play online with his friends he felt that he would have nothing enjoyable left in his life.

Wood notes that parents frequently focus on the time spent on game playing and treat it as a problem, but do not realize that it is a social activity for youth (Wood, 2008). At times, the root cause of the gaming lies elsewhere, and in Maritn's case, offline school bullying was the underlying issue.

One thing that is becoming clear is that for youth online gamers, MMORPGs are a very significant part of their life, at least in terms of time spent on it. Griffiths and his colleagues have established that the average time of play is about 2 years for adolescents (20 years and below) and 2 years and 3 months for older players (Griffiths, Davies, & Chappell, 2004). Youth also play MMORPGs more intensively (26 h weekly) than young adults (20–22 h weekly among players above 26 years). The average age of MMORPG players probably falls in the period of emerging adulthood, the typical age being around 25 years (Šmahel, Blinka, & Ledabyl, 2008; Yee, 2006). Men represent almost 90% of players and it is interesting that the average age of female players is higher (32 years) (Yee, 2006). Griffiths also found a more even gender distribution among older players whereas there were more males among younger players (Griffiths et al., 2004).

With regard to the incidence of addiction in online games, we turn to a study based on a world wide online sample of 548 players of MMORPGs (World of Warcraft and Everquest) (Šmahel et al., 2008), respondents' online addictive behavior score was assessed based on the work by Griffiths (2000c). We asked several questions related to the symptoms of the five factors of addictive behavior and calculated an addiction score. Our results showed that 5.5% of online players had a very high addiction score and 26.5% of participants had a high addiction score (Šmahel et al., 2008). Adolescents and emerging adults (up to 26 years) scored significantly higher in addictive behavior compared to older players (the difference between adolescents and emerging adults was not significant). Respondents with a low addiction score reported spending less than 20 h/week playing the game, whereas those with a very high addiction score reported spending an average of 41 h/week playing the game. The most problematic group included those with a high addiction score, but who at the same time did not consider themselves as addicted to playing: this corresponded to 6% of players in our study. These players had symptoms of addictive behavior, yet claimed that they were not addicted. In contrast, 45% of all players considered themselves addicted to the game, but over half of them displayed a low addiction score. With regard to self-perceived addiction measures, it is also possible that the youth in this study were saying, "I am addicted to something" (i.e. sport) simply as a fashion statement.

The social dimensions of MMORPGs are important with regard to their potential for addictive behavior (Wan & Chiou, 2006b). Players typically play in groups, join so-called "guilds" and communicate a lot with each when playing. Cooperation with other players is common and often required if someone wants to be successful in the game. This group-oriented environment found in MMORPGs corresponds to adolescents' and emerging adults' need to create and become members of groups (Bee, 1994; Dunphy, 1963). In contrast to girls, adolescent boys may feel compelled to compare themselves and measure strength as well as to increase their self-esteem and self-efficacy (e.g., Macek, 2003). MMORPGs entail such measuring of power and the urge to gain a good position in the rankings of the group. It is interesting that young adult males immerse themselves in MMORPGs – developmentally we would expect individuals in emerging adulthood to have less of a need to compare themselves in groups and measure their strength in virtual games, but this is not the case, and is deserving of more research.

It is also possible that playing online games will imbue players with an increased sense of self-efficacy, increasing their motivation to play fantasy role-playing games with consequences for addictive behavior. Wan and Chiou interviewed 10 adolescent Taiwanese players, who spent more than 48 h/week playing MMORPGs (Wan & Chiou, 2006b); using a psychoanalytical perspective, they speculated that the games offered players an environment with lower social control, so they did not have to hide behind defense mechanisms. On the contrary, they may have gained a feeling of control over events through their game character and fulfilled their need for self-presentation. However, if the adolescent gamer did not feel as powerful in the physical world, the self-efficacy, gained by the virtual character could make the individual fixated on the game, ultimately spiraling into some form of game addiction. Based on a case study of an 18-year-old hospitalized player, Allison and colleagues proposed a similar mechanism of addiction. They suggest that his excessive play sessions, which could last up to 18 h a day, were mostly a solution to his problems with self-esteem and social drawbacks (Allison, von Wahlde, Shockley, & Gabbard, 2006). The online character of this player was a "shaman capable of reviving the dead and calling lightning," which allowed him to create a full-fledged self in the game and helped to compensate for other deficits; for instance, although he had social phobias offline, he successfully socialized in the game. Both of the above mechanisms are speculative and based on a few subjects (10 interviews and a single case study). We need more research to understand whether the allure of online games helps gamers compensate for offline deficits and difficulties, and thus leading to excessive playing of online games.

We also need more research to understand the characteristics of youth who may be at risk for addictive behavior on the Internet. Among Canadian adolescents, it was found that emotional intelligence was a strong to moderate predictor of online gaming addiction, and of online gambling problems (Parker, Taylor, Eastabrook, Schell, & Wood, 2008). Youth with deficiencies in the ability to read, express, and elicit desired emotions may be more prone to partake in online-addiction-behaviors. In this study emotional intelligence and addictive behavior on the Internet were correlated for young adolescents ($r = -0.38$). The researchers also suggest that addictive behavior on the Internet, gaming, and gambling may be etiologically linked and might not be three separate phenomena.

Cyber Relationship Addictive Behavior

As the reader is aware, the Internet provides a variety of opportunities for people to meet and interact with others. The at-times anonymous character of online communication, which was especially true in the early years of the Internet, supports a quick exchange of personal information of an intimate nature and may even create an emotional bond of sorts between the communicating participants. Consequently users may be drawn to online communication and may even perceive a sense of social support, something that perhaps they feel is lacking in their offline lives (King, 1996; Young, 1997). Even youth who have good offline social relationships and use online communication tools to interact with offline friends, might find the instantaneous and seemingly 24/7 nature of such interactions appealing, and spend inordinate amounts of time interacting with online. Regardless of whether the communication partner is an online or offline partner, the issue here is the amount of time spent interacting and communicating. When time on such online communication intensifies to the point that an individual loses contact with other aspects of his/her life, we may consider the interaction as addictive behavior on the Internet.

An example of addiction to online communication is Becky, who began to create web pages when she was 15 years old (Hall & Parsons, 2001). After her parents divorced when she was 16, she started to isolate herself in online chat groups with other teens, whose parents were divorced. She felt that her online friends were more important than her school friends, and she started to spend almost all of her free time on the Internet with her online friends. Her off-line friends and schoolwork suffered from the excessive time she spent online. Becky's time spent online increased and she began faking illness to avoid school and to stay in front of the computer. Eventually Becky was in danger of not graduating with her senior class and it was at that time that her mother contacted a mental health counselor.

As with other kinds of problem behaviors, some characteristics of youth might heighten their risk for excessive online communication. Preliminary evidence suggests that addictive users may communicate more often than other online users. In one of the first studies on this topic, Young noted that non-addicted individuals (of all ages) most often use aspects of the Internet that allow them access to information, whereas users prone to online addictive behavior use applications that promote communication among users (Young, 1995, 1998c). Niemze et al. report that students ($n = 371$) inclined to addictive behavior on the Internet were friendlier and more open online compared to offline contexts; they have more friends on the Internet and share all their secrets with them (Niemz, Griffiths, & Banyard, 2005).

Loneliness is another user variable that may play a contributing role in excessive online communication. In the literature, there are two competing hypotheses regarding the relation between Internet use and loneliness: the first one proposes that Internet use leads to loneliness, while the second one states that lonely individuals are more likely to use the Internet in an excessive manner because of the expanded social networks provided in the online contexts (Morahan-Martin & Schumacher, 2003). Research by Kraut and colleagues on the first hypothesis was described earlier in Chapter 7 (Kraut et al., 1998, 2002). The second hypothesis presumes that loneliness is part of an individual's makeup (Morahan-Martin & Schumacher, 2003), an assumption that may not apply in all cases. Morahan-Martin and Schumacher's study on 277 undergraduate Internet users examined the relation between loneliness and Internet use and habits. Lonely individuals reported using the Internet more for emotional support, to meet new people, to interact with others, and behave online in a less inhibited way, and preferred online communication more, felt more open there, shared intimate secrets and stated that most of their friends were online friends. Lonely people also went online when they felt alone, depressed or anxious; they also more often reported developing Internet-related problems in their daily functioning. However, in their study of 699 youth, Leung (2002) obtained no significant relationship between loneliness and frequent online communication. The author suggests that online communication with friends is a popular activity among young people and may have little connection to loneliness, a claim for which we have little concrete evidence either way.

As we see, the outcomes of research concerning loneliness, online communication, and excessive Internet use are equivocal. Findings depend very much on the sample and the particular ways in which the authors defined addictive behavior. We think it is likely that loneliness is important as a risk factor in relation to addictive behavior to online communication because people who are lonely in the offline world may well have a greater tendency to seek interaction and social support online. We need more research to clarify the relation between online communication and addictive behavior on the Internet.

Sexual Compulsive Behavior and Sexual Addictive Behavior on the Internet

Similar to "Internet addiction," online sexual addiction is not an official category, but instead refers to recently emerging issues concerning excessive sexual behavior in online worlds. In the literature, terms such as "sexual addiction to the Internet" (Griffiths, 2001b) or "online sexually compulsive behavior" (Cooper, Putnam, Planchon, & Boies, 1999a) have been used to describe these behaviors. Online sexual compulsion can be viewed as preceding sexually addictive behavior on the Internet and compulsive behaviors online are most prevalent in adulthood and to a lesser extent in emerging adulthood. Currently, there is very little research on online addictive sexual behavior among adolescents and it is not clear to what extent adolescents engage in such addictive sexual behaviors. As described in Chapter 3, much of adolescent's online sexual behavior mostly takes the form of exploration and we therefore only provide a brief description of the characteristics of online sexual compulsive behavior, one that could help therapists and other clinicians in recognizing this type of behavior.

Cooper and colleagues (Cooper, Morahan-Martin, Mathy, & Maheu, 2002; Cooper et al., 1999a; Cooper, Scherer, Boies, & Gordon, 1999b) have defined sexually compulsive behavior as "an irresistible urge to perform irrational sexual behavior." This type of behavior is found among Internet users of different ages and gender and can be defined in terms of five basic characteristics.

(1) *Denial*: The individual underestimates or hides the sexual activity online.
(2) *Repeated unsuccessful discontinuation of this activity*: The individual tries repeatedly to cut down on sexual behavior but is not successful.
(3) *Excessive time*: The individual spends extreme amounts of time on online sexual activity/activities.
(4) *Negative effects of online sexual behavior*: The individual's online sexual activities lead to social, individual, and personal problems and conflicts.
(5) *Repeaing online sexual behavior:* The individual repeats the online sexual despite unfavorable consequences.

Cooper et al. (1999a) distinguish between three types of Internet users who are engaged in such online sexual activities. *Recreational and non-pathological users* satisfy their actual curiosity regarding available sexual materials, occasionally experimenting and thus satisfying their sexual needs. *Compulsive users* exhibit sexually compulsive traits and experience negative consequences because of their

activities. The Internet is just another domain for them in which to act out their problematic sexual behavior. Compulsive users may have already established patterns
of unconventional sexual practices, for example, preoccupation with pornography,
having multiple sexual encounters etc. Online sexual compulsivity develops in the
context of these other less typical activities. *Hazardous users* have no prior history of sexually compulsive behavior, but experience their first problems when
exploring the Internet. Cooper et al. (1999a) note that this latter group of users
are the most interesting because their problems may not have manifested without the Internet. The possible anonymity and accessibility of some Internet sexual
activities have "soaked them up" and altered their sexual behavior and habits. The
properties of the virtual environment seem to have provoked the manifestation of
sexually compulsive behavior and their addiction. Cooper describes the case of
Richard, a 20-year-old college student, who after accidentally getting exposed to
online pornography, developed compulsive patterns of masturbating while looking
at online pornography. As a result, he missed his school classes, withdrew from the
few friends he had, and developed a sleep disorder. His grades slipped, his depression increased, and he contacted a physician, who diagnosed him as depressive and
referred him to a psychologist. While we do not know the outcome of this case,
it certainly illustrates how accidental exposures might lead to addictions in people
without any prior history of unconventional sexual practices.

The groups most at risk are the second (Compulsive users) and third groups
(Hazardous users). Adolescents could probably be more often diagnosed in the third
group because their offline sexual behavior is not as developed as adults, and they
may have little to no experience with compulsive sexual behavior. The Internet, with
its potential for unintentional exposure, could be especially dangerous for them as
it could pave the way for the development of such compulsive behaviors.

Online Gambling

Gambling is defined as any activity in which an individual risks something of value
on the outcome of an uncertain event, whose results he or she does not have control
over (Cabot, 1999). In "online gambling", such activities occur on the Internet and
typically. Involves money, but individuals may also spend virtual currency in digital
worlds (e.g., the Linden Dollar in Second Life). The most typical forms of Internet
gambling are: online casinos, cards, sports pools, and the online lottery (Hardoon,
Derevensky, & Gupta, 2002; Manzin & Biloslavo, 2008). The issue of gambling and
online gambling is an important one and has law and policy implications that are
only tangentially relevant to this book. It can also be considered as risky behavior,
but because of its potential for addictive behavior, we briefly consider it in this
chapter.

From Fig. 9.3, we see that very few adolescents report gambling online. In the
WIP data, 2–4% of the respondents (12- to 18-year olds) reported that they gambled online weekly, at a rate that is considered as "regular gambling" (Hardoon

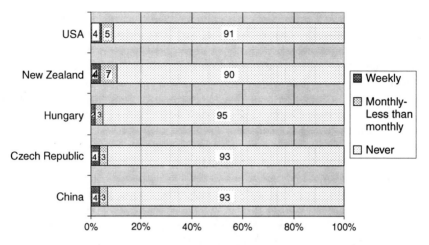

Fig. 9.3 Frequency of online betting/gambling among 12- to 18-year olds (WIP 2007 data)

et al., 2002). Similarly a 2001 survey of 2,336 11- to 19-year olds conducted in Ontario, Canada, revealed that 0.6% of adolescents gambled on the Internet regularly and 2.2% did so occasionally (Hardoon et al., 2002). In the same study, 66% of adolescents reported engaging in some type of gambling in the past year; the researchers determined that 4.9% of them were pathological gamblers and 8.0% were at risk gamblers. Because online gambling is relatively infrequent among adolescents and research is scarce, we do not know much about the impact or correlates of online gambling among youth who do so. However, we do know that pathological and at-risk youth gamblers report more problem behaviors. They were more likely to report a drug and/or alcohol problem for themselves, peers, and family members, have a learning disability, classify themselves as slow learners, have more family problems, and score higher in the clinical range assessing emotional problems (Hardoon et al., 2002). These correlates of gambling are very similar to those of addictive behavior on the Internet described earlier. Thus, it is very likely that youth who do gamble online will also report problems in other aspects of their lives.

Treatment of Addictive Behavior on the Internet

As the first mention of "Internet addiction" in the literature occurred only 14–15 years ago (Young, 1995, 1998c), clinicians, therapists, and researchers have had limited experience treating this new addictive behavior. Research evaluating the effectiveness of different treatments is even sparser. We also did not find any research that focused on treating adolescents. Here we describe treatment methods devised for the general population, although it is unclear whether we need strategies devised specifically for youth. In addition, since it is unclear whether an Internet user is addicted "to the Internet" per se, it is important to consider other potentially

problematic areas in the individual's life as well as the particular online application that is used excessively, and the environment within which addictive behavior
develops. Researchers generally agree that the goal of therapy is not to stop overall Internet use, but to interrupt the use of problematic applications, such as online
games, chat rooms, instant messengers, and sexual sites (Kim, 2007; Young, 2007).

Addictive behavior on the Internet can be treated using psychotherapy and also
pharmacotherapy administered by psychiatrists (Kim, 2007, 2008; Young, 2007).
Since pharmacotherapy is beyond the scope of this book, we focus on psychotherapy, and in particular, two treatment approaches that have been used for online
addictions: cognitive behavior therapy (Young, 1999, 2007) and reality therapy
(Kim, 2007, 2008).

Cognitive Behavioral Therapy

Cognitive behavioral therapy (CBT) is based on the premise that thoughts determine
feelings (Young, 1999, 2007) and entails training clients to monitor and identify
thoughts that trigger addictive actions and feelings. In the next step, the therapist
helps the client to develop new coping skills and ways to prevent addictive behavior
and possible relapse. CBT takes approximately 3 months and/or 12 weekly sessions
(Young, 2007).

CBT interventions help clients to limit the time spent online using the following
tools (Young, 1999): mapping the structure of the day and applying the opposite
structure, setting the goals of therapy, using external announcements (such as using
an alarm-clock to indicate that the time online is over), abstinence (if there is no
success in limiting time with dangerous applications, full abstinence could be used),
recommendation cards (write down the five biggest problems caused by Internet use
and stick it on the PC), and personal inventory (things or items that the user has cut
down on, or cut out, because of the time spent online). Young evaluated the effects of
cognitive behavior therapy on 114 clients (mean age for males = 38 years; mean age
of females = 46) and concluded that "upon 6-months follow-up, most clients were
able to maintain symptom management and continued recovery" (Young, 1999,
p. 677).

Reality Therapy

Reality therapy for Internet addiction is based on reality therapy as described by
Glasser (Glasser, 2000), and assumes that people are responsible for their lives, and
for what they do, feel, and think. It focuses on rational choices of behavior, which
can help Internet users to achieve their goal of limiting their Internet use. The program consists of 10 group sessions, described in detail in Kim (2007) and the reader
is referred to it to obtain more information about the treatment procedure. Kim also
evaluated the effects of reality therapy on a sample of 276 university students (2008)
and concluded that the "reality therapy group counseling program is very effective

to improve Internet addiction level of Internet addiction among University students and enhance their self-esteem related to Internet use" (p. 10).

Although there are only two main treatment therapy methods described in the current literature, practitioners can likely use other methods to treat adolescents' addictive behavior on the Internet. The first step for counselors and therapists is to understand a client's attraction to the Internet (Watson, 2005). If the addictive behavior has developed within the context of broader family problems, then marital or family therapy may be appropriate.

Conclusions

Addictive behavior on the Internet takes on many forms and has many labels such as, "excessive Internet use," "problematic Internet use", or simply "Internet addiction." Such excessive use is often accompanied by the symptoms associated with other addictions, such as preoccupations with a particular online application, withdrawal symptoms, and intrapersonal or interpersonal conflict. However, we do not believe that the empirical evidence justifies treating it as a clinical category and so concur with those who question whether we can really label excessive Internet use as "Internet addiction."

Regardless of whether problematic Internet use is a true addiction or not, parents should be concerned when the Internet becomes the single biggest activity in their teen's life. While spending long hours on the Internet alone is not indicative of addictive behavior, a red flag should be raised when the online activity interferes with other offline activities and creates conflict, such as when an adolescent neglects school because of Internet use, or when family relationships and offline friendships suffer due to Internet use. In these instances, it is important to identify the online activity, the particular needs that the activity may satisfy, and determine whether there might be any problems in other aspects of the teen's life. For example, excessive communication in teens when it comes to instant messengers or social networking sites may address their need for social support and contact (Niemz et al., 2005), but may also be the consequence of loneliness. Similarly, playing fantasy-based games (as many MMORPGs are) can both bestow power belonging in a peer and/or player group but can also provide an escape from the physical world to one based on fantasy.

Research to date has mostly looked at addictive online behavior as related to online games (MMORPGs), virtual relationships, and cybersex activities. Other types of applications may also be dangerous, such as P2P (peer to peer) networks for sharing and downloading files, gambling, auctions and online shopping sites that may also have financial impact (Young, 1998a, 1998c). Since there are so many different kinds of Internet applications that can lead to a variety of problematic uses, an understanding of the essence of addictive behavior is crucial. Is it a compensation for relationships in the real world? Alternatively, is it a way of nourishing a teen's self-esteem and self-efficacy? Such questions are often difficult for parents and teachers to answer, and we recommended referring adolescents prone to addictive Internet behavior to therapists or clinicians with experience treating excessive Internet use.

While we do not wish to downplay the dangers of online addictive behavior, our own anecdotal experiences suggest that extremes of Internet use may not always be harmful. In fact, one of us used to play MUDs while in college and several of his fellow students experienced all the previously described symptoms of addictive behavior, at times spending up to 14 h a day on the game. A very small number of them, who also had few offline relationships, eventually left school. However, for the rest, despite playing heavily for 4 or 5 years of their lives, the gaming ended up being just another phase in their lives. All of them now have jobs and families, live productive lives, mostly working as software programmers. Although there is no longitudinal research on online gamers, online applications are not drugs such as alcohol or cocaine, and the long-term influence of excessive Internet use may not be as serious as feared. Nonetheless, the effects of online addictive behavior should not be underestimated, and it is important to determine the reasons why an adolescent may be spending extreme amounts of time on any particular online activity. This is perhaps more important than the extreme levels of the activity itself.

References

Allison, S. E., von Wahlde, L., Shockley, T., & Gabbard, G. O. (2006). The development of the self in the era of the Internet and role-playing fantasy games. *The American Journal of Psychiatry, 163*, 381–385.

Beard, K. W. (2005). Internet addiction: A review of current assessment techniques and potential assessment questions. *CyberPsychology and Behavior, 8*, 7–14.

Beard, K. W., & Wolf, E. M. (2001). Modification in the proposed diagnostic criteria for Internet addiction. *CyberPsychology and Behavior, 4*, 377–383.

Bee, H. L. (1994). *Lifespan development*. New York, NY: HarperCollins Publishers.

Cabot, N. A. (1999). *The Internet gambling report II: An evolving conflict between technology, policy & law*. Las Vegas, NV: Trace.

Cao, F., & Su, L. (2007). Internet addiction among chinese adolescents: Prevalence and psychological features. *Child: Care, Health and Development, 33*, 275–281.

Charlton, J. P., & Danforth, I. D. W. (2004). Differentiating computer-related addictions and high engagement. In J. Morgan, C. A. Brebbia, J. Sanchez, & A. Voiskounsky (Eds.), *Human perspectives in the Internet society: Culture, psychology, gender* (pp. 59–68). Southampton: WIT Press.

Chou, C., Condron, L., & Belland, J. C. (2005). A review of the research on Internet addiction. *Educational Psychology Review, 17*, 363–368.

Cooper, A., Morahan-Martin, J., Mathy, R. M., & Maheu, M. (2002). Toward an increased understanding of user demographics in online sexual activities. *Journal of Sex and Marital Therapy, 28*, 105–129.

Cooper, A., Putnam, D. E., Planchon, L. A., & Boies, S. C. (1999a). Online sexual compulsivity: Getting tangled in the net. *Sexual Addiction and Compulsivity, 6*, 79–104.

Cooper, A., Scherer, C. R., Boies, S. C., & Gordon, B. L. (1999b). Sexuality on the Internet: From sexual exploration to pathological expression. *Professional Psychology: Research and Practice, 30*, 154–164.

Dunphy, D. C. (1963). The social structure of urban adolescent peer groups. *Sociometry, 26*, 230–246.

Glasser, W. (2000). *Reality therapy in action*. New York, NY: HarperCollins.

Goldsmith, T. D., & Shapira, N. A. (2006). Problematic Internet use. In E. Hollander & D. J. Stein (Eds.), *Clinical manual of impulse-control disorders* (pp. 291–308). Arlington, VA: American Psychiatric Publishing, Inc.

Griffiths, M. (2000a). Does Internet and computer "addiction" exist? Some case study evidence. *Cyberpsychology and Behavior, 3*, 211–218.

Griffiths, M. (2000b). Excessive Internet use: Implications for sexual behavior. *Cyberpsychology and Behavior, 3*, 537–552.

Griffiths, M. (2000c). Internet addiction – time to be taken seriously? *Addiction Research, 8*, 413–418.

Griffiths, M. (2001a). Online therapy: A cause for concern? *Psychologist, 14*, 244–248.

Griffiths, M. (2001b). Sex on the Internet: Observations and implications for Internet sex addiction. *Journal of Sex Research, 38*, 333–342.

Griffiths, M., Davies, M. N. O., & Chappell, D. (2004). Online computer gaming: A comparison of adolescent and adult gamers. *Journal of Adolescence, 27*, 87–96.

Grohol, J. M. (2005). Internet addiction guide. *PsychCentral, 2005*. Retrieved October 2, 2008, from http://psychcentral.com/netaddiction/

Grohol, J. M. (2007). Video games no addiction for now. *PsychCentral, 2007*. Retrieved October 2, 2008, from http://psychcentral.com/news/2007/06/26/video-games-no-addiction-for-now/

Hall, A. S., & Parsons, J. (2001). Internet addiction: College student case study using best practices in cognitive behavior therapy. *Journal of Mental Health Counseling, 23*, 312–327.

Hardoon, K., Derevensky, J., & Gupta, R. (2002). *An examination of the influence of familial, emotional, conduct and cognitive problems, and hyperactivity upon youth risk-taking and adolescent gambling problems*. A report to the Ontario Problem Gambling Research Centre. R & J Child Development Consultants, Inc., Montreal, QC.

Hinduja, S., & Patchin, J. W. (2007). Offline consequences of online victimization: School violence and delinquency. *Journal of School Violence, 6*, 89–112.

Johansson, A., & Gotestam, K. G. (2004). Internet addiction: Characteristics of a questionnaire and prevalence in norwegian youth (12–18 years). *Scandinavian Journal of Psychology, 45*, 223–229.

Kim, J.-U. (2007). A reality therapy group counseling program as an Internet addiction recovery method for college students in Korea. *International Journal of Reality Therapy, 26*, 3–9.

Kim, J.-U. (2008). The effect of a r/t group counseling program on the Internet addiction level and self-esteem of Internet addiction university students. *International Journal of Reality Therapy, 27*, 4–12.

King, S. A. (1996). *Is the Internet addictive, or are addicts using the Internet?*. Retrieved October 15, 2008, from http://webpages.charter.net/stormking/iad.html

Ko, C.-H., Yen, J.-Y., Chen, C.-C., Chen, S.-H., Wu, K., & Yen, C.-F. (2006). Tridimensional personality of adolescents with Internet addiction and substance use experience. *The Canadian Journal of Psychiatry/La Revue canadienne de psychiatrie, 51*, 887–894.

Ko, C.-H., Yen, J.-Y., Chen, C.-C., Chen, S.-H., & Yen, C.-F. (2005). Proposed diagnostic criteria of Internet addiction for adolescents. *Journal of Nervous and Mental Disease, 193*, 728–733.

Kraut, R., Kiesler, S., Boneva, B., Cummings, J., Helgeson, V., & Crawford, A. (2002). Internet paradox revisited. *Journal of Social Issues, 58*, 49–74.

Kraut, R., Patterson, M., Lundmark, V., Kiesler, S., Mukopadhyay, T., & Scherlis, W. (1998). Internet paradox: A social technology that reduces social involvement and psychological well-being? *American Psychologist, 53*, 1017–1031.

Kubey, R. W., Lavin, M. J., & Barrows, J. R. (2001). Internet use and collegiate academic performance decrements: Early findings. *Journal of Communication, 51*, 366–382.

Lemmens, J. S., Valkenburg, P., & Peter, J. (2009). Development and validation of a game addiction scale for adolescents. *Media Psychology, 12*, 77–95.

Lenhart, A., Kahne, J., Middaugh, E., Macgill, A. R., Evans, C., & Vitak, J. (2008). Teens, video games, and civics [Electronic version]. *Pew Internet & American Life Project*. Retrieved October 16, 2008, from http://pewinternet.org/pdfs/PIP_Teens_Games_and_Civics_Report_FINAL.pdf

Leung, L. (2002). Loneliness, self-disclosure, and icq ("I seek you") use. *Cyberpsychology and Behavior, 5*, 241–251.

Macartney, J. (2008). Internet addiction made an official disorder in china. *Times Online*. Retrieved October 15, 2009, from http://www.timesonline.co.uk/tol/news/world/asia/article5125324.ece

Macek, P. (2003). *Adolescence* (2nd ed.). Praha: Portál.

Manzin, M., & Biloslavo, R. (2008). Online gambling: Today's possibilities and tomorrow's opportunities. *Managing Global Transitions, 6*, 95–110.

Morahan-Martin, J. (2005). Internet abuse – Addiction? Disorder? Symptom? Alternative explanations? *Social Science Computer Review, 23*, 39–48.

Morahan-Martin, J., & Schumacher, P. (2000). Incidence and correlates of pathological Internet use among college students. *Computers in Human Behavior, 16*, 13–29.

Morahan-Martin, J., & Schumacher, P. (2003). Loneliness and social uses of the Internet. *Computers in Human Behavior, 19*, 659–671.

Niemz, K., Griffiths, M., & Banyard, P. (2005). Prevalence of pathological Internet use among university students and correlations with self-esteem, the general health questionnaire (GHQ), and disinhibition. *CyberPsychology and Behavior, 8*(6), 562–570.

Parker, J. D. A., Taylor, R. N., Eastabrook, J. M., Schell, S. L., & Wood, L. M. (2008). Problem gambling in adolescence: Relationships with Internet misuse, gaming abuse and emotional intelligence. *Personality and Individual Differences, 45*, 174–180.

Rau, P.-L. P., Peng, S.-Y., & Yang, C.-C. (2006). Time distortion for expert and novice online game players. *CyberPsychology and Behavior, 9*, 396–403.

Shapira, N. A., Goldsmith, T. D., Keck, P. E., Khosla, U. M., & McElroy, S. L. (2000). Psychiatric features of individuals with problematic Internet use. *Journal of Affective Disorders, 57*, 267–272.

Šmahel, D. (2003). *Psychologie a Internet: Děti dospělými, dospělí dětmi. [Psychology and Internet: Children being adults, adults being children.]*. Prague: Triton.

Šmahel, D., Blinka, L., & Ledabyl, O. (2008). Playing MMORPGs: Connections between addiction and identifying with a character. *Cyberpsychology & Behavior, 2008*, 480–490.

Šmahel, D., Blinka, L., & Sevcikova, A. (2009a). *Cyberbullying among Czech Internet users: Prevalence across age groups*. Paper presented at the EU Kids Online Conference. London, UK.

Šmahel, D., Sevcikova, A., Blinka, L., & Vesela, M. (2009b). Abhängigkeit und Internetapplikationen: Spiele, Kommunikation und Sex-Webseiten. [Addiction and Internet applications: Games, communication and sex web sites]. In B. U. Stetina & I. Kryspin-Exner (Eds.), *Gesundheit (spsychologie) und Neue Medien*. Berlin: Springer.

Šmahel, D., Vondrackova, P., Blinka, L., & Godoy-Etcheverry, S. (2009c). Comparing addictive behavior on the Internet in the Czech Republic, Chile and Sweden. In G. Cardosso, A. Cheong, & J. Cole (Eds.), *World Wide Internet: Changing societies, economies and cultures*. Macao: University of Macao.

Tsai, C.-C., & Lin, S. S. J. (2003). Internet addiction of adolescents in Taiwan: An interview study. *Cyberpsychology and Behavior, 6*, 649–652.

Wan, C.-S., & Chiou, W.-B. (2006a). Psychological motives and online games addiction: A test of flow theory and humanistic needs theory for Taiwanese adolescents. *CyberPsychology and Behavior, 9*, 317–324.

Wan, C.-S., & Chiou, W.-B. (2006b). Why are adolescents addicted to online gaming? An interview study in Taiwan. *CyberPsychology and Behavior, 9*, 762–766.

Watson, J. C. (2005). Internet addiction diagnosis and assessment: Implications for counselors. *Journal of Professional Counseling: Practice, Theory and Research, 33*, 17–30.

Widyanto, L., & Griffiths, M. (2007). Internet addiction: Does it really exist? (Revisited). In J. Gackenbach (Eds.), *Psychology and the Internet: Intrapersonal, interpersonal, and transpersonal implications* (2nd ed., pp. 141–163). San Diego, CA: Academic Press.

Wood, R. T. A. (2008). Problems with the concept of video game addiction: Some case study examples. *International Journal of Mental Health and Addiction, 6*, 169–178.

Yee, N. (2006). The demographics, motivations and derived experiences of users of massively-multiuser online graphical environments. *PRESENCE: Teleoperators and Virtual Environments, 15*, 309–329.

Yen, J.-Y., Yen, C.-F., Chen, C.-C., Chen, S.-H., & Ko, C.-H. (2007). Family factors of Internet addiction and substance use experience in Taiwanese adolescents. *CyberPsychology and Behavior, 10*, 323–329.

Young, K. S. (1995). Internet addiction: Symptoms, evaluation, and treatment. *Center for Online Addictions*. Retrieved October 6, 2008, from http://www.netaddiction.com/articles/symptoms.pdf

Young, K. S. (1997). *What makes the Internet addictive: Potential explanations for pathological Internet use*. Paper presented at the 105th annual conference of the American Psychological Association, Chicago. Retrieved October 15, 2008, from http://www.netaddiction.com/articles/habitforming.pdf

Young, K. S. (1998a). *Caught in the Net*. New York, NY: Wiley.

Young, K. S. (1998b). The center for online addiction – Frequently asked questions. *Center for online Addictions*. Retrieved October 6, 2008, from http://www.netaddiction.com/faq.htm

Young, K. S. (1998c). Internet addiction: The emergence of a new clinical disorder. *Cyberpsychology and Behavior, 1*, 237–244.

Young, K. S. (1999). Internet addiction: Symptoms, evaluation and treatment. In L. VandeCreek & T. Jackson (Eds.), *Innovations in clinical practice: A source book* (Vol. 17, pp. 19–31). Sarasota, FL: Professional Resource.

Young, K. S. (2007). Cognitive behavior therapy with Internet addicts: Treatment outcomes and implications. *Cyberpsychology and Behavior, 10*, 671–679.

Chapter 10
The Darker Sides of the Internet: Violence, Cyber Bullying, and Victimization

For almost as long as mass media have been around, so have concerns about young people's exposure to the darker sides of human nature portrayed within them. In Chapter 3, we examined one concern – pornography as well as sexually violent material online and the issues surrounding adolescents' exposure to such content. Here we examine some other concerns surrounding the Internet – its potential for violence, aggression, and victimization of young people. These concerns are not new. Several decades of research on earlier visual media forms like television and films and newer interactive media such as video games reveals that violent media content does lead to increases in violent and aggressive behavior (Anderson et al., 2003). The Internet, as we will show in this chapter, provides ready access to violent material. However, it is more than just a repository of content and we use it for communicating and interacting with others. With these new opportunities have come new challenges.

Consider the case of Megan Meier, a 13-year-old teenager in Missouri who committed suicide on October 17, 2006 by hanging herself in her closet. She had been the victim of online bullying or cyber bullying via her MySpace page. A month earlier, "Josh Evans," who said he was a 16-year-old home schooled boy and lived nearby, had befriended her on MySpace. After a month of friendly interactions, Josh unexpectedly turned the tables on her and on October 15, 2006 sent her a message saying he did not want to be friends with her. The two exchanged several more messages that were negative; they triggered a chain of unfortunate events that ended in Megan taking her own life. The tragedy in this instance of cyber bullying is that "Josh Evans" never existed, but instead was a fictional identity created by Lori Drew, the mother of a former friend of Megan. The bigger tragedy in this instance is that local prosecutors did not have a statute under which to file criminal charges against the adult responsible for the bullying. Subsequently a jury in Los Angeles convicted her of misdemeanor charges for violating MySpace's terms of service for providing false information in her profile. The judge subsequently overturned the conviction and the case is under appeal. That the case had to be pursued in Los Angeles, because the offices of MySpace are located in Los Angeles attests to the challenges involved in creating and enforcing laws that can adequately safeguard and protect young people from violence and harassment online. Although an adult

K. Subrahmanyam, D. Šmahel, *Digital Youth*, Advancing Responsible
Adolescent Development, DOI 10.1007/978-1-4419-6278-2_10,
© Springer Science+Business Media, LLC 2011

perpetrated the cyber bullying in this instance, it nonetheless calls attention to the Internet's potential for aggressive and hostile interactions at the hands of peers and adults.

This chapter examines the many different forms of online violence and aggression. To provide some perspective, we start by briefly reviewing the findings of extant research on violence in media (e.g., television, video games, etc). The bulk of the chapter will then focus on three categories of online aggression: (1) violence in websites and other online content, (2) interactive online games with violent content, (3) online interactions that are aggression-tinged, including cyber bullying and online sexual solicitation and victimization. For each, we describe the online landscape or interaction and then examine its impact on adolescents' lives.

Effects of Violent Media Content

We start by briefly considering what researchers have already learned about the effects of violence in television, movies, music videos, and video games. There are several excellent research reviews on this topic (Anderson, 2004; Anderson et al., 2003; Kirsh, 2006) and one review by several leading scholars concluded thus (Anderson et al., 2003, p. 1):

> Research on violent television and films, videogames, and music reveals unequivocal evidence that media violence increases the likelihood of aggressive and violent behavior in both immediate and long-term contexts. The effects appear larger for milder than for more severe forms of aggression, but the effects on severe forms of violence are also substantial ($r = .13$ to $.32$) when compared with effects of other violence risk factors or medical effects deemed important by the medical community (e.g., effect of aspirin on heart attacks).

Anderson and colleagues defined aggressive and violent behavior "as any behavior that is intended to harm another person." They reviewed studies that investigated the impact of media violence on a variety of aggressive behaviors including verbal aggression (e.g., name-calling), relational aggression (aggressive behaviors that are enacted behind the target's back, e.g., spreading rumors), and physical aggression (which involve physical actions such as hitting, pushing or shoving). In addition they included research that examined the influence on aggressive ideation (ideas that promote aggression) and aggressive emotions (emotional reactions related to aggressive behavior) (Anderson et al., 2003). From a developmental perspective, two conclusions that emerged from this review are relevant. First, "high levels of exposure to violent TV programs in childhood can promote aggression in later childhood, adolescence, and even young adulthood" (Anderson et al., 2003). Although longitudinal studies on the effect of violent video games were not conclusive, they suggested a link between playing violent video games and increases in aggressive behavior. Second, at least for television, the effects of televised violence on behavior are stronger for younger users. Together they imply that consuming violent media early in life does have cumulative effects and the younger the user, the stronger those effects are likely to be.

Violence in Web Sites and Other Online Content

Given the sheer vastness and dynamic nature of the Internet and World Wide Web, it would be futile to attempt to detail all the different kinds of violent sites that are on it. So instead, we will focus our attention on violent content that is most relevant with regard to young people. Some of the most common ways that violent content appears online is via web sites with violent and aggressive themes, web sites that advocate violence and aggression, and web sites that sometimes provide detailed directions for committing violent actions. The Columbine incident in Littleton, Colorado on April 20, 1999 illustrates the potential negative effects of such content. Two teens, Eric Harris and Dylan Klebold, entered their high school with pistols, shotguns, and homemade bombs. They killed 12 people and wounded several others before killing themselves. It was found later that the shooters had obtained detailed bomb-making instructions online and Harris even had bomb-making instructions on his web site (Pooley, 1999). Almost 10 years later, such information continues to be available online. In October 2008, a Google search for "bomb making instructions" yielded several links to press stories about bomb making as well to sites containing detailed information about making bombs. Such online information is readily available to anyone with access to a computer connected to the Internet.

Even web sites with violent themes vary amongst themselves with regard to whether or not they advocate such behavior. Web sites focused on suicide are a case in point. A Google search on "committing suicide" from a US IP address yielded hardly any sites with information on suicide methods. More often, the sites argued against ending one's life, provided resources that people contemplating suicide could use in order to not commit suicide, and even listed all the things that could go wrong when attempting suicide. In fact, we came across a bulletin board, where a poster complained that most sites he/she had visited provide details of all the things that could go wrong when attempting suicide! However, in a similar search on the Czech Internet we found serious discussions in the Czech language about how best to commit suicide.

Another category of violent-themed sites is those that contain violent gore content such as pictures of torture and mutilation. The Canadian web site *Be Web Aware* (http://www.bewebaware.ca/english) has identified two examples that belong to this category including "gorezone.com" and "rotten.com." Some of the violence on such sites may also contain degrading acts and sexual violence including extreme acts of misogyny and sadism. Although most have a disclaimer stating that they contain mature content and ask users to proceed only if they are over 18 years of age, nonetheless they can be readily found and easily accessed.

Online music also merit attention with regard to violence especially as youth use the Internet as an important source for music and music videos (Aikat, 2004). Content analyses of music videos reveal that rap and to a lesser extent, hip-hop music, contain considerable talk about explicit violence, guns, and weapons (DuRant et al., 1997; Jones, 1997). According to Aikat, music videos are available on sites such as BET.com, Country.com, MTV.com, and VH1.com; because the content on such sites linked to television networks and a vast cable audience, it is important to examine their role in distributing violent and aggression-themed material. In a recent content analysis of online music videos, violent acts included assaults (property and armed assaults), fights, and hostile chases. Weapons were used in 76% of such acts and the most commonly found weapons included guns (22%), explosives (18%), bladed weapons (16%), household items (8%), and vehicles (4%) (Aikat, 2004). Among online music videos, Hard Rock, Hip Hop/Rap, and Pop/Top 40 were the music genres that contained the most amount of violent content.

Another online forum where we find violent and aggressive messages against individuals and groups is that of hate sites. According to Tynes (2005), online hate "includes hate speech and so-called persuasive rhetoric;" hate speech generally contains messages of racial inferiority and targets members of historically persecuted groups. One content analysis of extremist sites found the most commonly depicted types of extremism were: White Nationalist (20%), Skinhead (19%), Christian Identity (13%), Holocaust Denial (13%), and Neo-Nazi (11%) (Gerstenfeld, Grant, & Chiang, 2003). Tynes writes that hate speech targets adherents and potential members as well as targets of the hatred such as African–Americans, Jewish people, and members of other minority groups. Often run by racist organizations (e.g., Ku Klux Klan, Skinheads, Aryan Nations), hate sites are augmented by chat rooms as well as bulletin boards that serve to extend their negative discourse. Given the fluid nature of the web, it is impossible to know how many such sites there are at any given moment in time. Tynes (2005) cites a 2004 count, which determined that within the USA, there were 497 web sites espousing hatred toward others. Hate messages may also be sent via e-mails (considered as spam by most recipients) and text messages. For instance, the following text message was found to have been exchanged by convicted gang rapists in Sydney, Australia: "When you are feeling down…bash a Christian or Cathoic to lift up." The rape crimes were considered hate crimes as the perpetrators were Australians of Lebanese Muslim descent, who selected their victims on the basis of their ethnicity (Cappi, 2007).

The web site of the Media Awareness Network points out that we can find milder forms of online hate in sites such as "uglypeople.com," which appear to legitimize cruel satire targeting other individuals. At a more global level, terrorist groups use the Internet extensively for their operations and in particular to reach young people; some organizations have sites with content ostensibly for youth, but also promote messages of suicide terrorism to glorify suicide bombers, presumably to recruit new members (Weimann, 2008). More insidious, they offer free online games that promote radical, extremist messages and violent content. Weimann writes about one such game:

> One such game is the "Quest for Bush," aka "Night of Bush Capturing," a free online game released by the Global Islamic Media Front, a media outlet of Al Qaeda. Armed with a rifle, a shotgun or a grenade launcher, players navigate missions that include "Jihad Growing Up," "Americans' Hell" and "Bush Hunted Like a Rat." In the final stage, the player's task is to kill President Bush.

Finally, there are violent messages in online user-generated media such as YouTube. Again, it is impossible to arrive at a realistic estimate of how widespread such content is. We provide a few examples here, and while anecdotal, they nonetheless illustrate our point. A recent Los Angeles Times report noted that a prolific 24-year-old graffiti tagger called "Buket" was arrested after the police began investigating him when videos of his vandalism were posted on YouTube and tagger-related blogs (Blankstein, 2008). There have been two recent instances of Finnish youth going on a killing rampage where the killers had posted violent clips on YouTube prior to the incident. For example, in the September 2007 incident, YouTube postings showed a young man calling for a revolution and firing a semiautomatic handgun. Although such violent incidents are relatively rare, they nonetheless highlight the fact that technology has now made it very easy for individuals to both post such violent messages as well as access them. Research is only just beginning on adolescents' exposure to the different kinds of violent content that we described in this section. Next, we describe what we know about adolescents' exposure to violence theme web sites and online hate and the potential consequences of such exposure.

Adolescents and Violence-Themed Web Sites

Researchers interested in the effects of mediated violence began with content analyses of television and video games targeting youth to determine the prevalence of violent messages within them. Using the same line of reasoning, one place to start is by determining the amount and kinds of violent content in web sites and on applications such as YouTube, chat groups, and by assessing the extent to which adolescents access and create them. Unfortunately, to date, except for hate sites, researchers have not done a content analysis for the other online sources described earlier. Even if the Internet were a static entity, it would be a Herculean task to catalog and list the different kinds and numbers of violence-laced web sites available online. However, the constantly evolving and changing nature of the Internet makes the task even more challenging.

An even more vexing issue centers on the extent and nature of adolescents' exposure to such violent content. The few available estimates are vastly different. An Australian study of 11- to 17-year olds found that 47% had been exposed to offensive or disgusting material such as pornography, and nudity, violent images of death and accidents (Aisbett, Authority, & Insights, 2001; Fleming, Greentree, Cocotti-Muller, Elias, & Morrison, 2006). One male participant provided a graphic image of a "blood pattern made from shooting upwards through a human head." In another survey, also of Australian youth, between 13 and 16 years of age, 77% of males and 55% of females reported that they were exposed to violent images online (Fleming et al., 2006). Despite the discrepancies in the estimate, together they indicate that many teens report exposure to online violence.

Often, exposure may be inadvertent such as finding it unexpectedly when searching online, or receiving the links to it from unknown people (Aisbett et al., 2001). Inadvertent exposure might occur more often than intentional exposure. In The UK Children Go Online project (Livingstone, Bober, & Helsper, 2005), among youth between 9 and 19 years of age who went online at least once a week, 22% of respondents ended up on a site showing violent images by accident and 12% visited sites with violent images on purpose. In general, boys and older children were more likely to experience the risk of violent content online; boys were also more likely to seek violent sites on purpose. When exposure is inadvertent, youth report being upset when they encountered such material. Some report feeling "shocked" and "degraded," and a few were concerned that a parent might find them with such content on their computer screen (Aisbett et al., 2001).

Impact of violence-themed web sites. We know even less about the potential impact of exposure to violent online content online and the review of the literature on media violence that we referred to earlier had this to say (Anderson et al., 2003):

> The basic theoretical principles concerning the effects of exposure to media violence should be applicable to Internet media. We found no published studies that address how exposure to Web-based media violence affects aggressive and violent behavior, attitudes, beliefs, and emotions. However, because of the visual and interactive nature of Web material, we expect the effects to be very similar to those of other visual and interactive media. The Web materials with violence tend to be video games, film clips, and music videos, and there is no reason to believe that delivering these materials into the home via the Internet, rather than through other media, would reduce their effects.

Five years later, we were still not able to find a single experimental study that evaluated the effects of online violent content online on youth.

Keep in mind that concerns about the potential effects of violent online content on youth viewers presume the "media effects" perspective described in Chapter 2. However, the notion that effects flow from the medium to the user assumes that the media landscape is relatively circumscribed and users are passive recipients, who have little choice in the media content that they consume. These assumptions were likely true in the first couple of decades of film and television. However, they no longer hold true, even for television, and especially not for the Internet. Recall that in the survey by Livingstone and colleagues (2005), only 12% of youth reported visiting online sites with violent content on purpose. Although this represents a seemingly small proportion of youth, those who seek out violent content might actually be more vulnerable and consequently more susceptible to its effects as well.

This was in fact the conclusion arrived to by Slater (2003) and Slater, et al. (2003). Using a longitudinal survey of over 2,000 6th and 7th grade students (mean age $= 12.34$ years) across the US, Slater et al. (2003) assessed participants' aggressiveness as well as use of media violence including viewing action films, playing violent computer and video games, and visiting violence-oriented Internet sites. They used multilevel modeling to examine growth curves in individual subjects' aggressiveness and use of violent media. Controlling for covariates (gender, sensation-seeking, general Internet use, and age), they found that violent media use predicted aggressive behavior both concurrently as well as at a subsequent point in time. In contrast, aggressive behavior only predicted violent media use concurrently. In another survey study of 8th grade students (median age = 14 years) in the USA, Slater (2003) used hierarchical regression analyses to determine that gender, sensation seeking, aggression, and frequency of Internet use strongly predicted use of violent web site content. Alienation from school and family explained the use of web sites with violence-oriented content over and beyond a general interest in violent media. Alienation also mediated the effects of sensation seeking and aggression. Slater concluded that "websites containing violence may represent a potentially more socially destructive interest, given the support for destructive behavior and availability of information such as bomb-making instructions on some websites" (p. 117). In particular, he speculated that such sites might provide a refuge for young people, who are alienated from school and family, and provide an alternative socialization context compared to the negative peer associations commonly seen among such individuals. Thus, violence-oriented web sites may not be harmful for a majority of adolescents, but may be particularly dangerous for a minority among them, especially those, who are alienated from their immediate contexts, are sensation seekers, and are generally at risk for problem behaviors.

Adolescents and Online Hate

There is now a small but significant body of research that has documented the forms and extent of online hate, and its intersection with young people – specifically how young people are targeted by these sites, the persuasive effects of hateful content on young people, and the at-risk youth who may be susceptible to hate-filled messages (Tynes, 2005).

Despite the challenges of dynamic and unconstrained online spaces, a few studies have attempted to collect a list of hate forums as well as analyze their content (Gerstenfeld et al., 2003; Schafer, 2002; Zhou, Qin, Lai, & Chen, 2007). For instance, Schafer provides a list and URL of 132 extremist sites; although many of the links are no longer active, a few did lead to sites that were still active at the time when we wrote this in 2009 (Schafer, 2002). Gerstenfeld and colleagues identified and analyzed 157 extremist web sites (Gerstenfeld et al., 2003). Zhou and colleagues used a web mining approach to create a collection of 110 US domestic extremist forums, which together contained more than 640,000 documents (Zhou et al., 2007). At a much larger scale, the Simon Wiesenthal Center's guide to extremist sites, Digital Terrorism and Hate (2007), is based on 7,000 problematic web sites, blogs, newsgroups, YouTube, and other on-demand video sites (Simon Wiesenthal Center, 2007). The popular online tools for hate groups include web sites, e-mail, chat rooms, multi-user domains (MUDs), discussion boards, music, video games, audio tapes and videotapes, games, and literature (Tynes, 2005). According to Tynes, chat rooms and discussion boards may play an important role, as they are interactive and facilitate the creation of a global community of hate.

   More relevant to us is how these online forums target youth in order to both spread their message to impressionable young people and recruit them to their cause. Tynes (2005) has identified the following strategies used by hate sites to appeal to and recruit young people: Creation of web pages as well as sections within larger sites that are specifically suited for children and adolescents; organizing web pages so they may appear legitimate to youth (e.g., the web site www.martinlutherking.org looks like a legitimate site, but contains many hateful messages instead); using multimedia such as regular games, video games, and music; assigning websites with ambiguous titles that may seem legitimate to young people (www.stormfront.org) as well as various "foot-in-the-door" techniques such as warnings, disclaimers, objectives/purposes, social approaches, and counterargument strategies. To target youth, such sites may word ideas to be more understandable to young people, and may even feature messages by youth directed to other youth.

   Research suggests that even college students sometimes do not recognize the true messages of extremist sites (Leets, 2001). Purveyors of hate use techniques that capitalize on young people's still developing cognitive skills and limited abilities and experience to evaluate the credibility of online information in order to suck them into their world of hate. Of even more concern is how extremist groups use innocent-looking multimedia tools to lure young people, who might otherwise not even be willing to consider their hateful ideology. Consider Schafer's finding that White supremacist organizations allow users to listen online and buy "White power music," which contains violent, hateful, and profane lyrics set to a heavy metal tune (Schafer, 2002). Such music might serve as bridge between the ideologies of extremist groups and youth, who are first attracted to the music, and then get lured into the ideology when they delve more deeply into the sub-culture that surrounds the music (e.g., attending live performances and interacting with other fans).

   An experimental study on the persuasiveness of hate messages such as those found on White supremacist web pages indicates that they can be effective under certain conditions (Lee & Leets, 2002). Since this is one of the few experimental studies on this topic, we discuss it in some detail. The study was conducted online and involved 108 adolescents (between 13- and 17 years of age), who viewed graphics and read text on web pages. The researchers informed participants that they were evaluating web pages, and some content might be offensive to them. A pre-test assessed participant's initial attitudes toward the messages conveyed in the web page; a week later participants viewed the actual message and the researchers measured their attitude change immediately after exposure. They also measured participants' attitudes in a follow-up 2 weeks later to test for attitude decay. The stimulus on the web page viewed by the participants comprised graphics and passages on topics commonly found on hate sites such as interracial dating, White pride and heritage, immigration, joining a White supremacist group, etc. The narrative elements (e.g., character motivation, plots, and settings) and message explicitness (e.g., "To be born WHITE is an honor and privilege" for an explicit message versus "Rich heritage is an honor and privilege" for an implicit message) of the passages were manipulated. The researchers measured participants' acceptance of the presented messages, their favorability rating of the concepts, impressions of the web page, and prejudice and receptivity to the advocated message.

Initially, the high narrative implicit message was more persuasive. However, the effects of low narrative explicit messages were more stable 2 weeks later. Moreover, participants' receptivity mediated the effectiveness of the message. Although high narrative messages were more persuasive regardless of an individuals' receptivity, participants who did not agree with prejudiced messages to begin with were more able to resist low-narrative, explicit messages (Lee & Leets, 2002). The study shows that hate-filled messages such as those found on web sites can influence young people's attitudes and such effects may last up to 2 weeks later. This study has important implications that we should consider further. First, they suggest that even brief exposure to negative messages such as those found on online hate sites can have somewhat persistent changes in young Internet users' attitudes. Second, and even more important, they suggest that youth who are already susceptible to such messages may be at most risk for such changes. Recall that they were not able to resist low narrative explicit messages, which were also the ones that had more stable effects. Anecdotally it seems that low narrative explicit messages may be more common online. Given the interactive nature of the Internet, at-risk individuals may choose to only visit hate sites with the cumulative impact of such intentional exposure leading to lasting changes.

Who are the youth and who may be at risk for such messages? We suggest that some youth might be more susceptible to hate messages compared to others. We saw earlier that youth, who seek sensation and are alienated from school and home, may be more vulnerable to violence-laced content online (Slater, 2003). Similarly, Tynes has identified other risk factors for involvement in hate: youth in economically distressed areas, youth from single-parent homes, youth who have experienced psychological distress from blocked goal attainment and lack of established social norms, and lastly individuals who have experienced economic, racial, genetic (e.g., interracial dating), and gender-based threats (Tynes, 2005).

Nonetheless, there is some evidence that despite the various strategies used by extremist hate groups, and the persuasiveness of hate messages, the Internet might not be a very effective medium to recruit people to their cause. For instance, Turpin-Petrosino surveyed high school and college students to examine their attitudes toward hate groups (Turpin-Petrosino, 2002). Although there were respondents who were minorities, the researcher only analyzed the responses of White participants, as they were interested in attitudes toward White hate groups. Turpin-Petrosino found that out of 567 respondents, only 96 reported contacts with hate groups and only 10 (approximately 2% of the entire sample) of those were reported to be Internet contacts with White supremacist groups and 4 of those reported supporting the groups. Although less than 2% of the entire sample reported Internet-based contacts with hate groups, a majority (70%) of them were high school students. The study was conducted nearly 6–7 years ago and since then, the Internet has become very diffuse with increased multi-media capabilities. We therefore need more research to confirm these trends, and to identify youth who are most likely to be recruited to the causes espoused by online extremist sites.

Violence in Online Games

Violence has always existed in interactive single-player games that generally involve a player against the computer. Here we consider the issue of violence in massively multiplayer online games (MMOs) and massively multiplayer online role playing games (MMORPGs), a sub-class of MMOs. Players in both MMOs and MMORPGs play with and against thousands of other players in fantasy worlds; in MMORPGs, they play while taking on roles specific to the particular game world within which they are playing (see Fig. 10.1). The expanded opportunities for player to player interactions that these games provide have also given rise to new ways of aggressive and antisocial interactions that are the focus of this section; the role of MMORPGs role in online addiction was discussed in the previous chapter.

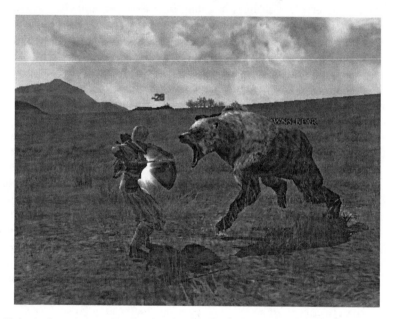

Fig. 10.1. A players' avatar fighting a creature: from the 'The Lord of the Rings Online'

According to Cho (2004), in addition to the more traditional player versus non-player-character violence, other forms of violence in multiplayer online games include "player killing" (violence against players by other players), and milder forms of aggressive acts such as verbal abuse initiated by players against other players, grief play, where players cause inconvenience or hurt to other players, stealing another person's character or avatar, and victimization of poorer characters in the game. Player killing (PK) or Player versus player (PvP) is a big issue within MMOs and has even given rise to Player Killer Killing or PK Killing, where players target and kill players who engage in PK or griefing of other players. PK is an integral part of several MMORPGs (such as in *World of Warcraft* or WoW as it is called), but is forbidden in several other games (such as *Lord of the Rings Online* – LOTRO). Games not only differ in whether PK is allowed, but also in the extent to which PK occurs, the particular game contexts (e.g., servers) where they may occur, and the specific forms that they can assume. For example, in some games, PK is allowed only in some areas, so the player entering the area already knows that he/she will be exposed to such behavior.

Adolescents and Violence in Online Games

As before, we first briefly consider research on the effect of playing violent video games. Based on a meta-analysis (a statistical analysis of other studies' statistical effects), Anderson concluded that playing violent video games was associated with increases in "aggressive behavior, aggressive cognition, aggressive affect, and physiological arousal," as well as decreases in "helping behavior." Stronger effects were obtained from methodologically stronger studies compared to methodologically weaker studies. Anderson points out that the size of the effect of violent video game exposure on aggressive behavior is larger than that of condom use on HIV risk or passive workplace smoke exposure on lung cancer (Anderson, 2004). Consequently, even small effects can translate into large societal consequences, if significant numbers of youth spend considerable amounts of time interacting with violent media. It would be surprising if playing MMORPGs did not have similar effects as players engage in simulated people-to-people aggression, ranging from annoying others to killing them.

Regrettably, there is very little systematic research on the nature and prevalence of violence in this context, the extent to which adolescents are both exposed to it and participate in it, and on the potential effects of such violence on adolescent gamers. The few studies on the topic are on participants of different ages and have contradictory findings making it difficult to draw any clear inferences from them. A link between playing violent online games and aggression was found by Wei, who surveyed online gamers between 11 and 22 years of age at an Internet café in a city in Central China (Wei, 2007). Those who played violent games online showed greater tolerance of violence, a lower empathetic attitude, and more aggressive behavior; playing online games had the strongest relation on attitudes toward violence.

However, Funk, Baldacci, Pasold, and Baumgardner (2004) found no relation between exposure to real-life and media violence (video games, television, movies, and the Internet) and empathy and attitudes toward violence among 4th and 5th graders (mean age of 9.99 years). They assessed participants' exposure to violence by asking them about the time they spent in each of the four categories (e.g., video games or television) and their favorite activities within each category. Funk and colleagues measured Internet activity by asking children about their gaming (playing one-person games with and without violence, playing multiplayer games with and without violence) and non-gaming activities (e.g., chatting, instant messaging, shopping, looking for information, etc). Only video game violence was associated with lowered empathy and both video game and movie violence were associated with stronger pro-violence attitudes. Along similar lines, Williams and Skoric found no effect of playing an online violent fantasy game on aggressive cognitions and behaviors (Williams & Skoric, 2005). Participants were first-time MMORPG players, who had prior video game playing experience and were tested before and after the study treatment, which lasted a month. They reported playing the game for an average of 56 h over the course of the study. Although their ages ranged from 14 to 68 years, we include it here because the literature on the topic is so sparse. One reason for the study's finding might be that the game used for the treatment, *Asheron's Call 2*, rarely involves conflict between players, although players do have to kill evil monsters.

One reason that the findings on MMORPGs are so different from that of video games could be the very nature of the online game environment, particularly in MMORPGs. Unlike many video games, MMORPGs have very complex and varied game worlds in terms of terrain, flora, fauna, and inhabitants (Yee, 2006). Yee also points out that players take part in increasingly complex activities that "revolve around character advancement and translate into a functional advantage in terms of the mechanics of the world, whether this is combat capability, social status, avatar appearance, geographic knowledge, equipment quality, or even cooking skills." MMORPGs can also be very cooperative, community-based, supportive games: In our survey of 548 players from all over the world, 94% agreed that "The game enables me to cooperate with other players," and 81% agreed that "I can join a guild and feel a sense of belonging to it." (Šmahel, unpublished data). In all likelihood, the violent aspects of MMROPGs are counterbalanced by their group-based, cooperative culture. The complexity of the social world and activities that players engage within it might help put the violence and aggression in context leading to the lack of a consistent finding about the playing of violent online games. At the same time, we saw from Slater's work (Slater, 2003; Slater et al., 2003) that some youth are more susceptible to aggressive content in media. For these adolescents, playing violent MMORPGs, particularly when excessive, may put them at risk.

Aggressive Interactions in Online Contexts

As we noted at the start of this chapter, the Internet's potential to meet and engage with others has given rise to a range of negative and aggressive interactions. Reports of young people being victimized via electronic technologies such as social networking sites, cell phones, text messages, instant messages, and e-mail have become commonplace. Here we consider two main kinds of such interactions that adolescents encounter online (1) cyber bullying perpetrated by peers and (2) online sexual solicitation and victimizaiton perpetrated by predatory strangers/adults.

Cyber Bullying

Cyber bullying "is broadly defined as the use of the Internet or other digital communication devices to insult or threaten someone" (Juvonen & Gross, 2008). According to Raskauskas and Stoltz, cyber bullying includes taunting, insulting, threatening, harassing, and intimidation behavior using text messaging, e-mails, defaming web sites, and online slam books (online spaces to post anonymous comments about peers). The purpose of these actions seems to be to "circulate rumors, secrets, insults, and even death threats to harass, manipulate, and harm their victims" (Raskauskas & Stoltz, 2007). The following account provided by a 14-year-old girl illustrates how youth use text messaging to bully their peers:

> I went on this trip with my family. When I came back everyone at school was avoiding me. They moved away when I came by and whispered and pointed at me. Finally a friend told me that my friend (name omitted) had sent text messages to everyone that I had been out of school because I'd had an abortion. I was so embarrassed. Raskauskas & Stoltz (2007, p. 565)

Cyber bullying also includes impersonating others online, posting personal information about others, and forwarding private e-mail and instant message conversations. More recently with the advent of cameras on cell phones, we are seeing instances where young people take pictures of their peers in compromising situations (e.g., gym shower, drunk at a party) and distribute it via e-mails or worse upload it on YouTube (Raskauskas & Stoltz, 2007). Cyber bullying can also involve hacking into servers and releasing users' private information, as in the case on the Czech server "libimseti.cz" ("Ilikeyou.cz"), where hackers downloaded private pictures from the profiles of thousands of girls and published them on the Internet.[1] Thus virtually all forms of electronic media have come to be used creatively by young people to bully and harass their peers.

Research on cyber bullying among adolescents. From studies on cyber bullying among youth (Juvonen & Gross, 2008; NCH, 2005; Raskauskas & Stoltz, 2007), we have learnt that cyber bullying typically occurs in the form of name calling or threats in online contexts such as chat rooms as well as via online tools such as e-mail, instant messaging, or text messaging. Sharing of private online communications (e.g., cutting and pasting instant messages, forwarding e-mails) and password theft are other forms of online harassment (Juvonen & Gross, 2008). New forms of cyber harassment have emerged as technologies have changed. For instance, in a 2005 survey in the UK conducted around the time when cell phone cameras first came out, 10% of the surveyed adolescents reported feeling embarrassed, uncomfortable, or threatened by a picture that someone took of them with a cell phone camera. Young people are typically early adopters of technology and in the past, have come up with new ways of interacting within them (Greenfield & Subrahmanyam, 2003); as new technologies become available, we expect that youth will find ways of using them to bully and harass their peers online. Consequently, we focus less on the particular forms of cyber bullying, and more on aspects that are less likely to change with the technology, such as the characteristics of bullies and victims, relation between offline and online bullying, and the consequences of such victimization.

---

[1] http://www.zive.cz/Bleskovky/Hacker-stahl-tisice-intimnich-fotek-ze-seznamky-Libimseticz/sc-4-a-144169/default.aspx

Cyber bullying has become fairly commonplace in the lives of adolescents and in one survey study, more than two-thirds reported that they were aware of such incidents (Beran & Li, 2005). As with other aspects of Internet use, estimates regarding the prevalence of cyber bullying vary widely, and between 11% (Kowalski & Limber, 2007) and 72% (Juvonen & Gross, 2008) of adolescents report being victims within the U.S. A 2005 survey in the UK found a prevalence rate of 20% (NCH, 2005). In a representative sample from the Czech WIP 2008, 16% of 12- to 15-year olds reported being cyber bullied at least sometimes, and 4% several times per month; 20% of 16- to 19-year olds reported being cyber bullied at least sometimes and 3% several times a month (Sevcikova & Šmahel, 2009). The highest share of victims across all age groups was among the 12- to 19-year-old respondents.

We can attribute some of the differences in prevalence estimates to study methodology, specifically participant recruitment. For instance, in a face-to-face survey of 84 13-to 18-year olds in the USA, Raskauskas and Stoltz found that 49% reported being a victim of cyber bullying. On an online survey of 1,378 adolescents, 34% reported being victims of online harassment (Hinduja & Patchin, 2008). Finally, another large-online survey ($n = 1454$) of 12- to 17 year olds conducted at a popular teen Internet site in 2005 found a much higher rate of harassment – 72% for the previous year (Juvonen & Gross, 2008). Notwithstanding that the three studies had different samples and recruited participants in different ways, the discrepancy in their estimates are large enough to warrant further investigation. However, together they draw attention to the latest thorn in adolescents' peer relationships as they migrate to online contexts.

The good news is that despite the relatively high numbers of adolescents who report that they have been bullied via electronic tools, at an individual level it appears that they experience it only infrequently. For instance, in the Juvonen and Gross study, a little less than half of the victims (41%) reported experiencing one to three incidents and only 19% had experienced seven or more incidents of online bullying in the prior year. Despite all the attention that cyber bullying has received, teens may actually experience school-based bullying more frequently than online bullying (Juvonen & Gross, 2008). Furthermore, in spite of the purported anonymity afforded by electronic tools, victims of cyber bullying think they know who is bullying them and the majority report that harassers are peers from their offline lives such as school and other offline contexts. Less than half the participants reported that they were bullied by someone they only knew from their online interactions (Juvonen & Gross, 2008).

Characteristics of bullies and victims. In order to direct intervention efforts appropriately, it is important to develop profiles of potential bullies as well as victims. The second Youth Internet Safety Survey (YISS-2) conducted in 2005 in the USA revealed that both girls and boys were targets, although girls were more likely to receive distressing harassment (Wolak, Mitchell, & Finkelhor, 2006). Research conducted in the USA and Czech have found that male and female adolescents are equally likely to be offender and victim (Hinduja & Patchin, 2008; Sevcikova & Šmahel, 2009). This is contrary to traditional face-to-face bullying, where males have generally been the perpetrators, particularly when the bullying gets physical

(Hinduja & Patchin, 2008). One reason for the evening out of gender differences may be that much of cyber bullying involves relational aggression, generally preferred by girls (Hinduja & Patchin, 2008; Juvonen & Gross, 2008). Evidence also indicates that there is no difference in the likelihood of being a bully or a victim based on a youth's race; but the sample in the study that reported this finding comprised 80% Whites, making it somewhat inconclusive (Hinduja & Patchin, 2008).

Other aspects of adolescents' online and offline behaviors are related to cyber bullying. Both the extent of adolescents' Internet use and the kinds of online applications they use are associated with the risk of online bullying. Heavier teen Internet users are not only more likely to be bullied (Hinduja & Patchin, 2008), they are also more likely to be repeatedly intimidated online (Juvonen & Gross, 2008). Some online communication tools may put teens at greater risk for being bullied – Juvonen and Gross report that those who used instant messaging and webcams were between one and a half to three times more likely to be repeatedly bullied than those who did not (Juvonen & Gross, 2008). In addition to online behavior, adolescents' offline behavior, particularly problematic ones are related to cyber bullying. Teens who reported recent school problems, assaultive behaviors, and substance use were more likely to be both offenders and victims of cyber bullying (Hinduja & Patchin, 2008).

Cyber bullies are also more likely to report poor parent–child relationships, substance use, and delinquency (Ybarra & Mitchell, 2004). Youth (10- to 17-year olds) with symptoms of depression were more likely to report that they had been harassed. Among boys, those reporting major depression were three times more likely to be harassed than those reporting mild to no depression (Ybarra, 2004). As with other correlational studies, it is impossible to know the direction of causality. The author suggests that "future studies should focus on establishing the temporality of events, that is, whether young people report depressive symptoms in response to the negative Internet experience, or whether symptomatology confers risks for later negative online incidents."

Perhaps the most important clue to determining which teens are most likely to be online bullies or victims is to identify victims and perpetrators in the offline world. There is now a small body of work, which suggests that there is an overlap between online versus in-school bullying. In one online survey, 85% of respondents who reported at least one incident of on-line bullying within the last year also reported one incident of in-school bullying in the same period (Juvonen & Gross, 2008). More importantly, youth who reported that they had bullied their peers offline were 2.5 times more likely to report that they had bullied their peers online (Hinduja & Patchin, 2008). This finding is contrary to initial speculation that youth who were victims of offline bullying would use the anonymity of the Internet as a cover to get back at their tormentors. The in-person survey study by Raskauskas and Stoltz (2007) further clarifies the connection between a youth's role as a bully offline and online. Although a subset of traditional bullies were victims in the virtual world, there was no indication that victims of bullying in the real world were retaliating by becoming bullies on the Internet or via text messages. Nor was there any indication that bullying began electronically and was thence transferred to the real world.

Together with the finding that offline problem behaviors are associated with cyber bullying, these results lead us to concur with (Juvonen & Gross, 2008) that we need to stop seeing the Internet and other electronic tools as the problem. Instead, we should start viewing them as "tools" that adolescents may use for both positive and pro-social as well negative and more anti-social uses. Two findings from the foregoing studies provide support for our proposal that young people's offline and online worlds are connected. First, behavior commonly associated with offline schoolyards has slowly found their place within online contexts. Second, and more important, we see the transfer of offline behaviors and roles to online contexts.

Consequences of online bullying. There is now a solid body of research which confirms that being involved in traditional bullying, whether as the bully or as the victim, does not portend well for the individual teen (Raskauskas & Stoltz, 2007). Indications are that online bullying has similar negative outcomes. In Raskauskas and Stoltz' study, adolescent victims reported feeling negatively impacted via emotional and social disruptions. Victims of online bullying report feeling angry, upset, embarrassed, sad, or hopeless, and powerless because they feel that they were unable to stop the harassment (Beran & Li, 2005; Finkelhor, Mitchell, & Wolak, 2000; Raskauskas & Stoltz, 2007). Research also suggests that victims of bullying are more likely to report school problems and delinquent behavior (Hinduja & Patchin, 2007; Ybarra, Diener-West, & Leaf, 2007). For instance, Ybarra, et al. (2007) found that youth who were harassed online were more likely to report receiving two or more detentions or suspensions and being truant from school. Despite these very real consequences for victims, perpetrators of bullying do not seem to understand the cost of their actions. In Raskauskas and Stoltz's study (2007), bullies reported that they engage in online bullying for fun to get back at others, and to feel better about themselves. Given the overlap between online and offline bullying, it is likely that the same teens are being bullied at school and online and it appears that the effects of online and school-based bullying may be additive. Juvonen and Gross found that being bullied online and at school each independently increased the victim's social anxiety, presumably leading to elevated levels of distress (Juvonen & Gross, 2008).

As we noted earlier, many bullies seem to think that they are having fun or getting back at their peers and do not recognize the far reaching consequences of their actions. It is significant that victims of online harassment are eight times more likely to report that they carried a weapon to school in the past 30 days (Ybarra, et al., 2007) This finding should be of concern to parents and school officials as some incidents of school violence have reportedly involved youth who were victims of bullying at school. It is important to recognize the potentially deadly effects of bullying, whether offline (in and out of school) or online, and the strategies that can be used to combat such peer harassment are described in Chapter 11.

Sexual Solicitation

One of the dramatic changes wrought by the Internet is that it has enabled youth to connect with strangers. We have discussed the potential benefits of such contacts, but unfortunately, it has also placed adolescents at risk for sexual solicitation and sexual exploitation by adult sexual predators. Online sexual solicitation includes unwanted requests to talk about sex as well as requests for personal sexual information and to do something sexual (Mitchell, Wolak, & Finkelhor, 2008; Ybarra & Mitchell, 2008). Such inappropriate, and often illegal sexual contact can either occur entirely online such as when a youth is asked to engage in "cybersex" or it may involve a face-to-face component, where the initial contact with the youth is made online, and then a face-to-face meeting is set up, wherein the youth is sexually exploited or assaulted (Mitchell, Finkelhor, & Wolak, 2002). In their national study, Wolak, Mitchell, and Finkelhor found that 39% of the solicitors were 18 years or older and were largely unknown in person to the victim (Wolak et al., 2006). The majority of unwanted sexual solicitations are actually perpetrated by strangers, who are closer in age to youth (Mitchell et al., 2002; Wolak et al., 2006). The following example offered by a 15-year-old boy illustrates sexual solicitation by a similar-aged peer: "A girl in her teens asked me to get naked on 'cam' but I just ignored her" (Mitchell et al., 2008). Even though youth sexual solicitation may actually occur more frequently, given the developmental and safety implications, the available research has largely focused on sexual solicitation perpetrated by older adults, who may lure adolescents into sexually exploitative relationships with them.

The second Youth Internet Safety Survey (YISS-2), conducted in 2005 in the USA, found that only 4% of respondents had experienced aggressive sexual solicitations (Wolak et al., 2006). However in The Growing Up With Media Survey on 10- to 15-year-old youth, 15% reported an unwanted sexual solicitation incident in the past year (Ybarra & Mitchell, 2008). These numbers are much lower compared to those found during the Internet's early years. Research has confirmed that over a 5-year period, reports of unwanted sexual solicitation and harassment have declined probably as a result of better education and more effective law enforcement (Mitchell, Wolak, & Finkelhor, 2007). Sexual solicitation may occur more frequently via instant messaging (43%) and in chat rooms (32%), compared to social networking sites (4%) (Ybarra & Mitchell, 2008); the latter sites have privacy controls that, if used, seem able to limit the risks for sexual victimization. As with cyber bullying, the particular tool used by perpetrators is less important as they are likely to change with the technology.

Despite these small numbers, it is important to identify the characteristics of offenders and of the youth, who are most likely to be the targets of such victimization. Older teens between 14- and 17 years of age are most at-risk for sexual solicitation; solicitors are also more likely to be male (Mitchell et al., 2002). The YISS-2 survey showed that youth who engaged in a pattern of risky online behaviors in their interactions with strangers were more at risk for unwanted sexual solicitation or harassment. These behaviors included aggressive actions in the form of rude or nasty comments, embarrassing others, meeting people in multiple ways (e.g., on an online dating site, when instant messaging), and talking about sex with strangers (Ybarra, Mitchell, Finkelhor, & Wolak, 2007). Youth at risk for the most aggressive solicitations were female, used chat rooms, used the Internet with a cell phone, talked to people they met online, talked about sex online, and experienced offline physical or sexual abuse (Mitchell, Finkelhor, & Wolak, 2007). In general, it appears that adolescents involved in sexual solicitation as perpetrators or victims have psychosocial problems, including substance use, problematic offline aggressive behaviors (physical and sexual), and poor emotional bonds with caregivers and poor monitoring by caregivers (Ybarra, Espelage, & Mitchell, 2007). As with cyber bullying, online victimization is accompanied by physical and psychological costs and victims of unwanted sexual solicitation report emotional distress, depressive symptoms, and offline victimization (Finkelhor et al., 2000).

Conclusions

In the previous chapters, we showed that adolescents are using the Internet and other technologies for information and interaction, and are doing so to help them with the developmental tasks facing them. Unfortunately, as we showed in this chapter, the Internet also exposes them to content and interactions laced with violence and aggression. We provided several examples of the former such as in web sites, music, hate sites, and games and described the main kinds of victimization including cyber bullying and online sexual solicitation. However, given the fast changing nature of new technologies, the particular forms of violent content and harassment we described will likely change as users adapt to the affordances of newer digital tools. It is important not to lose sight of the fact that ultimately technology is but a tool, and in the hands of a user, can be used for either good or ill (Juvonen & Gross, 2008).

While adolescents' easy access to violence-themed content via web sites or online hate sites is of concern, we suggest that efforts to understand and limit access to such content should not be directed indiscriminately at all teens, but must target those who are most likely to seek violent messages, be persuaded by them, or be associated with online victimization. From extant research, we know that alienated youth, sensation seekers, and generally those at-risk are most likely to access violent media. We must direct our efforts, both research and intervention, toward those youth who are susceptible to hate messages and so are most likely to be persuaded by them. Similarly, we described the constellation of youth characteristics associated with perpetrators and victims of cyber bullying and sexual solicitation. Youth who seek out violent or hateful content, bully peers, or are victims of harassment seem to have difficulties in other areas of their offline lives. We therefore suggest that when teachers, physicians, counselors, and other health professionals interact with youth, who are troubled in other areas (e.g., conflict at home, sexual or physical abuse, or engaging in high risk behaviors), they probe for online activities or victimization that might place them at further risk. In the next chapter, we describe the specific strategies that can safeguard adolescents from inappropriate and harmful online content and interactions to ensure that they have positive and safe experiences in digital worlds.

There is much that we do not know about negative online content and interactions, in particular their short- and long-term effects on attitudes and behavior at different points in development, and it is critical for high quality experimental studies to address this gap in our understanding of young people's online worlds.

References

Aikat, D. O. (2004). *Violent content in online music videos: Chararcteristics of violine in online videos on bet.com, countrh.com, mtv.com and vh1.com.* Paper presented at the Annual Meeting of the International Communication Association, New Orleans. Retrieved November 15, 2008, from http://www.allacademic.com/meta/p113373_index.html

Aisbett, K., Authority, A. B., & Insights, E. (2001). *The Internet at home: A report on Internet use in the home.* Retrieved January 16, 2009, from http://www.acma.gov.au/webwr/aba/newspubs/documents/internetathome.pdf

Anderson, C. A. (2004). An update on the effects of playing violent video games. *Journal of Adolescence, 27,* 113–122.

Anderson, C. A., Berkowitz, L., Donnerstein, E., Huesmann, L. R., Johnson, J. D., Linz, D., et al. (2003). The influence of media violence on youth. *Psychological Science in the Public Interest, 4,* 81–110.

Beran, T., & Li, Q. (2005). Cyber-harassment: A study of a new method for an old behavior. *Journal of Educational Computing Research, 32,* 265–277.

Blankstein, A. (2008). Alleged tagger seen on YouTube is arrested. *Los Angeles Times.* http://articles.latimes.com/2008/may/28/local/me-buket28

Cappi, M. (2007). *A never ending war.* Victoria, Canada: Trafford Publishing.

Cho, I. (2004). *Computer games – Violence in multiplayer games.* Retrieved October 20, 2008, from http://wiki.media-culture.org.au/index.php/Video_games_Violence_in_multiplayer_games

DuRant, R. H., Rich, M., Emans, S. J., Rome, E. S., Allred, E., & Woods, E. R. (1997). Violence and weapon carrying in music videos. A content analysis. *Archives of Pediatrics and Adolescent Medicine, 151,* 443–448.

Finkelhor, D., Mitchell, K. J., & Wolak, J. (2000). *Online victimization: A report on the nation's youth.* Alexandria, VA: National Center for Missing and Exploited Children.

Fleming, M. J., Greentree, S., Cocotti-Muller, D., Elias, K. A., & Morrison, S. (2006). Safety in cyberspace: Adolescents' safety and exposure online. *Youth & Society, 38,* 135–154.

Funk, J. B., Baldacci, H. B., Pasold, T., & Baumgardner, J. (2004). Violence exposure in real-life, video games, television, movies, and the Internet: Is there desensitization? *Journal of Adolescence, 27,* 23–39.

Gerstenfeld, P. B., Grant, D. R., & Chiang, C. P. (2003). Hate online: A content analysis of extremist Internet sites. *Analyses of Social Issues and Public Policy, 3,* 29–44.

Greenfield, P. M., & Subrahmanyam, K. (2003). Online discourse in a teen chatroom: New codes and new modes of coherence in a visual medium. *Journal of Applied Developmental Psychology, 24,* 713–738.

Hinduja, S., & Patchin, J. W. (2007). Offline consequences of online victimization: School violence and delinquency. *Journal of School Violence, 6,* 89–112.

Hinduja, S., & Patchin, J. W. (2008). Cyberbullying: An exploratory analysis of factors related to offending and victimization. *Deviant Behavior, 29,* 129–156.

Jones, K. (1997). Are rap videos more violent? Style differences and the prevalence of sex and violence in the age of MTV. *Howard Journal of Communication, 8*, 343–356.

Juvonen, J., & Gross, E. F. (2008). Extending the school grounds? Bullying experiences in cyberspace. *The Journal of School Health, 78*, 496–505.

Kirsh, S. J. (2006). *Children, adolescents, and media violence: A critical look at the research.* Thousand Oaks, CA: Sage.

Kowalski, R. M., & Limber, S. P. (2007). Electronic bullying among middle school students. *Journal of Adolescent Health, 41*, 22–30.

Lee, E., & Leets, L. (2002). Persuasive storytelling by hate groups online: Examining its effects on adolescents. *American Behavioral Scientist, 45*, 927–957.

Leets, L. (2001). Responses to Internet hate sites: Is speech too free in cyberspace? *Communication Law & Policy, 6*, 287–317.

Livingstone, S., Bober, M., & Helsper, E. (2005). *Internet literacy among children and young people: Findings from the UK Children Go Online project.* Retrieved January 16, 2009, from http://eprints.lse.ac.uk/397/1/UKCGOonlineLiteracy.pdf

Mitchell, K. J., Finkelhor, D., & Wolak, J. (2002). Online victimization of youth. In D. Levinson (Ed.), *Encyclopedia of crime and punishment* (Vol. 3, pp. 1109–1112). Thousand Oaks, CA: Sage.

Mitchell, K. J., Finkelhor, D., & Wolak, J. (2007). Youth Internet users at risk for the most serious online sexual solicitations. *American Journal of Preventive Medicine, 32*, 532–537.

Mitchell, K. J., Wolak, J., & Finkelhor, D. (2007). Trends in youth reports of sexual solicitations, harassment and unwanted exposure to pornography on the Internet. *Journal of Adolescent Health, 40*, 116–126.

Mitchell, K. J., Wolak, J., & Finkelhor, D. (2008). Are blogs putting youth at risk for online sexual solicitation or harassment? *Child Abuse & Neglect, 32*, 277–294.

NCH. (2005). *Putting u in the picture: Mobile bullying survey 2005.* Retrieved August 7, 2007, from http://www.nch.org.uk/uploads/documents/Mobile_bullying_%20report.pdf

Pooley, E. (1999). Portrait of a deadly bond. *Time, 26*. Retrieved May 10, 2009, from http://www.time.com/time/magazine/article/0,9171,990917,00.html

Raskauskas, J., & Stoltz, A. D. (2007). Involvement in traditional and electronic bullying among adolescents. *Developmental Psychology, 43*, 564–575.

Schafer, J. A. (2002). Spinning the web of hate. Web-based hate propagation by extremist organizations. *Journal of Criminal Justice and Popular Culture, 9*, 69–88.

Sevcikova, A., & Šmahel, D. (2009). Cyberbullying among Czech Internet users: Comparison across age groups. *Zeitschrift für Psychologie [Journal of Psychology], 4*, 227–229.

Simon Wiesenthal Center. (2007). *Digital terrorism and hate 2007.* From http://fswc.ca/publications.aspx

Slater, M. D. (2003). Alienation, aggression, and sensation seeking as predictors of adolescent use of violent film, computer, and website content. *The Journal of Communication, 53*, 105–121.

Slater, M. D., Henry, K. L., Swaim, R. C., & Anderson, L. L. (2003). Violent media content and aggressiveness in adolescents: A downward spiral model. *Communication Research, 30*, 713–736.

Turpin-Petrosino, C. (2002). Hateful sirens... Who hears their song? An examination of student attitudes toward hate groups and affiliation potential. *Journal of Social Issues, 58*, 281–301.

Tynes, B. M. (2005). Children, adolescents and the culture of online hate. In N. E. Dodd, D. E. Singer, & R. F. Wilson (Eds.), *Handbook of children, culture and violence* (pp. 267–289). Thousand Oaks, CA: Sage.

Wei, R. (2007). Effects of playing violent videogames on Chinese adolescents' pro-violence attitudes, attitudes toward others, and aggressive behavior. *CyberPsychology & Behavior, 10*, 371–380.

Weimann, G. (2008). *Online terrorists prey on the vulnerable.* Retrieved October 20, 2008, from http://yaleglobal.yale.edu/display.article?id=10453

Williams, D., & Skoric, M. (2005). Internet fantasy violence: A test of aggression in an online game. *Communication Monographs, 72*, 217–233.

Wolak, J., Mitchell, K. J., & Finkelhor, D. (2006). *Online victimization of youth: 5 years later.* Retrieved August 9, 2007, from http://www.unh.edu/ccrc/pdf/CV138.pdf

Ybarra, M. L. (2004). Linkages between depressive symptomatology and Internet harassment among young regular Internet users. *CyberPsychology & Behavior, 7,* 247–257.

Ybarra, M. L., Diener-West, M., & Leaf, P. J. (2007). Examining the overlap in Internet harassment and school bullying: Implications for school intervention. *Journal of Adolescent Health, 41,* 42–50.

Ybarra, M. L., Espelage, D. L., & Mitchell, K. J. (2007). The co-occurrence of Internet harassment and unwanted sexual solicitation victimization and perpetration: Associations with psychosocial indicators. *Journal of Adolescent Health, 41,* S31–S41.

Ybarra, M. L., & Mitchell, K. J. (2004). Youth engaging in online harassment: Associations with caregiver–child relationships, Internet use, and personal characteristics. *Journal of Adolescence, 27,* 319–336.

Ybarra, M. L., & Mitchell, K. J. (2008). How risky are social networking sites? A comparison of places online where youth sexual solicitation and harassment occurs. *Pediatrics, 121,* e350–e357.

Ybarra, M. L., Mitchell, K. J., Finkelhor, D., & Wolak, J. (2007). Internet prevention messages: Targeting the right online behaviors. *Archives of Pediatrics and Adolescent Medicine, 161,* 138–145.

Yee, N. (2006). The demographics, motivations, and derived experiences of users of massively multi-user online graphical environments. *PRESENCE: Teleoperators and Virtual Environments, 15,* 309–329.

Zhou, Y., Qin, J., Lai, G., & Chen, H. (2007). *Collection of US extremist online forums: A web mining approach.* Proceedings of the 40th Hawaii International Conference on System Sciences (Vol. 40, p. 1184). Waikoloa, HI. Retrieved October 12, 2010, from http://ieeexplore.ieee.org/xpls/abs_all.jsp?arnumber=4076513&tag=1

Chapter 11
Promoting Positive and Safe Digital Worlds: What Parents and Teachers Can Do to Empower Youth

As the reader is by now undoubtedly aware digital worlds present a mass of contradictions for users. For youth, they offer opportunities for interaction and access to vast amounts of information and resources, but as we saw in the previous chapter, they also have their unsavory aspects, such as pornography, violent, and other inappropriate content that can be readily accessed, as well as potential for victimization at the hands of peers and adults. Understandably parents, practitioners, and policy makers are confused and uncertain as to how to respond to young people's online forays. Consider David's (the second author) experience while teaching a distance learning course on psychology and the Internet. Despite the course taking place in the relatively liberal Czech Republic, students, who were also parents of teens, had many concerns about inappropriate content (e.g., pornography, online violence) and interactions (e.g., cybersex, sexting) that their teens might encounter and more importantly, were unsure as to whether they should limit and restrict their child activities with digital media.

Such questions and worries may prompt parents to either prohibit their teen from using digital tools (e.g., the Internet) or applications (e.g., social networking sites, texting) or monitor their child too closely while using them (Tynes, 2007). Considering how deeply enmeshed technology is in young people's lives and the fact that adolescences is a time when youth are developing autonomy and independence, these are neither practical or feasible, nor even wise options. Limiting and restricting adolescents' access to digital media could well be akin to throwing the baby out with the bathwater. A smarter and more productive approach is to focus our efforts on protecting and empowering youth so they can use technology positively and safely, and in ways that will promote their well being.

This chapter describes what we can do to ensure that youth have positive and safe experiences in digital worlds by safeguarding them from inappropriate and harmful online content (e.g., pornography and violence) and victimization by peers (e.g., cyber bullying) and adult predators (sexual solicitation). Doing so will require the concerted and proactive actions of government, industry, parents, and schools (Chisholm, 2006; Dombrowski, Lemasney, Ahia, & Dickson, 2004; Oswell, 1999; Tynes, 2007), and in the next sections, we examine their roles in this endeavor. For each stakeholder, we first present strategies that they can adopt to protect youth

K. Subrahmanyam, D. Šmahel, *Digital Youth*, Advancing Responsible
Adolescent Development, DOI 10.1007/978-1-4419-6278-2_11,
© Springer Science+Business Media, LLC 2011

from inappropriate content and then present those that they can use to protect from victimization; since we can use many of the same strategies against both threats, the latter category only includes those measures that are unique to online victimization. Much of our discussion is also in the context of the USA, but where available, we provide information from other countries and contexts as well.

The Role of Government and Industry

Safeguarding Youth from Inappropriate Content

To understand the role of government and industry in safeguarding youth, we need to reconsider some aspects of adolescents' digital worlds. As we noted in Chapter 1, the digital landscape is getting more complex and there is a blurring of the distinctions between hardware, content, and applications. Adolescents use a variety of hardware, including computers, cell phones, and other mobile hand-held devices, to access online content and interactions. With the emergence of the Web 2.0, user-generated content and opportunities for interaction are becoming a more central part of young people's digital worlds. As a result, it is also getting more difficult to identify the face of industry, which now not only includes Internet service providers and commercial content providers, but also a host of online social forums or contexts and individual content creators themselves. For instance, mobile devices may allow access to content provided by cell phone companies or third parties, or even via the World Wide Web. Figuring out the relationship between government and industry is therefore not easy, and the changing nature of this relationship is reflected in the way the European Union has moved from a model of industry self-regulation in the 1990s to the current preference for co-regulation between government, industry, and user groups (EICN, 2005; Oswell, 1999).

Within the USA, the Federal Communication Commission does not regulate Internet content (Schwabach, 2005); the main challenge for government regulation is that most online content is protected as free speech by the First Amendment. In fact, the Child Online Protection Act (COPA)[1], which was passed to protect minors from harmful online material, was struck down in July 2008 because of threats to the First Amendment (ACLU v. Mukasey, 2008). With regard to violent content, Weissblum has discussed the incitement of violence on the Internet in the context of the Columbine school shooting incident in Littleton, CO, in which the teenage perpetrators were reported to have obtained information about making bombs from online web sites (Weissblum, 2000). Even though most online content is treated as speech and is protected by the First Amendment, online speech is not protected if it creates a "clear and present danger" of imminent lawless action. Weissblum notes that "this action must be imminent, and there must be both intent to produce, and

---

[1]The COPA should not be confused with the COPPA, which is the Children's Online Privacy Protection Act of 1998 and regulates the collection of personal information (such as name, address) from minor children younger than 13 years of age.

a likelihood of producing, imminent disorder." However, the advocacy of violence alone is not regarded as incitement to imminent lawless action and consequently is protected by the First Amendment. Similarly, pornography per se is not considered illegal (although obscene material and child pornography are) and the courts have generally suggested that the use of filtering or blocking software are constitutionally more acceptable ways of regulating minors' access to such material (Schwabach, 2005).

The legal arguments at the heart of these issues are beyond the scope of this book. Suffice to say that there are both legal as well as practical challenges to regulating violent, pornographic, and other online content that are potentially harmful to minors, and different governments have adopted different approaches. Given this reality, and the changing nature of technology itself, we submit that the onus of protecting youth from such content falls more squarely upon parents and others (e.g., teachers and physicians) who work with youth.

Safeguarding Youth from Online Victimization

Unlike aggressive and other negative online content that may be protected by free speech laws, aggressive online interactions (e.g., sexual solicitation, bullying, and harassment) are not. They have serious physical and psychological effects and in some cases, may even threaten the life and safety of youth. Consequently, at the legislative level, most countries have passed a variety of laws to protect children from such behaviors, with varying degrees of success. Within the USA, the Children's Online Privacy Protection Act of 1998 (COPPA) protects young children's privacy by requiring that commercial web site operators obtain parent consent prior to "collecting, using, or disclosing personal information from children under 13" (Federal Trade Commision, 1999). Child exploitation statutes have criminalized online sexual coercion, exploitation, solicitation, and abuse and perpetrators may be prosecuted at the Federal or State levels for child abuse, exploitation, and sexual solicitation (Dombrowski et al., 2004). Furthermore, there are laws that mandate web site providers, Internet service providers, and other similar parties to report evidence of child pornography and sexual exploitation to the "Cyber Tip Line" (http://www.cybertipline.com) at the National Center for Missing and Exploited Children (NCMEC) (Dombrowski, Gischlar, & Durst, 2007; Dombrowski et al., 2004). Other countries such as the UK, Canada, and Australia, have also similarly passed laws that protect children from online grooming and pornography; most also have mechanisms to report online predatory behavior although the particular means may vary (e.g., web site vs. phone) (Dombrowski et al., 2007).

Legislation by itself cannot be effective and we need aggressive enforcement, including investigation and prosecution of online sexual predators. Within the USA, one such coordinated effort is the Project Safe Childhood (PSC) initiative, launched by the US Department of Justice in 2006 to "combat the proliferation of technology-facilitated sexual exploitation crimes against children." It involves the coordinated action by several agencies and organizations including US Attorneys, the Child Exploitation and Obscenity Section of the Department's

Criminal Division, Internet Crimes Against Children (ICAC) task force, federal partners, including the FBI, US Postal Inspection Service, Immigration and Customs Enforcement and the US Marshals Service as well as advocacy organizations (such as the NCMEC), and state and local law enforcement officials (Department of Justice, 2008). Similarly, in Europe, Insafe (http://www.saferinternet.org) seeks to promote the Internet safety of citizens, particularly youth and children, by creating a national level-based network of concerned actors including children, government, educators, parents, media, and industry. It provides information and resources for parents, teachers and others, promotes awareness campaigns, coordinated actions, as well as Internet help lines, and hotlines. "Safer Internet Programme,"[2] also in Europe, seeks to empower and protect online youth by awareness-raising initiatives and by fighting illegal and harmful online content. One project of this program is "EU Kids Online,"[3] which coordinates a public and searchable database of European research on children's online activities[4] that can be an important resource for parents, educators, and practitioners concerned about this issue. In 2010, project "EU Kids Online II" carried out a robust comparative research in 25 European countries focusing on online risks for children aged 9 to 16 years. The research report is available on the aforementioned project web page (from October 2010).

Legislating online bullying and victimization is much more challenging and less successful as well. The Megan Meier case described in Chapter 10 illustrates some of the difficulties involved. Prosecutors at the local level did not prosecute the case, as they could not find relevant statutes under which to pursue it. It was not until a year later that Federal authorities in Los Angeles (the location of the web site operator) pursued action against Lori Drew (the adult behind the incident). Even then, the prosecution was not for harassment per se, but for a violation of the Terms of Service agreement with MySpace as she had used a fictitious name to open an account. Federal prosecutors charged Ms. Drew with violating the Federal Computer Fraud and Abuse Act showing how difficult it is to prosecute the intent to harm another. Some states such as Missouri, where this incident occurred, have since modified harassment laws to include Internet harassment. However, we think that these newer laws will be used only if the harassment leads to murder, suicide, or other equally dire consequences.

The Role of Parents

Safeguarding Youth from Inappropriate Content

Most youth first start using the Internet at home, which remains an important context where much of their online activity takes place. Parents therefore have a critical role

---

[2] http://ec.europa.eu/information_society/activities/sip/index_en.htm

[3] http://www.lse.ac.uk/collections/EUKidsOnline/

[4] http://webdb.lse.ac.uk/eukidsonline/search.asp

to empower and safeguard their teen while they are online. Parents' success in this regard will depend on both what they know about objectionable online content and their teens' access to such material, and what they actually do to monitor and limit such access.

It turns out that parents are not very knowledgeable about the extent to which their adolescent accesses and views negative content. When teens and their parents were surveyed, it was found that parents underestimated their teens' accidental and intentional exposure to content such as violent online games, sexually explicit sites, online interactions with strangers, and online gambling (Cho & Cheon, 2005). Such discrepancy between parents and teens' reports about the latter's offline and online behavior is not that uncommon; for instance, in Chapter 8, we noted that parents were in the dark as to whether or not their teens, who had visited an eating disorder clinic, had visited pro-anorexia sites.

Parental mediation strategies. Within the parenting literature, parents' strategies and actions to help their children deal with unwanted media content is referred to as *mediation techniques* (Eastin, Greenberg, & Hofshire, 2006; Nathanson, 2001). Research on television and radio has led researchers to identify three mediation styles, *factual mediation, evaluative mediation,* and *restrictive mediation.* With regard to the Internet, a fourth kind, *technological mediation,* has been described (Eastin et al., 2006). We describe each of these mediation techniques next, with examples of how they can be used by parents to help their teens deal with unwanted online content.

Factual mediation techniques seek to provide users with facts about the content and production of media such as plot and character development, light and sound effects. With regard to Internet content, factual mediation does not transfer very readily, especially to aggressive material; it has also not been studied in the context of the Internet (Eastin et al., 2006). Specific examples of factual mediation with regard to online content come from the teaching of Internet literacy skills, such as the evaluation, credibility, and crediting of sources. These strategies are more critical to young people's handling of information for schoolwork and health-related content, and were addressed in Chapters 6 and 8, respectively.

Evaluative mediation techniques entail parent and child co-viewing and discussion to evaluate and interpret media content. Specific evaluative mediation techniques that parents can adopt to help children deal with online content include the following (Eastin et al., 2006; Tynes, 2007):

(1) Jointly visiting websites and other online content with their children.
(2) Having frank and open discussions with their teen about online content, and specifically addressing violent, hateful, and other more harmful kinds of content.
(3) Evaluating with their teen online websites and other formats (e.g., music videos, YouTube videos) for violent images, hateful themes, and other negative content.

Restrictive mediation consists of rules regarding media use, specifically parental rules as to the "where," "when," and the "what" content their teens access online

(Eastin et al., 2006; Wang, Bianchi, & Raley, 2005). Specific examples of this strategy include the following:

(1) Placing the computer in a public space.
(2) Having rules about the time spent online.
(3) Having content restrictions, in other words, having rules about the kind of content that a teen can consume.

Technological mediation refers to parents' use of technological strategies to mediate their children's use of the Internet. Examples include software to track application usage and browser history, filtering software, installation of a firewall (Dombrowski et al., 2004; Eastin et al., 2006). Of particular note, parents can install filtering software on their children's computers in order to limit exposure to violent and potentially disturbing content. Many different kinds of filters are available, such as those that allow access to selected web sites, or block access to sites with questionable content, or block sites that contain forbidden words (Ins@fe, 2009). Such electronic monitoring has its limits – filters are not foolproof and often will block access to legitimate sites. Moreover, even if parents use filters on home computers and laptops, their teens might still be able to access inappropriate content outside the home on a computer in a friend's home or even in a public place such as a library.

Use and effectiveness of parental mediation strategies. Like so many other aspects of Internet use, we do not have a clear picture of the extent to which parents use the different techniques described above. The little we know is from parental self-report, and as we shall see below, they are often at odds with what teens say about their parents' actions. In a US study, 33% of parents reported using filtering or blocking software, and 5% even reported discontinuing its use (Mitchell, Finkelhor, & Wolak, 2005). Similarly, in the Czech Republic, 27% of parents reported using such software (World Internet Project, 2008, unpublished data). Parents were also more likely to use such software if they were very concerned about exposure to sexual material, suggesting that there may be much less use of blocking software to limit access to violent content. But it's hard to know how much faith one can have in these numbers: Just as parents are often in the dark about their teens' exposure to undesirable content, they also seem to overestimate the extent to which they actually monitor their Internet use. In the data from the Czech Republic described earlier, only 11% of 12- to 18-year olds reported that their parents installed some kind of filtering software on their computer. In another study, 40% of the parents and their teens disagreed as to whether they had rules about Internet use; in the majority of the cases, the parents reported having rules, whereas the teens reported that there were none (Wang et al., 2005). Worth noting also is that parents' estimates of online dangers do not always match their actions in terms of setting limits or monitoring their teens (e.g., viewing their MySpace profile) (Rosen, Cheever, & Carrier, 2008).

Research on the effectiveness of parental mediation is both sparse and equivocal. One US study examined the effects of parental monitoring on adolescents' exposure to pornography in a national sample of 1,500 youth between 10- and

17 years of age (Wolak, Mitchell, & Finkelhor, 2007). Two types of prevention efforts were associated with lowered risks of unwanted exposure to online pornography and we describe them next. The first included the use of filtering, blocking, or monitoring software, which had a "modest protective effect" on both accidental as well as intentional exposure to pornographic material. Not all technological solutions were equally effective and the use of pop-up advertisement blockers and e-mail spam filters had no effect on exposure to online pornography. In fact, the study's authors warn that "filtering and blocking software alone cannot be relied on for a high level of protection against unwanted exposure and other approaches are needed" (p. 254). The second effort, which was associated with reducing unwanted exposure to pornography, entailed parents attending a law enforcement presentation about Internet safety. Such programs provide specific information about how pornography is disseminated online, how it can be accessed on a computer, and how to avoid it. They are more effective for reducing unwanted exposure, compared to intentional exposure. A surprising result of this study was that adolescents, who talked to their parents or other adults about online pornography, actually had higher odds of exposure to unwanted pornography. To account for this finding, the authors speculate that the parent–adolescent conversations may have occurred after the unwanted exposure rather than before. The fact that there was no association between intentional exposure to pornography and parent–teen conversations on this issue suggests that this may indeed be the case. In contrast, a Dutch study found no association between parental monitoring and adolescents' exposure to online pornography (Peter & Valkenburg, 2006). However, only one item ("My parents know when I am surfing the Internet") was used to assess the extent of parental mediation and this may be why no relation was found between parental actions and adolescents' exposure to online content.

Factors affecting parental mediation of online content. Parental and child demographics, parenting style, and family cohesion variables all influence the extent and particular kind of mediation techniques that parents use to monitor their teen's Internet use. As one would expect, parents of younger teens report higher levels of monitoring compared to parents of older teens (Eastin et al., 2006; Wang et al., 2005). In addition, parents with less education are more likely to use monitoring software than parents with higher education because more highly educated parents might have greater experience with computers and the Internet and so may have more confidence in their ability to monitor their teens' Internet use without using monitoring software (Wang et al., 2005).

Not surprisingly, parental mediation and monitoring is related to parenting style. Authoritative parents[5] are more likely to set limits (e.g., time limits and not allowing computers in the bedroom) and to use both evaluative and restrictive mediation techniques compared to authoritarian and neglectful parents (Eastin et al., 2006; Rosen et al., 2008). Ironically, technological blocking was generally the least-used

---

[5] See Chapter 6 for a brief description of authoritative parents.

technique compared to time restrictions, content restrictions, and co-viewing. It was also used most often by authoritative parents, and less so by authoritarian and neglectful ones (Eastin et al., 2006). Lastly, family variables may also be related to parents' mediation of their teen's exposure to online content. One study found that shared web activities between parent and teen, and parents' perceived family cohesion enhanced parental perceived control over Internet use, which in turn led to decreased exposure of Internet content (Cho & Cheon, 2005). Family cohesiveness may generally be related to teens' online activities – Mesch (2008) found that among Israeli adolescents, those who reported higher commitment to their families were also less likely to consume online pornography and be involved in aggressive behavior.

The family's role in promoting positive and healthy online experiences for adolescents cannot be overstated. Indeed, in her testimony to the Congressional Committee on Government Reform (Greenfield, 2004), Greenfield suggested that a warm parent–child relationship and communication may be the most important non-technical means that parents can use to help youth face a sexualized media environment.

Safeguarding Youth from Online Victimization

Parents have an important role when it comes to protecting and educating youth so they are able to deal with the aggressive acts of their peers and predatory adults. They must maintain open lines of communication with their teens and use evaluative and restrictive mediation techniques to teach them about online safety. Specific strategies they can use include the following (Dombrowski et al., 2007; Tynes, 2007):

(1) Parents should have conversations with their teens about their online activities and interaction partners. Although most teens appear to interact with people from their offline lives (see Chapter 5), this is not true for everyone. Therefore, it is important for parents to talk to their child about the dangers of making friends with people they have never met offline, particularly if they are adults. Dombrowski and colleagues also recommend that parents talk to their teens about the dangers of sexual predators and do so at a developmentally appropriate level. More generally, parents should discuss the dangers of meeting face to face with people, only known online. They should discuss common precautions when a teen meets with such online friends, particularly peers; examples include taking a friend along, or meeting in a public space. Parents should also discuss the problem of cyber bullying and encourage their child to talk to them or to a trusted adult at school if they are the victims of online bullying.

(2) Related to the above, parents should have constructive conversations with teens about what they can do to safeguard their privacy online (see Chapter 6 for

more on teens' understanding of privacy). For instance, they should discuss with them that information posted on online forums may be publicly available, others may intercept information sent over the Internet, and that one should not disclose personal information about oneself (e.g., age, location, etc) over the Internet. Given the requirements of COPPA and concerns about online privacy in general, most online forums such as blogs and social networking sites allow users to choose from a variety of privacy settings. For instance, Facebook users can chose profile settings so that limited profile information (e.g., details about the user) is revealed in a search; it allows users to provide restricted access to their profiles, so their Facebook friends are not able to access all parts of their profile. Parents should learn about these options and educate and encourage their teen to use these settings (Tynes, 2007).

(3) Approving screen names: Parents and guardians should explain to teens that screen names are the equivalent of their online faces. They should know and approve of their screen names and should dissuade teens from using sexually suggestive ones, as sexual predators may be more likely to target teens with sexually provocative screen names (Dombrowski et al., 2007).

(4) Parents should also help their teens to develop what Tynes calls an exit strategy (Tynes, 2007). They should help youth to recognize the behavior of predators and should talk to them about strategies they can adopt when they feel threatened by an online conversation/interaction partner; for instance, they should end the interaction immediately and block the person as well. These strategies are also useful when a peer is harassing a teen. If the individual continues to contact the youth or the threatening behavior continues, they should advise the teen to report it to parents and appropriate authorities. In the case of bullying and harassment, parents should advise teens to complain to the Internet Service Provider of the harasser. Teens should be advised that if they are sexually solicited online by an adult or someone they think is an adult, they should report it immediately to the "CyberTipline" mentioned earlier (Tynes, 2007).

In addition to the technological mediation strategies that have already been discussed (e.g., monitoring browser history and application tracking and usage) (Dombrowski et al., 2007), parents can use the following technical tools to protect youth from online victimization, particularly at the hands of predatory adults:

1. Installing a firewall and anti-virus or anti-Trojan software to prevent unauthorized access into computer systems and to prevent access to private information.
2. Installation of a key logger or a chat logger to monitor communication with third parties: These programs record all key strokes typed on a computer, or record plain-text communication via a chat client.
3. Encryption for chat clients (e.g., AOL's Instant Messenger) that protects youth from predators who may use Ethernet sniffers to spy on their online communication.

4. Privacy filtration to block the transmission of personal information over the Internet; parents can use such programs to specify the kinds of information that can or cannot be transmitted over the computer.

No doubt, more such tools will be developed to counteract the aggressive actions of sexual predators. However, we should keep in mind that technological measures have their limitations: they require parents to be technologically proficient, they do not protect youth when they access computers outside the home, and peers and predators with technological skills might find ways to counteract them. Most importantly, they do raise concerns of privacy and trust, at the very time that adolescents desire more autonomy and their relationships with their parents may be changing.

The Role of Schools

Safeguarding Youth from Inappropriate Content

With regard to protecting youth from inappropriate content online, many states in the USA have laws mandating that schools prevent minors from gaining access to sexually explicit, obscene, and harmful material. In addition, the US Congress has enacted The Children's Internet Protection Act (CIPA), which imposes similar requirements when schools receive federal funding for technology and Internet access (FCC, 2009). Generally, schools use filtering and blocking software to comply with these laws. It should be noted that only obscene content, child pornography, and content "harmful to minors" is explicitly addressed by the law, but most school districts use electronic filters to also block sites that contain violence, as well as sites that provide access to social networking sites, games, shopping, and gambling.

Safeguarding Youth from Online Victimization

Schools and educators can help protect youth from harassing and threatening interactions online by adopting the evaluative and restrictive mediation strategies described earlier. However, cyber bullying presents special challenges for schools – it may occur when a youth is on school premises, but can also happen when the youth is at home and at virtually any time of the day, making it difficult for schools to regulate it. Moreover, since offline and online bullying are related, cyber bullying that occurs outside of school may later on be related to incidents at school. Legally it is difficult for schools to control behavior that occurs outside of school and as such there is little consensus on how they should respond. Developing effective policy to combat cyber bullying will necessarily require the collaboration of all important parties – policy makers (e.g., school board), school officials, parents, and youth (Brown, Jackson, & Cassidy, 2006).

Conclusions

Thus far, we have discussed the different strategies that government, law enforcement, parents, and schools can adopt to help make youth have positive and safe online experiences. Parents have an especially important role to play in safeguarding youth and we need more research to ascertain the extent to which they consistently adopt different mediation techniques, their effectiveness, and the factors that mediate their efficacy. There is some evidence that when, parents, and teachers take a more proactive role, there are immediate benefits with regard to protecting youth from harmful interactions. In one study of adolescent girls, 70% reported that their parents had discussed online safety with them and 35% reported that their teachers had done this as well; furthermore, it appeared that direct supervision, periodic monitoring, and ongoing discussion with adults was associated with less risky behaviors online, such as disclosing personal information, and offline meetings (Berson, Berson, & Ferron, 2002). Importantly, teen girls who discussed online safety with their teachers and parents were less likely to report having agreed to meet with a stranger they had met online. Teacher discussions were especially important for teens who did not have such a discussion with their parents.

The parental role in cyber bullying may be hampered because they are generally unaware of cyber bullying as many youth do not tell their parents about their bullying behavior or when they are bullied (Dehue, Bolman, & Vollink, 2008; Juvonen & Gross, 2008). In Juvonen and Gross's study, 90% of participants reported not telling their parents when they were bullied mainly because they were afraid that they would get into trouble with their parents and might have their Internet use restricted. Similarly, when it comes to using technological strategies, a quarter of the youth who had been bullied online had never blocked the bullies' screen name (Juvonen & Gross, 2008). While not conclusive, these findings do suggest that even the most sophisticated strategies and tools will not work unless parents, teachers, and other health professionals discuss online safety with teens, teach them about using technological strategies to protect themselves, and reiterate that informing adults about unpleasant experiences or interactions will not lead to repercussions.

Finally yet importantly, parents' decision to monitor their teen's online activities and exposure is itself not an easy one. Parents have to grapple with the competing demands of giving their teens freedom, respecting their online privacy, and ensuring their online safety. Ultimately, the decision to monitor and to limit teens' online activities and the content they accesses is an individual one, and depends on cultural norms as well as family beliefs and parenting practices. Not only are there enormous differences in attitudes about sexuality and permissiveness between individuals in different countries, there are also differences between parents and families within a particular country. There are also individual differences among adolescents in the amount of freedom they can handle and how much they have to be monitored. Consequently, there is no single, correct way of handling adolescents' exposure to inappropriate online content and interactions. Parents and families will have to make individual decisions concerning whether and how much to monitor their teens' online activities.

References

ACLU v. Mukasey. (2008). *Aclu v. Mukasey – Opinion of the court*. From http://www.aclu.org/pdfs/freespeech/copa_20080722.pdf

Berson, I. R., Berson, M. J., & Ferron, J. M. (2002). Emerging risks of violence in the digital age: Lessons for educators from an online study of adolescent girls in the United States. *Journal of School Violence, 1*, 51–72.

Brown, K., Jackson, M., & Cassidy, W. (2006). Cyber-bullying: Developing policy to direct responses that are equitable and effective in addressing this special form of bullying. *Canadian Journal of Educational Administration and Policy, 57*, 8–11.

Chisholm, J. F. (2006). Cyberspace violence against girls and adolescent females. *Annals of the New York Academy of Sciences, 1087*, 74–89.

Cho, C. H., & Cheon, H. J. (2005). Children's exposure to negative Internet content: Effects of family context. *Journal of Broadcasting & Electronic Media, 49*, 488–509.

Dehue, F., Bolman, C., & Vollink, T. (2008). Cyberbullying: Youngsters' experiences and parental perception. *CyberPsychology & Behavior, 11*, 217–223.

Department of Justice. (2008). *Fact sheet: Project safe childhood*. Retrieved January 19, 2009, from http://www.ojp.usdoj.gov/newsroom/pressreleases/2008/psc08-999.htm

Dombrowski, S. C., Gischlar, K. L., & Durst, T. (2007). Safeguarding young people from cyber pornography and cyber sexual predation: A major dilemma of the Internet. *Child Abuse Review, 16*, 153–170.

Dombrowski, S. C., Lemasney, J. W., Ahia, C. E., & Dickson, S. A. (2004). Protecting children from online sexual predators: Technological, psychoeducational, and legal considerations. *Professional Psychology, Research and Practice, 35*, 65–73.

Eastin, M. S., Greenberg, B. S., & Hofschire, L. (2006). Parenting the Internet. *Journal of Communication, 56*, 486–504.

EICN. (2005). *Protecting minors from exposure to harmful content on mobile phones*. Retrieved January 16, 2009, from http://www.foruminternet.org/specialistes/international/multi-fr-rapports-et-guides-en-reports-and-guides-multi/protecting-minors-from-exposure-to-harmful-content-on-mobile-phones.html

FCC. (2009). *Children's Internet protection act*. Retrieved October 11, 2009, from http://www.fcc.gov/cgb/consumerfacts/cipa.html

Federal Trade Commision. (1999). *New rule will protect privacy of children online*. Retrieved January 18, 2009, from http://www.ftc.gov/opa/1999/10/childfinal.shtm

Greenfield, P. M. (2004). Inadvertent exposure to pornography on the Internet: Implications of peer-to-peer file-sharing networks for child development and families. *Journal of Applied Developmental Psychology: An International Lifespan Journal, 25*, 741–750.

Ins@fe. (2009). *Filtering, labels, parenting controls*. Retrieved January 15, 2009, from http://www.saferinternet.org/ww/en/pub/insafe/safety_issues/faqs/filtering.htm

Juvonen, J., & Gross, E. F. (2008). Extending the school grounds? Bullying experiences in cyberspace. *The Journal of School Health, 78*, 496–505.

Mesch, G. S. (2008). Social bonds and Internet pornographic exposure among adolescents. *Journal of Adolescence, 32*, 601–618.

Mitchell, K. J., Finkelhor, D., & Wolak, J. (2005). Protecting youth online: Family use of filtering and blocking software. *Child Abuse & Neglect, 29*, 753–765.

Nathanson, A. I. (2001). Mediation of children's television viewing: Working toward conceptual clarity and common understanding. *Communication Yearbook, 25*, 115–151.

Oswell, D. (1999). The dark side of cyberspace: Internet content regulation and child protection. *Convergence, 5*, 42–62.

Peter, J., & Valkenburg, P. M. (2006). Adolescents' exposure to sexually explicit material on the Internet. *Communication Research, 33*, 178–204.

Rosen, L. D., Cheever, N. A., & Carrier, L. M. (2008). The association of parenting style and child age with parental limit setting and adolescent myspace behavior. *Journal of Applied Developmental Psychology, 29*, 459–471.

Schwabach, A. (Ed.). (2005). *Internet and the law: Technology, society, and compromises.* Santa Barbara, CA: ABC-CLIO.

Tynes, B. M. (2007). Internet safety gone wild? Sacrificing the educational and psychosocial benefits of online social environments. *Journal of Adolescent Research, 22,* 575–584.

Wang, R., Bianchi, S. M., & Raley, S. B. (2005). Teenagers' Internet use and family rules: A research note. *Journal of Marriage and Family, 67,* 1249–1258.

Weissblum, L. (2000). Incitement to violence on the world wide web: Can web publishers seek first amendment refuge? 6 Mich. Telecomm. *Tech. L. Rev. 35.* Retrieved November 17, 2008 from http://www.mttlr.org/volsix/weissblum.html

Wolak, J., Mitchell, K. J., & Finkelhor, D. (2007). Unwanted and wanted exposure to online pornography in a national sample of youth Internet users. *Pediatrics, 119,* 247–257.

Chapter 12
Adolescents' Digital Worlds: Conclusions and Future Steps

Today's youth, as digital natives, have lived virtually their entire lives surrounded by digital media, especially computers and the Internet (Rideout, Vandewater, & Wartella, 2003; Roberts & Foehr, 2008). Not surprisingly, their interactions with technology have raised questions and concerns. Research has begun to uncover the many different ways that technology intersects young people's lives. Our goal for this book was to sift through this body of work and present a balanced and comprehensive account of youth digital worlds and their implications for adolescent development. In this concluding chapter, we revisit some of the themes encountered throughout the book, consider their implications, and identify questions and gaps in our understanding that future research must address.

Media in Adolescents' Lives

Media – new and old – are clearly a big part of young people's lives. Contrary to fears, their media use may not necessarily be coming at the expense of interactions with peers. As we saw in Fig. 1.1, across a number of different countries, the time youth spent socializing with friends was comparable to the time they spent watching television or going online. Further, even though their combined screen time (that is television and the Internet combined) is more than the time they spend in offline interactions, much of their online time involves interaction and communication. Recall Fig. 1.2, which showed that the communication activities on the Internet were most frequent, followed by entertainment and school-related information-based activities. Thus, it is important to recognize that a significant aspect of young people's digital worlds is their extensive use of digitally mediated communication forms (Subrahmanyam & Greenfield, 2008).

Despite the widespread popularity of digital communication tools among youth, there are many inter-group differences in how they are used. For instance, US youth use chat rooms much more infrequently compared to youth in Singapore or the Czech Republic (Fig. 1.7). Among social networking sites, Facebook tends to be more popular among White youth and MySpace among Latino youth (Hargittai, 2007; Subrahmanyam, Reich, Waechter, & Espinoza, 2008). Finally, youth bloggers

K. Subrahmanyam, D. Šmahel, *Digital Youth*, Advancing Responsible Adolescent Development, DOI 10.1007/978-1-4419-6278-2_12,
© Springer Science+Business Media, LLC 2011

are overwhelmingly female (Subrahmanyam, Garcia, Harsono, Li, & Lipana, 2009) whereas online gamers tend to be male (Griffiths, Davies, & Chappell, 2004). There are also differences in what youth do within different online contexts. Chat rooms, with their more anonymous and disembodied contexts were used by youth for sexuality and partner selection (Šmahel & Subrahmanyam, 2007; Subrahmanyam, Šmahel, & Greenfield, 2006), whereas social networking sites and instant messaging are used primarily to interact and connect with offline friends (Gross, 2004; Reich, Subrahmanyam, & Espinoza, 2009). In sum, digital contexts are incredibly varied and adolescents use them in a variety of way – to be less or more anonymous, to interact with close friends or acquaintances, to play games, and for their schoolwork. It is important to keep these differences in mind when examining the role of digital media in development, the issue we address next.

Understanding the Role of Digital Media in Development

Online and Offline Worlds Are Psychologically Connected

In Chapter 2, we presented our co-construction model of adolescents' online behavior (Subrahmanyam et al., 2006). We argued that online contexts are interactive, dynamic, and constantly changing and young online users play an important part in constructing and co-constructing their online environments. Based on this co-construction framework, we proposed that adolescents' online and offline worlds might be psychologically connected and that we would find important offline themes in their online activities and interactions. In developmental theory, we refer to the important themes of a particular life phase as developmental issues or tasks. To demonstrate that young people's offline and online lives are connected, we organized the first part of the book around core adolescent issues; accordingly, in Chapters 3–5 we showed that adolescents bring concerns such as sexuality, identity, and intimacy into their digital worlds.

In Chapter 3, we described some of the different ways that youth take advantage of digital contexts to adjust to their changing bodies and develop their sexual selves. We showed that youth use digital tools such as, nicknames, avatars, and explicit text messages and pictures for sexual exploration as well as to construct and present their sexual selves (National Campaign to Prevent Teen and Unplanned Pregnancy & Cosmogirl.com, 2008; Subrahmanyam, Greenfield, & Tynes, 2004; Subrahmanyam et al., 2006). We also described teens' participation in cybersex (Šmahel, 2003) and their access of sexually explicit material/pornography (Peter & Valkenburg, 2006; Ybarra, 2004).

Similarly, in Chapter 4, we saw that adolescents take advantage of online tools such as nicknames, avatars, profiles, blog entries, photos, videos, and language codes for identity exploration and self-presentation (Huffaker & Calvert, 2005; Subrahmanyam et al., 2009; Subrahmanyam et al., 2006). Contrary to early speculation, adolescents neither abandon their offline identities nor engage in identity experiments, but instead, bring their offline selves, including their gender and ethnic identities, with them to their digital worlds (Gross, 2004; Huffaker & Calvert, 2005; Subramanian, 2010; Tynes, 2007).

Finally, in Chapter 5, we showed how adolescents use digital tools in the service of their developing capacity for intimacy and their offline relationships. We saw that they use online communication applications such as instant messaging, social networking sites, and text messaging to connect with their friends, romantic partners, and family members (Gross, 2004; Kaare, Brandtzaeg, Heim, & Endestad, 2007; Reich et al., 2009). Online tools have not only increased the frequency and intensity of adolescents' peer contact, it has also widened it to include both intimate as well as less intimate peers. Moreover, contrary to concerns that youth use the Internet to interact and develop relationships with strangers, they mostly use it to connect with people whom they already know offline (Gross, 2004; Reich et al., 2009).

Adolescents' online behavior and interactions not only reflect core concerns and issues, they also support the more negative aspects of their lives. Offline characteristics seem to predict some kinds of problematic online behaviors. In Chapter 3, we saw that higher sensation-seeking adolescents view sexually explicit media more frequently (Brown & L'Engle, 2009). Intentional exposure to pornography is associated with delinquent behaviors, substance abuse, depression, and reduced emotional relations with parents and immediate family members (Ybarra & Mitchell, 2005). In Chapter 10, we saw that alienated youth, sensation seekers, and generally those at-risk were most likely to access violent media (Slater, 2003); moreover, youth who were sympathetic to prejudiced messages were also more likely to be persuaded by them (Lee & Leets, 2002). We also saw in Chapters 9 and 10 that troubled youth (e.g., conflict at home, sexual or physical abuse, or engaging in high risk behaviors such as substance abuse) were at risk for online bullying, victimization, sexual solicitation, harassment, and addictive behavior (Hinduja & Patchin, 2008; Ko et al., 2006; Mitchell, Finkelhor, & Wolak, 2007). The evidence suggests that online youth who seek out violent or hateful content, bully peers, or are victims of harassment have difficulties in other areas of their offline lives. Unfortunately, connectedness holds for both the positives and negatives in adolescents' lives and consequently digital worlds represent both opportunities and risks for them. In later sections, we address the issue of online opportunities and risks, and in particular the challenge of ensuring that adolescents take advantage of the opportunities while at the same time safeguarding them from some of the risks.

Psychological Connectedness Does Not Mean Identical

Even though adolescents' online lives seem to center around offline issues and people, from our descriptions of online behaviors it should be clear to the reader that they are not identical to their offline versions. This is not very surprising when one considers that online communication environments are very different from offline ones and have very unique capabilities and affordances. In Chapter 1, we identified relevant features of digital contexts, such as their potential for anonymity, disembodied users, text-based communication, disinhibited behavior, and self-disclosure. Some features (e.g., disembodied users and text-based environments) present challenges to online communication, whereas others (e.g., potential for anonymity and self-disclosure) provide special opportunities, but also some risks. As young users have brought their offline concerns to their online worlds, they have adapted to these features of digital contexts. In doing so, they have created very different and at times even exaggerated forms of behaviors compared to their offline counterparts.

Consider young people's use of chat rooms for sexual exploration and identity construction, which we described in Chapters 3 and 4. Within anonymous online teen chat rooms, participants were able to have free and frank discussions about sex, and engage in identity expression as well as self-presentation (Subrahmanyam et al., 2006). The disembodied and anonymous space of chat rooms disinhibited users and encouraged them to self-disclose, but at the same time, also made it harder for them to share information about their identity (e.g., age and gender) and interest in sexualized interactions, elements that are essential to further their offline concern with sexuality and identity. Young participants adapted by resorting to sexualized (e.g., *RomancBab4U*) and gendered (*Lilprincess72988*) nicknames as well as explicit identity utterances using the a/s/l slot filler format. Similarly, adolescents use text-based blog-entries to create narratives about their self (Subrahmanyam et al., 2009) and take advantage of photos, music, and other profile elements of social networking sites for identity-expression and self-presentation (Manago, Graham, Greenfield, & Salimkhan, 2008).

Online versions of traditional behaviors are at times much more exaggerated as well. In our analysis of online teen chat rooms, we found that there was one sexual remark per minute, two identity declarations per minute, and two partner requests per minute (Šmahel & Subrahmanyam, 2007; Subrahmanyam et al., 2006). While we do not have hard data as to the frequency of these behaviors in teens' face-to-face interactions, we would be surprised if they occurred at such elevated rates. Another example is the very exaggerated nature of teen interactions on social networking sites discussed in Chapter 5. Recall that high school students who used social networking sites reported between 0 and 793 "friends," on their SNS profile (Reich et al., 2009). An important question that we will consider in a subsequent section is whether such exaggerated versions of online behaviors may be fundamentally transforming core processes.

Psychological connectedness seems to also extend to online gender presentation and gender differences in online activities. We saw in Chapter 4 that adolescents use various online tools such as nicknames and user pictures to present their offline gender (Manago et al., 2008; Schmitt, Dayanim, & Matthias, 2008; Subrahmanyam et al., 2009; Subrahmanyam et al., 2006). As noted earlier, there are gender differences with regard to blogging and gaming, which parallel offline differences in keeping dairies, playing video games, and more generally in young people's play, reading, and television preferences (Durkin & Barber, 2002; Griffiths et al., 2004; Subrahmanyam & Greenfield, 1998; Subrahmanyam et al., 2009).

Developmental trends in digital worlds parallel offline ones, and provide further support for our contention that offline and online worlds are psychologically connected. In our research on online teen chat rooms, we found that chat users who self-declared as older were also more likely to make explicit sexual utterances and more actively searched for a partner (Šmahel & Subrahmanyam, 2007; Subrahmanyam et al., 2006). Similarly, boys and older adolescents were more likely to report accidental exposure as well as much higher rates of intentional exposure to sexually explicit material (Flood & Hamilton, 2003; Lo & Wei, 2005; Wallmyr & Welin, 2006). In their study on home pages, Schmitt, and colleagues found that girls and older adolescents provided more information about themselves (Schmitt et al., 2008). While many offline gender differences seem to be projected online, at times traditional gender trends may also be reversed: within online chat rooms, we found that females searched more often for partners than males (Šmahel & Subrahmanyam, 2007). A content analysis of teen blogs found no gender differences in the use of aggressive or forceful language and passive or compliant language (Huffaker & Calvert, 2005). Together the pattern of results indicate that although traditional offline gender differences are often replicated online, nonetheless, online contexts might disinhibit users and lead to some shifting or even reversals of gender roles. In sum, although adolescents' online and offline worlds are psychologically connected, the connectedness has its limits. Online and offline worlds are not mirror images of each other. Online behaviors often take on new and different forms, and may even be exaggerated or reverse offline trends in behaviors.

Implications of Connectedness for Development

In light of the findings that young people bring the issues and people in their offline lives to their online contexts, it is important to consider whether addressing core issues in online contexts might change and affect the course of these important developmental issues. Take the case of sexuality, which we addressed in Chapter 3. We described some of the ways that young people present their sexual selves via sexualized nicknames, the electronic exchange of sexual content using explicit texts, as well as nude or semi-nude personal pictures (National Campaign to Prevent Teen and Unplanned Pregnancy & Cosmogirl.com, 2008; Subrahmanyam et al., 2006). Cybersex or sexual communication and accessing of sexually explicit material are other means of sexual exploration (Šmahel, 2006). Digital contexts have clearly made it possible for young people to engage in such sexual self-presentation and sexual exploration as they work to establish their sexuality, a core adolescent task. We have also argued that one advantage of online contexts is that some of this exploration can occur in the relative safety of the young person's home. Gay teens may also use the Internet for information, support, and to meet potential partners and this may even be contributing to the trend that youth are disclosing their homosexual identity at younger ages compared to previous years (Alexander, 2002; Savin-Williams, 2005).

At the same time, we do not fully understand the potentially negative implications of these activities. For example, extant research suggests that exposure to pornography may be associated with more permissive attitudes as well as greater sexual arousal and preoccupation with sex (Brown & L'Engle, 2009; Peter & Valkenburg, 2008). We need research to disentangle whether online exposure to pornography triggers the more permissive and casual attitude toward sex or whether certain youth are simply more likely to gravitate toward pornography. Until we address questions about the causal direction of influence, a legitimate concern is that digital contexts with their potential for easy access to sexualized content and activities may be contributing to the precocious sexual socialization of youth. Complicating matters, some exposure to sexualized content is accidental and unintended and thus could have different kinds of effects compared to intentional exposure. We also need more research on the effects of online sexual socialization on actual rates of teenage sexual activity, self-esteem, well-being, and romantic relationship formation, both during the teen years and beyond.

Similar issues are pertinent with regard to adolescents' online construction of identity and intimacy. While it is clear that youth take advantage of the numerous and varied opportunities for self-exploration and self-presentation that are available, we do not know the impact of such activities on their identity development. Being able to test different aspects of their self-online and receive feedback from peers might facilitate identity construction. Most youth do not assume alternative identities online, and the virtual personas they construct may actually help to solidify their sense of self. However, they may also interfere with identity construction processes, especially if the adolescent is also having trouble in other dimensions, such as with their peers and parents.

Digital worlds also have implications for the development of intimacy and interconnection and as well as for ethics and morality, the two other adolescent issues that we examined in Chapters 5 and 6. In both cases, we described how technology has wrought changes in the way that adolescents deal with these tasks. Less clear is whether these changes are more superficial in nature or whether they are fundamentally and radically changing the way youth learn to form intimate relations and to do the right thing. For instance, we saw that digital tools such as instant messaging and text messaging enable adolescents to connect with offline peers at all times of the day, even late into the night. On social networking sites, many adolescents have a large number of "friends," and much of their interactions with this network of friends occur in the public space for their entire network to see and follow. These larger networks provide a wider circle of friends from whom youth can draw support and from whom they can learn how to negotiate their social world. In fact, the words "friend" and "friendship" themselves may be undergoing subtle transformations, which is why we enclosed them in quotes in the first place. The relevant question then is whether these changes in the way youth interact with their offline peers is fundamentally altering and transforming the way adolescents form intimate relationships. Equally important, do digitally mediated peer relationships offer similar levels of social support and protective benefits (e.g., buffer against stress) compared to earlier generations of offline peer relationships?

Technology is similarly relevant to adolescents' interaction with their families. Again, it is too early to conclude that it is fundamentally transforming family relationships, but it may nonetheless be subtly affecting family dynamics. Digital tools make it possible for adolescents to both have increased contact with their parents and family members, while at the same shutting them and increasing their contact with their peers. Technology might help to accelerate teen autonomy and is a source of conflict within the family (Mesch, 2006). Furthermore, youth are frequently the technology experts in the family reversing traditional family roles, wherein the parent is more knowledgeable and has more expertise. Technology is likely contributing to the renegotiation of family relationships, and it is an empirical question whether these renegotiations will affect adolescent well-being and outcomes.

Digital worlds are also significant to adolescents' developing sense of ethics and morality. They present special challenges to doing the right thing and adolescents have to learn that moral rules and principles apply to online contexts just as much as they do to offline ones. Also, youth often test their values, norms, and moral rules within disinhibiting online environments, such as discussion boards and online games (Šmahel, 2003). For example, online actions such as lying, cheating, and stealing online often do not lead to repercussions. Additionally, there is psychological distance between users, their online representations, and the actions of their online representations and we do not understand how this distance may mediate the development of morals and ethics. Given all of these issues, the challenge for researchers is to understand the relation between adolescents' online activities and their sense of morality and ethics.

Youth Digital Worlds: Opportunities and Risks

In Chapter 1, we noted the ambivalence and questions surrounding young people's use of digital technologies, which were similar to the suspicions about earlier media forms, such as film and television. To address these questions, the second part of the book examined the practical implications of digital worlds for adolescents: the effect of technology on well-being, use of technology for health and wellness, and the potential for addiction, aggression, and victimization. Again, it was evident that the Internet and other digital tools are not inherently good or bad. They are ultimately tools and like every other tool, they can lead to good or bad outcomes depending on how we use them. Here we summarize some of the opportunities and risks that digital worlds present for young people.

Perhaps no other issue has evinced as much interest as that concerning the effects of youth technology use on well-being, and in particular, whether Internet use leads to lowered well-being. In Chapter 7, we described the extant research on this topic and concluded that increased use of digital tools does not automatically lead to lowered psychological well-being. Instead, the Internet's effects may depend on the particular online activities, interaction partners, as well the adolescent users' own psychological and social resources, such as extroversion and self-esteem

(Eijnden, Meerkerk, Vermulst, Spijkerman, & Engels, 2008; Kraut et al., 2002; Subrahmanyam & Lin, 2007; Sun et al., 2005). Along similar lines, technology use, when excessive or inappropriate (e.g., texting while driving) can lead to injuries (e.g., texting tenosynovitis or car crashes), sleep loss, and quite possibly heightened arousal (Storr, de Vere Beavis, & Stringer, 2007; Van den Bulck, 2003). Sleep loss is associated with mood regulation and school problems (Chapter 7) (Fredriksen, Reddy, Way, & Rhodes, 2004; Tarokh & Carskadon, 2008) and addictive behavior (Chapter 9) (Ng & Wiemer-Hastings, 2005), and sustained arousal accruing from technology use may have long-term negative effects as well (Sundar & Wagner, 2002).

For teens, digital tools can help to enhance health and illness as we showed in Chapter 8. Youth use Internet forums such as websites and bulletin boards for information about general health & sexuality (e.g., pregnancy/birth control, body image, and personal grooming) (Suzuki & Calzo, 2004) and about specific concerns such as cancer (Suzuki & Kato, 2003), eating disorders (Wilson, Peebles, Hardy, & Litt, 2006), and self-injurious behavior (Whitlock, Powers, & Eckenrode, 2006). Advantages of online resources include their around the clock availability and potential for anonymity, which can be useful to obtain answers to sensitive questions. However, there are challenges as well. Youth are not very good at searching for information (Skinner, Biscope, Poland, & Goldberg, 2003) or at evaluating the credibility of online sources (Eysenbach, 2008). This is important because online information is all not of equal quality and some information may even be incorrect and harmful. In fact, many discussion groups dedicated to particular issues, such as eating disorders may not have professional therapists or clinicians to answer user questions. There is also the very real concern that online sites focused on problems such as eating disorders or self-injury might even normalize these potentially deadly behaviors (Whitlock et al., 2006). Similarly, digital technologies can be used to deliver interventions to enhance health and wellness, such as for obesity and eating disorders (Doyle et al., 2008; Williamson et al., 2005), and to ease parent-teen conflicts (Carpenter, Frankel, Marina, Duan, & Smalley, 2004). Unfortunately, such interventions have had limited success, primarily due to low log-on rates and more research is needed to identify program characteristics that can enhance effectiveness.

Another aspect of digital worlds that provides both opportunities and risks is the potential for interaction. As we have already pointed out in this chapter, adolescents use digital tools to interact and communicate. Much of their online communication is with their offline peers and a large part of these interactions is about every day issues – school, friends, gossip, and hanging out (Gross, 2004). We have suggested that these interactions help them with the task of establishing intimacy. Even interactions with strangers may be helpful as we saw in Gross's cyberball study (Gross, 2009) (Chapter 7). In that study, teen participants who experienced social exclusion showed greater recovery from the resulting negative affect when they engaged in instant messaging with an unknown peer compared to solitary game play. However, as we saw in Chapter 10, online interactions also present risks such as cyber bullying and harassment by peers (Juvonen & Gross, 2008; Raskauskas & Stoltz, 2007), as well as sexual solicitation and victimization by predatory adults (Wolak, Mitchell, & Finkelhor, 2006; Ybarra, Espelage, & Mitchell, 2007). Similarly, Chapter 6 showed that some youth take advantage of digital contexts to construct new modes of engaging with their local and distant communities (Chapter 6) (Cassell, Huffaker, Tversky, & Ferriman, 2006; Montgomery, 2007). However, there are others who may be at risk for excessive or problematic online behavior (Chapter 9) (Ko et al., 2006) or may seek and be persuaded by online aggressive content (such as in hate sites and music videos) (Lee & Leets, 2002) (Chapter 10).

The foregoing highlights some of the negative aspects of digital technologies. Regrettably, parents, policy makers, and other observers often assume that all youth are equally at risk. This is not so and earlier in this chapter we provided examples to demonstrate that adolescents' offline characteristics (e.g., age, gender, sensation seeking, depression, self-esteem) seem to predict some kinds of problematic online behaviors (e.g., pornography, aggressive content, addictive behavior) (Brown & L'Engle, 2009; Lee & Leets, 2002; Peter & Valkenburg, 2008; Slater, 2003; Ybarra & Mitchell, 2005). Similarly, we saw in Chapter 10 that teens at risk for cyber bullying tend to be victims of repeated school-based offline bullying, spend more time online, use certain online applications such as instant messaging and webcams (Hinduja & Patchin, 2008; Juvonen & Gross, 2008). They also report offline problems such as at school, assaultive behaviors, and substance use (Hinduja & Patchin, 2008). We also saw in Chapter 9 that youth with addictive behavior on the Internet had problems in other areas of their life, such as in their academics, family relations, physical health (sleep deprivation due to long hours of Internet use), mental health (depression), finances (cost of accrued Internet expenses), substance abuse, and cyber bullying (Griffiths, 2000; Ko et al., 2006; Kraut et al., 1998; Kubey, Lavin, & Barrows, 2001; Tsai & Lin, 2003; Young, 1998).

In sum, we recommend adopting new perspectives when assessing the practical and policy implications of digital worlds on youth. We have to recognize that digital worlds present both opportunities as well as challenges/risks to them and be open to finding opportunities where we least expect to find them, such as in the case of stranger interaction. Future research efforts should uncover the characteristics of youth most likely to be susceptible to online risks, while at the same time mindful that effects of online activities might also be different for these groups of youngsters.

Promoting Positive and Safe Online Digital Worlds

The foregoing section illustrates that digital worlds contain opportunities as well as risks for young people and here we summarize what we can do to ensure that they have access to positive and safe digital worlds. This will require a two-pronged approach, comprising protecting and safeguarding youth from the risks while at the same time empowering them so they can and do benefit from the opportunities.

Chapter 11 detailed the various strategies that we can adopt to protect youth from inappropriate and harmful online content (e.g., pornography and violence) and victimization by peers (e.g., cyber bullying) and adult predators (sexual solicitation). It reiterated that protecting and safeguarding youth in digital worlds will require the concerted and proactive actions of all stakeholders – government, industry, schools, parents and even youth themselves. Parents, guardians, and others who work closely with youth (e.g., teachers, clinicians, and physicians) have to be the first and most important line of defense. This is especially so when it comes to safeguarding children from aggressive and other inappropriate content as it is realistically and legally impossible for government or other agencies (e.g., law enforcement) to monitor and regulate the vast amount of digital content that is available. Parents have at their disposal numerous mediation strategies, including technological (e.g., blocking and filtering software) and non-technological (e.g., evaluative and restrictive mediation) ones (Eastin, Greenberg, & Hofschire, 2006) and these were outlined in Chapter 11. However, for parental mediation to be successful, parents have to become more knowledgeable than they currently are about online dangers, their teen's online activities, and the various solutions themselves. Also needed is systematic research on the use and effectiveness of parental mediation strategies, as well as parent education programs based on this research.

Equally important is educating and empowering youth so they learn to navigate digital worlds safely and are equipped with strategies to adopt when they do encounter challenges. We saw in Chapter 11 that many youth who are victims of cyber bullying do not inform their parents or even use a simple technological strategy such as blocking their bullies' screen names (Dehue, Bolman, & Vollink, 2008; Juvonen & Gross, 2008). At various points in the book, we also identified problematic aspects of young people's technology use as well as gaps in their knowledge and understanding of digital literacy and here we briefly highlight some of the more pressing ones. In Chapter 7, we described the potential for harm from excessive and inappropriate use of computer/laptops and mobile devices and the need for education about using them moderately and safely. Chapter 8 demonstrated that adolescents are not very good at searching for health information; they may also not consistently pay attention to the credibility of online health resources. Finally, Chapter 6 discussed adolescents' incomplete understanding of moral and ethical issues within digital worlds. They mostly do the right thing with regard to safeguarding their own privacy, but frequently engage in cyber plagiarism and digital piracy, as they do not have a good appreciation of the ethical, moral, and legal issues intrinsic to digital objects. In light of the above, there is an urgent need to investigate the developmental trajectory in young people's understanding of digital literacy and to design training programs informed by this line of inquiry.

Digital Worlds and Development: Future Steps for Research

In 2006, the journal Developmental Psychology published a special section on children, adolescents, and the Internet. It was one of the first such collections of research on this topic, and the goal of the editors was to survey "the state of a new field of inquiry in developmental psychology" (Greenfield & Yan, 2006). This was also our goal when we set out to write this book and as we did so, we were heartened to note that we have started to make progress in this direction. However, there are many gaps in our understanding of technology and development, and we have already identified some of the more pressing research questions. In this final section, we offer further considerations that researchers should keep in mind as they investigate these questions.

First is the issue of age; extant research on youth and technology has generally lumped adolescents of all ages in one group. However, the period of adolescence is not a monolithic one, and we can distinguish between early (10- to 13-years), middle (14- to 17-years), and late adolescence (18- to 21-years). Different developmental tasks may be more or less salient during these different periods. Adolescents in the different phases may also deal very differently with the same task, since they have very different social rights and privileges. For instance, early adolescents are adjusting to their developing sexuality and often have less autonomy compared to older adolescents, who may be sexually mature and more autonomous (e.g., having their driver's license), but still be formulating their identity. Consequently, adolescents of different ages will likely behave differently in online contexts, and their online activities may influence them differently. For this reason, whenever possible we provided participants' ages when describing empirical studies and we urge the reader to keep that in mind when interpreting the results. Future studies must also compare adolescents of different ages when examining the role of digital worlds in adolescent development. There is also very little research on the role of technology in the lives of 9- to 11-year-old youth, who are in the transition between childhood and adolescence. As youth are adopting technologies at younger and younger ages, it is important for research on digital worlds to include these very young adolescents.

We also do not have a good understanding of the role of the context in adolescents' digital worlds. From research in developmental psychology, we know that contextual variables influence offline behavior and development and probably influence their online counterparts. Readers may recall some of the differences in the use of online applications among youth from the seven countries in the World Internet Project (Chapter 1): consider that in 2007, two thirds of Czech adolescents visited anonymous chat rooms, but approximately a third of US and Canadian adolescents did so. Such differences in the use of digital worlds very likely lead to differences in online behavior as different online contexts seem to give rise to different kinds of activities. For instance, young people have more sexualized interactions with strangers in chat rooms but tend to connect with offline friends when using social networking sites.

Differences in online behavior may also arise from offline differences in cultural norms and values. In Chapter 5, we described a study on online romantic relationship formation among young adolescents in Mauritius (Rambaree, 2008). Mauritius is much more conservative and parents and other adults do not approve of dating or romantic relationships in early adolescence. Within this context, the Internet had become a new and secret environment for adolescents to experience dating. Here we see continuity in a core concern – interest in forming a relationship with a romantic partner; but because of cultural values, the online context afforded behaviors not found online. Teens from different contexts might behave very differently online and their online behaviors might have very different outcomes. It is important for researchers to examine the role of the larger cultural context when studying the role of new media in development.

A third consideration for future research is that digital media are varied and dynamic entities. In Chapter 1, we noted some of the challenges we faced when we first began to study digital worlds. Digital tools are constantly changing and evolving and researchers must keep track of changes in teens' use of online tools and applications. In addition, they must keep in mind that as new and different digital worlds emerge, they give rise to very different online behaviors and consequently new research topics and questions. For instance, digital contexts such as MMORPGs are relatively new, and ever since they became popular and were found to be associated with addictive behavior (Chapter 9), online addictive behavior has become an often researched theme. Mobile phones and hand-held devices are another ubiquitous tool. They allow users to connect to the Internet, to be online at all times, seemingly never alone, and are very likely are creating new patterns of youth peer interactions. At the time when we wrote this book, we could find very few US and European studies on young people's use of mobile devices and it is important to include these devices when studying young people's technology use. However, it is important to keep in mind that mobile devices are much more diffuse in Asian countries such as Japan and South Korea[1] and there is correspondingly more research from these countries on these tools.

Not only do technologies change with time, so do young people's interactions with them. How users interact with an online application initially may be very different with how they use it over time. Studies that obtain a single snapshot of a user's online activities will not capture the changes that occur with prolonged use and most of the existing research has done just this. Longitudinal studies are one way to address this; cross-sequential studies are even better because they also allow us to test for cohort effects as the technologies themselves change and evolve over time.

In conclusion, a pressing question for future research is whether adolescents' online activities centered on core developmental issues are fundamentally transforming the offline developmental processes themselves. For instance, does online exposure to sexually explicit pornographic material increase rates of youth sexual activity? Do adolescents' large number of "friends" on social networking sites and their very public interactions with these friends transform the nature of their friendships and level of intimacy? How does online self-presentation influence young people's developing sense of self? Because much of the existing findings relating online and offline behaviors are correlational, such questions about the direction of influence remain unanswered. Future research must use longitudinal as well as experimental designs to determine whether the transferring of core developmental

---

[1] See Information Society Statistical Profiles 2009 – Asia and the Pacific – at http://www.itu.int/en/pages/default.aspx

issues to online contexts may be fundamentally transforming adolescents' construction of their sexual selves, self-presentation and identity, and their peer and family relationships.

References

Alexander, J. (2002). Introduction to the special issue: Queer webs: Representations of LGBT people and communities on the World Wide Web. *International Journal of Sexuality and Gender Studies, 7*, 77–84.

Brown, D. J., & L'Engle, L. K. (2009). X-rated: Sexual attitudes and behaviors associated with U.S. early adolescents' exposure to sexually explicit media. *Communication Research, 36*, 129–151.

Carpenter, E. M., Frankel, F., Marina, M., Duan, N., & Smalley, S. L. (2004). Internet treatment delivery of parent-adolescent conflict training for families with an ADHD teen: A feasibility study. *Child and Family Behavior Therapy, 26*, 1–20.

Cassell, J., Huffaker, D., Tversky, D., & Ferriman, K. (2006). The language of online leadership: Gender and youth engagement on the Internet. *Developmental Psychology, 42*, 436–449.

Dehue, F., Bolman, C., & Vollink, T. (2008). Cyberbullying: Youngsters' experiences and parental perception. *CyberPsychology and Behavior, 11*, 217–223.

Doyle, A. C., Goldschmidt, A., Huang, C., Winzelberg, A. J., Taylor, C. B., & Wilfley, D. E. (2008). Reduction of overweight and eating disorder symptoms via the Internet in adolescents: A randomized controlled trial. *Journal of Adolescent Health, 43*, 172–179.

Durkin, K., & Barber, B. (2002). Not so doomed: Computer game play and positive adolescent development. *Journal of Applied Developmental Psychology, 23*, 373–392.

Eastin, M. S., Greenberg, B. S., & Hofschire, L. (2006). Parenting the Internet. *Journal of Communication, 56*, 486–504.

Eijnden, R., Meerkerk, G. J., Vermulst, A. A., Spijkerman, R., & Engels, R. (2008). Online communication, compulsive Internet use, and psychosocial well-being among adolescents: A longitudinal study. *Developmental Psychology, 44*, 655–665.

Eysenbach, G. (2008). Credibility of health information and digital media: New perspectives and implications for youth. In M. J. Metzger & A. J. Flanagin (Eds.), *Digital media, youth, and credibility* (pp. 123–154). Cambridge, MA: MIT Press.

Flood, M., & Hamilton, C. (2003). Regulating youth access to pornography. *Discussion Paper Number 53*. From https://www.tai.org.au/documents/dp_fulltext/DP53.pdf

Fredriksen, K., Reddy, R., Way, N., & Rhodes, J. (2004). Sleepless in Chicago: Tracking the effects of sleep loss over the middle school years. *Child Development, 74*, 84–95.

Greenfield, P. M., & Yan, Z. (2006). Children, adolescents, and the Internet: A new field of inquiry in developmental psychology. *Developmental Psychology, 42*, 391–394.

Griffiths, M. (2000). Does Internet and computer "Addiction" exist? Some case study evidence. *Cyberpsychology and Behavior, 3*, 211–218.

Griffiths, M. D., Davies, M. N. O., & Chappell, D. (2004). Online computer gaming: A comparison of adolescent and adult gamers. *Journal of Adolescence, 27*, 87–96.

Gross, E. F. (2004). Adolescent Internet use: What we expect, what teens report. *Journal of Applied Developmental Psychology, 25*, 633–649.

Gross, E. F. (2009). Logging on, bouncing back: An experimental investigation of online communication following social exclusion. *Developmental Psychology, 45*, 1787–1793.

Hargittai, E. (2007). Whose space? Differences among users and non-users of social network sites. *Journal of Computer-Mediated Communication, 13, Article 14*. Retrieved November 27, 2009, from http://jcmc.indiana.edu/vol13/issue1/hargittai.html

Hinduja, S., & Patchin, J. W. (2008). Cyberbullying: An exploratory analysis of factors related to offending and victimization. *Deviant Behavior, 29*, 129–156.

Huffaker, D. A., & Calvert, S. L. (2005). Gender, identity, and language use in teenage blogs. *Journal of Computer-Mediated Communication, 10,* 1. Retrieved October 15, 2009, from http://jcmc.indiana.edu/vol10/issue2/huffaker.html

Juvonen, J., & Gross, E. F. (2008). Extending the school grounds? Bullying experiences in cyberspace. *The Journal of School Health, 78,* 496–505.

Kaare, B. H., Brandtzaeg, P. B., Heim, J., & Endestad, T. (2007). In the borderland between family orientation and peer culture: The use of communication technologies among Norwegian tweens. *New Media and Society, 9,* 603–624.

Ko, C.-H., Yen, J.-Y., Chen, C.-C., Chen, S.-H., Wu, K., & Yen, C.-F. (2006). Tridimensional personality of adolescents with Internet addiction and substance use experience. *The Canadian Journal of Psychiatry/La Revue canadienne de psychiatrie, 51,* 887–894.

Kraut, R. E., Kiesler, S., Boneva, B., Cummings, J., Helgeson, V., & Crawford, A. (2002). Internet paradox revisited. *Journal of Social Issues, 58,* 49–74.

Kraut, R. E., Patterson, M., Lundmark, V., Kiesler, S., Mukopadhyay, T., & Scherlis, W. (1998). Internet paradox: A social technology that reduces social involvement and psychological well-being? *American Psychologist, 53,* 1017–1031.

Kubey, R. W., Lavin, M. J., & Barrows, J. R. (2001). Internet use and collegiate academic performance decrements: Early findings. *Journal of Communication, 51,* 366–382.

Lee, E., & Leets, L. (2002). Persuasive storytelling by hate groups online: Examining its effects on adolescents. *American Behavioral Scientist, 45,* 927–957.

Lo, V., & Wei, R. (2005). Exposure to Internet pornography and taiwanese adolescents' sexual attitudes and behavior. *Journal of Broadcasting and Electronic Media, 49,* 221–237.

Manago, A. M., Graham, M. B., Greenfield, P. M., & Salimkhan, G. (2008). Self-presentation and gender on MySpace. *Journal of Applied Developmental Psychology, 29,* 446–458.

Mesch, G. S. (2006). Family relations and the Internet: Exploring a family boundaries approach. *Journal of Family Communication, 6,* 119–138.

Mitchell, K. J., Finkelhor, D., & Wolak, J. (2007). Youth Internet users at risk for the most serious online sexual solicitations. *American Journal of Preventive Medicine, 32,* 532–537.

Montgomery, K. C. (2007). Youth and digital democracy: Intersections of practice, policy, and the marketplace. In W. L. Bennett (Ed.), *The John D. and Catherine T. MacArthur Foundation Series on Digital media and learning* (pp. 25–49). Cambridge, MA: MIT Press.

National Campaign to Prevent Teen and Unplanned Pregnancy, & Cosmogirl.com. (2008). *Sex and tech: Results from a survey of teens and young adults.* Retrieved July 16, 2009, from http://www.thenationalcampaign.org/sextech/PDF/SexTech_Summary.pdf

Ng, B. D., & Wiemer-Hastings, P. (2005). Addiction to the Internet and online gaming. *CyberPsychology and Behavior, 8,* 110–113.

Peter, J., & Valkenburg, P. M. (2006). Adolescents'exposure to sexually explicit material on the Internet. *Communication Research, 33,* 178–204.

Peter, J., & Valkenburg, P. M. (2008). Adolescents' exposure to sexually explicit Internet material and sexual preoccupancy: A three-wave panel study. *Media Psychology, 11,* 207–234.

Rambaree, K. (2008). Internet-mediated dating/romance of Mauritian early adolescents: A grounded theory analysis. *International Journal of Emerging Technologies and Society, 6,* 34–59.

Raskauskas, J., & Stoltz, A. D. (2007). Involvement in traditional and electronic bullying among adolescents. *Developmental Psychology, 43,* 564–575.

Reich, S. M., Subrahmanyam, K., & Espinoza, G. E. (2009, April 3). *Adolescents' use of social networking sites – Should we be concerned?* Paper presented at the Society for Research on Child Development, Denver, CO.

Rideout, V. J., Vandewater, E. A., & Wartella, E. A. (2003). *Zero to six: Electronic media in the lives of infants, toddlers and preschoolers.* Retrieved November 10, 2009, from http://www.kff.org/entmedia/3378.cfm

Roberts, D. F., & Foehr, U. G. (2008). Trends in media use. *The Future of Children, 18,* 11–37.

Savin-Williams, R. C. (2005). *The new gay teenager.* Cambridge: Harvard University Press.

Schmitt, K. L., Dayanim, S., & Matthias, S. (2008). Personal homepage construction as an expression of social development. *Developmental Psychology, 44*, 496–506.

Skinner, H., Biscope, S., Poland, B., & Goldberg, E. (2003). How adolescents use technology for health information: Implications for health professionals from focus group studies. *Journal of Medical Internet Research, 5*, e32.

Slater, M. D. (2003). Alienation, aggression, and sensation seeking as predictors of adolescent use of violent film, computer, and website content. *The Journal of Communication, 53*, 105–121.

Šmahel, D. (2003). *Psychologie a Internet: Děti dospělými, dospělí dětmi. [Psychology and Internet: Children being adults, adults being children.]*. Prague: Triton.

Šmahel, D. (2006). *Czech adolescents' partnership relations and sexuality in the Internet environment.* Paper presented at the Society for Research on Adolescence Biennial Meeting, San Francisco. From http://www.terapie.cz/materials/smahel-SRA-SF-2006.pdf

Šmahel, D., & Subrahmanyam, K. (2007). 'Any girls want to chat press 911': Partner selection in monitored and unmonitored teen chat rooms. *CyberPsychology and Behavior, 10*, 346–353.

Storr, E. F., de Vere Beavis, F. O., & Stringer, M. D. (2007). Case notes: Texting tenosynovitis. *New Zealand Medical Journal, 120*, 107–108.

Subrahmanyam, K., Garcia, E. C., Harsono, S. L., Li, J., & Lipana, L. (2009). In their words: Connecting online weblogs to developmental processes. *British Journal of Developmental Psychology, 27*, 219–245.

Subrahmanyam, K., & Greenfield, P. M. (1998). Computer games for girls: What makes them play? In J. Cassell & H. Jenkins (Eds.), *From Barbie to Mortal Kombat: Gender and computer games* (pp. 46–71). Cambridge, MA: The MIT Press.

Subrahmanyam, K., & Greenfield, P. M. (2008). Communicating online: Adolescent relationships and the media. *The Future of Children, 18*, 119 –146.

Subrahmanyam, K., Greenfield, P. M., & Tynes, B. M. (2004). Constructing sexuality and identity in an online teen chat room. *Journal of Applied Developmental Psychology: An International Lifespan Journal, 25*, 651–666.

Subrahmanyam, K., & Lin, G. (2007). Adolescents on the Net: Internet use and well-being. *Adolescence, 42*, 659–677.

Subrahmanyam, K., Reich, S. M., Waechter, N., & Espinoza, G. (2008). Online and offline social networks: Use of social networking sites by emerging adults. *Journal of Applied Developmental Psychology, 29*, 420–433.

Subrahmanyam, K., Šmahel, D., & Greenfield, P. M. (2006). Connecting developmental constructions to the Internet: Identity presentation and sexual exploration in online teen chat rooms. *Developmental Psychology, 42*, 395–406.

Subramanian, M. (2010). New Modes of Communication: Web Representations and Blogs. *Encyclopedia of Women and Islamic Cultures*. United States: South Asians.

Sun, P., Unger, J. B., Palmer, P. H., Gallaher, P., Chou, C. P., Baexconde-Garbanati, L., et al. (2005). Internet accessibility and usage among urban adolescents in Southern California: Implications for web-based heath research. *CyberPsychology and Behavior, 8*, 441–453.

Sundar, S. S., & Wagner, C. B. (2002). The world wide wait: Exploring physiological and behavioral effects of download speed. *Media Psychology, 4*, 173–206.

Suzuki, L. K., & Calzo, J. P. (2004). The search for peer advice in cyberspace: An examination of online teen bulletin boards about health and sexuality. *Journal of Applied Developmental Psychology, 25*, 685–698.

Suzuki, L. K., & Kato, P. M. (2003). Psychosocial support for patients in pediatric oncology: The influences of parents, schools, peers, and technology. *Journal of Pediatric Oncology Nursing, 20*, 159–174.

Tarokh, L., & Carskadon, M. A. (2008). Sleep in adolescents. In L. R. Squire (Ed.), *Encyclopedia of neuroscience* (pp. 1015–1022). Oxford: Academic Press.

Tsai, C.-C., & Lin, S. S. J. (2003). Internet addiction of adolescents in Taiwan: An interview study. *Cyberpsychology and Behavior, 6*, 649–652.

Tynes, B. M. (2007). Role taking in online "Classrooms": What adolescents are learning about race and ethnicity. *Developmental Psychology, 43,* 1312–1320.

Van den Bulck, J. (2003). Text messaging as a cause of sleep interruption in adolescents, evidence from a cross-sectional study. *Journal of Sleep Research, 12,* 263–263.

Wallmyr, G., & Welin, C. (2006). Young people, pornography, and sexuality: Sources and attitudes. *The Journal of School Nursing, 22,* 290–295.

Whitlock, J. L., Powers, J. L., & Eckenrode, J. (2006). The virtual cutting edge: The Internet and adolescent-self-injury. *Developmental Psychology, 42,* 407–417.

Williamson, D. A., Martin, P. D., White, M. A., Newton, R. W., Walden, H., York-Crowe, E., et al. (2005). Efficacy of an Internet-based behavioral weight loss program for overweight adolescent African-American girls. *Eating and Weight Disorders, 10,* 193–203.

Wilson, J. L., Peebles, R., Hardy, K. K., & Litt, I. F. (2006). Surfing for thinness: A pilot study of pro-eating disorder web site usage in adolescents with eating disorders. *Pediatrics, 118,* e1635–e1643.

Wolak, J., Mitchell, K. J., & Finkelhor, D. (2006). *Online victimization of youth: Five years later.* Retrieved August 9, 2007, from http://www.unh.edu/ccrc/pdf/CV138.pdf

Ybarra, M. L. (2004). Linkages between depressive symptomatology and Internet harassment among young regular Internet users. *CyberPsychology and Behavior, 7,* 247–257.

Ybarra, M. L., Espelage, D. L., & Mitchell, K. J. (2007). The co-occurrence of Internet harassment and unwanted sexual solicitation victimization and perpetration: Associations with psychosocial indicators. *Journal of Adolescent Health, 41,* 31–41.

Ybarra, M. L., & Mitchell, K. J. (2005). Exposure to Internet pornography among children and adolescents: A national survey. *CyberPsychology and Behavior, 8,* 473–486.

Young, K. S. (1998). *Caught in the Net.* New York, NY: Wiley.

Index

A

Abortion, 44, 191
Academic honesty, 111
Addiction
  internet, 158–160, 162–165, 170, 172–174
  online, 157–159, 165, 168, 173, 188
Addictive behavior
  diagnostic criteria, 163
  treatment of, 172–174
Adolescent crowds, 32
After-school settings, 83
Age restrictions, 108
Aggression, 107, 179–182, 185, 189–190, 193, 221
Aggressive behavior, 104, 179–180, 185, 189, 196, 208
Aggressive ideation, 180
Aggressiveness, 91, 184
Alienation, 185
Amphetamine, 152
Anonymity, 2, 14, 35, 43, 47, 63, 76, 85, 91, 147, 171, 192–193, 218, 222
Anorexia, 12, 144, 150–151, 159, 205
Appearance, 32, 43, 63, 75, 107, 124, 151, 163, 190
Armed assaults, 182
a/s/l code, 64–65
At-risk individuals, 187
Audience, 73, 92, 116
Authoritative parents, 106, 207–208
Autonomy developing, 31, 82, 146, 201
Avatars, 9, 11, 44, 62, 65–67, 75, 216

B

Bipolar disorder, 164
Birth control methods, 44
Blocking software, 207

Blog, 2, 7–8, 16, 19, 33, 45, 60, 62, 64, 66–69, 92–93, 105, 107, 114, 137, 143–144, 183, 185, 209, 216, 218–219
Blogging, 7–8, 218
Body image, 144, 222
Bomb-making instructions, 181, 185
Bulimia, 150–151
Bulletin boards, 11–12, 14, 21, 35–36, 41, 43–44, 63, 72, 137, 146–148, 182, 222
Bullies, 191–194, 211, 224

C

Cancer, "cancer teens", 145, 147–149
Cell phone, 1–3, 43, 46, 87, 95–97, 99–100, 116, 129, 153, 190–191, 196, 202
Chat rooms, 2, 10–11, 13–14, 16, 19–21, 33–36, 41, 43–46, 48, 53, 63–65, 68–69, 71–72, 74, 76, 82–83, 86, 88, 91–92, 107, 132–134, 136–138, 146, 148, 164, 173, 182, 185, 191, 195–196, 215–216, 218–219, 225
Childhood, 82, 180, 203, 225
Child Online Protection Act (COPA), 202
Child pornography, 46, 203, 210
Circadian rhythms, 129
Circle of friends, 86, 99, 220
Civic actions, 117–118
Civic discourse, 117
Civic engagement, 103–119
Close friends, 31, 82, 88, 99, 132, 134, 136–137, 216
Co-construction model, 33–36, 134, 216
Cognitive behavioral therapy (CBT), 173
Commitment, 31, 60–61, 70–71, 92, 208
Common values, 117
Communication
  mother-adolescent, 130

K. Subrahmanyam, D. Šmahel, *Digital Youth*, Advancing Responsible
Adolescent Development, DOI 10.1007/978-1-4419-6278-2,
© Springer Science+Business Media, LLC 2011

Communication (*cont.*)
 non-verbal, 17
 text-based, 8, 14–15, 16, 218
Communities, 22, 53–54, 63, 103, 113–115,
 118, 136, 150, 223
Compulsive behavior, 158, 170–171
Compulsive users, 170–171
Computer, 1–2, 9, 12–13, 15–18, 22, 32, 43,
 59, 65, 74, 97–98, 104, 110–113,
 117, 124–125, 127, 130–131, 136,
 157, 165–166, 169, 181, 184,
 188, 202, 204, 206–207, 209–210,
 215, 224
Computer-based property, 113
Conflicts with parents, 88, 98
Consequences of online bullying, 194
Contact with peers, 86, 148
Contraception, 145
Conversational coherence, 20
Coping strategy, 148
Copying, 109–112
Copyright rights, 112
Co-viewing, 205, 208
Cryptomnesia, 110
Cultural context (of romantic relationships/
 dating), 30, 59, 94
Cultural icons, 75
Cultural patterns, 90
Cyberball task, 136
Cyber bullying, 165, 190–194
Cyber harassment, 191
Cyber plagiarism, 104, 109–111
Cybersex, 47, 53, 219
Cybertipline, 209

D
Daily logs, 132
Dangerous online content, 150–152
Dating, 28–29, 42, 47, 81, 90, 92–94, 109, 145,
 186–187, 196, 225
Deliberation, 117
Delinquent behaviors, 50, 217
Depression, 50, 89, 130–133, 135, 145, 148,
 164, 171, 193, 217, 223
Destructive behavior, 185
Developing sexuality, 30, 42, 90, 225
Developmental, 3, 10, 20–22, 28–34, 36,
 41–43, 45, 48–49, 54, 59, 61, 68, 76,
 81, 84, 87, 99, 103, 113, 118, 180,
 195–196, 208, 216, 219, 224–226
Developmental processes, 20, 33, 226
Developmental stages, 87
Developmental tasks, 28–31, 33–34, 81,
 103, 225

Dialogues, 117
Digital immigrants, 1, 19–20, 98
Digital media, 1, 13–14, 20, 22, 32–33, 36, 62,
 201, 216–221, 226
Digital natives, 1, 16, 19, 98, 100, 113, 215
Direct Connect, 112
Discussion groups, 82, 98, 160, 222
Disembodied users, 2, 13–14, 85, 91, 218
Disinhibited behavior, 2, 13, 16, 218
Displacement hypothesis, 123, 126, 128
Download speed, 126
Drug prescription, 150, 152
Drug usage, 82, 152, 159

E
Early adolescence, 16, 225
Early adopters, 1, 3, 19, 146, 191
Eating disorders, 145, 148, 150–151, 153, 222
Educational internet usage, 98
Ego identity, 60–61, 70
Elections, 109, 113–115
Electronic gadgets, 19
Emerging adulthood, 30–31, 50, 62,
 166–167, 170
Emoticons, 13, 16–17
Emotion, 12, 16–17, 29, 31, 46, 50, 62, 68,
 91–92, 131, 148, 159, 162, 165,
 168–169, 172, 180, 184, 194, 217
Emotional independence, 29
Emotional intelligence, 168
Emotional support, 12, 148, 159, 169
Empathetic attitude, 189
Energy expenditure, 128
Energy intake, 128
Entertainment, 2, 5, 34, 105, 114,
 135, 215
Equality, 82, 117
Erotic/romantic contacts, 48, 82
Ethical behavior, 104
Ethical boundaries, 109
Ethnic identity, 62, 72–73, 137
Ethnicity, 50, 72–73, 138, 145, 182
Evaluative mediation, 205
Excessive behavior, 158
Excessive sleepiness, 129
Exposure to sexually explicit content,
 47–48
Extremism, 182
Extremist web sites, 185
Extroverted/introverted teens, 134

F
Facebook, 6, 8, 20, 69, 72–73, 87, 93–94,
 114–116, 135, 209, 215

Face-to-face interactions, 4, 64, 85–86, 218
Factual mediation, 205
Faking, 107–108
Family
    cohesion, 98–99, 207–208
    interaction, 61, 97
    life, 29, 96–97
    members, 6, 30, 50, 81–100, 137, 163, 172,
        217, 221
    relationships, 97–99
    roles, 98, 221
Fast food consumption, 127
Feminine nickname/masculine nickname,
    45, 64
Filter blogs, 7
Filtering software, 106, 206, 224
Flaming, 105–106
Flirt, 74, 83–84
"Foot-in-the-door" techniques, 186
Friendship
    closeness, 87
    duration, 82, 90
    quality, 87
Functional impairment, 164

G
Game
    addictions, 10
    players, 166–167
Gay communities, 53–54
Gaze, 14, 43, 89, 123
Gender, 6, 10, 21, 31–32, 34–35, 42–43, 45,
        50–51, 59, 62–65, 67–69, 72–73,
        75, 82–83, 89, 92, 107, 134, 145,
        160–161, 167, 170, 185, 187, 193,
        217–219, 223
Gesture, 14, 43, 89, 123
Global community, 116–117
Gratification theory, 34

H
Hacking, 104, 191
Hardware, 2–3, 202
Harm avoidance, 165
Hate forums, 185
Hazardous users, 171
Health
    information, 21, 34, 144–150
    questions, 149
Heavy internet usage, 99, 164
High engagement, 158
High-risk communicators, 89
Hobby, 88
Honesty, 16, 31, 82, 111

I
Ideal self, 69
Identifying information, 14, 45, 105
Identity
    achievement, 30, 61, 71
    construction, 32, 60, 63–76, 218, 220
    experimenting, 16, 74
    formulation, 32
    presentation, 10, 91
Illegal downloading, 13, 104, 109, 111–113
Illness, 143–154, 158, 169, 222
Inadequate exhibitionism, 91
Inappropriate content, 47, 202–208, 210, 224
Independence from parents, 29, 97
Instant messaging, 2, 5, 8–9, 11, 13, 15, 17–20,
        22, 34, 36, 45, 81, 83–88, 93–94,
        96, 105, 107, 133–134, 136–138,
        189, 191, 193, 195–196, 216–217,
        220, 222–223
Interactive technologies, 2, 19, 27, 127
Internet
    addiction
        components (dimensions),
            162–163, 165
        prevalence, 159–161
    expert, 98–99
    -related arousal, 126
    safety, 133, 192, 195, 204, 207
Intimacy, 22, 28, 30–31, 33–34, 81–100,
        216–217, 220, 222, 226
Intimate problems, 87, 89
Intimate relationships, 16, 31, 81, 99, 220
Isolated youth, 148

K
Kazaa, 112
Key logger, 209
K(nowledge)-logs, 7

L
Lack of sleep, chronic, 129
Late adolescence, 30–31, 50, 90, 225
Legislating (bullying, victimization), 204
Leisure activities, 32
Life satisfaction, 135
LimeWire, 112
Loneliness, 34, 130–134, 169
Lurking, 44, 138, 147
Lying online, 75

M
MAMA, 71

Massively Multiplayer Online Role Playing
    Games (MMORPG), 2, 9, 36, 63,
    65, 75, 166–167, 174, 188–190, 226
Media effects model, 33, 123, 134
Mediation styles, 205
Mediation techniques, 205, 207–208, 211
Micro blogging, 8
Middle adolescence, 16, 31, 42
Mobile phone, 1, 6, 13, 44, 85, 97, 99, 113,
    129, 226
Monitoring software, 207
Moral reasoning, 113
Mother-adolescent communication, 130
Multiple selves, 61
Multitasking/media-multitasking, 2, 17–19
Multi-user domains (MUDs), 36, 59, 74,
    164, 185
Music
    burning, 112
    downloading, 12–13, 112
    videos, 3, 84, 112, 180–182, 184–185,
        205, 223
Mutilation, 181
MySpace, 6, 17, 20, 59, 69, 84, 88, 97, 105,
    107, 114, 179, 204, 206, 215

N
Narratives, 8, 62, 68, 218
Negative stereotypes, 138
Netspeak, 15
Nicknames, 10, 41, 44–45, 64–67, 75, 216,
    218–219
Nintendinitis, 125
Non-verbal communication, 17
Novelty seeking, 165
Nude/semi-nude pictures, 46
Nudity, 182
Nutrition, 144, 148

O
Obesity, 126–128, 153, 222
Obscene language, 41
Offline cultural idols, 69
Offline identity, 14, 71
Offline life, 36, 50, 70–71, 94
Offline/online friendship, 81, 88–90, 114, 174
Offline peers, 86, 148, 220, 222
Offline sources, 134
One-night stand, 52
Online applications, 2, 4–13, 16, 19–20, 22,
    36, 45, 64, 82, 131, 146, 148, 173,
    193, 223, 225
Online attraction, 91
Online cheating, 108–109

Online gaming, 9–10, 98, 158, 165–168, 171
Online hate, 182–183, 185, 187, 196
Online health resources, 144–152, 224
Online information falsifying, 107–108
Online intervention, 153
Online marketing, 105
Online personas, 75
Online piracy, digital/software piracy, 111–113
Online pretending, 60
Online privacy, 105–106, 209, 211
    maintaining/safeguarding, 103,
        105–106, 224
Online sexual addiction, 170
Online sexually compulsive behavior, 170
Online stealing, 108–109
Online/virtual relationships, 42, 47, 76, 81,
    88–90, 92–93, 134, 158, 165, 174
Openness, 16, 31, 82
Overfat, 127
Overweight, 126–127, 151–153

P
Parent's safeguarding role, 204–210
Parent-adolescent closeness, 98, 207
Parental mediation strategies
    effectiveness of, 206–207
    factors affecting, 207–208
Parental monitoring, 206–207
Parent-teen conflict, 98
Partner
    intimacy, 93
    requests, 88, 92, 218
    selection, 10, 92, 216
Passivity, 91
Peer
    cliques, 82
    crowds, 82
    group, 18, 42, 81–90
        relationships, 81–90
    network, 86, 114, 174
    pressure, 138
Peer-to-peer (P2P), 111–112, 174
Personal homepages, 67–68
Personal identifying information, 105
Personal identity, 62–63
Personality development, 76
Personal journals, 7
Pharmacotherapy, 173
Physical activities, 123–124, 127–128
Physical aggression, 180
Physical appearance, 43, 63, 124, 163
Physical attractiveness, 63, 91
Physical injuries, 125

Physical well-being, 124–129
Physiological arousal, 126, 189
Plagiarizing, 104, 109
Player killing, 188
Political awareness, 118
Politics, 12, 114–115
Pop culture, 67
Pornography/online pornography, 41–55,
      171, 183, 201, 203, 206–208, 210,
      216–217, 220, 223
Predators, 10, 105, 195, 201, 203,
      208–210, 224
Pregnancy/birth control, 44, 144–145, 222
Pre-marital sex, 44
Privacy settings, 209
Private settings, 83
Pro-anorexia sites (pro-ana sites), 144,
      150–151, 205
Problematic internet use, 158, 165, 167, 173
Pro-eating disorder (ED) sites, pro-ED sites,
      12, 144, 150–151, 159, 205
Protected online content, 22
Proximity, 91, 93
Psychological well-being, 50, 108,
      130–138, 221
Psychosocial moratorium, 60
Psychotherapy, 173
Psychotic disorder, 164

R
Race, 21, 35, 43, 63, 72–73, 109, 138, 193
Racial prejudice, 73, 138
Racist attitudes, 138
Reality therapy, 173–174
Reciprocity, 82
Relational aggression, 180, 193
Relationship
      with parents, 94–99, 217
      with strangers, 88–90
Restricted/urestricted sites, 88
Restrictive mediation, 205, 207–208, 210, 224
Reward dependence, 165
"Rich-get-richer" model, 131
Risk assesment, 106
Role playing games (RPG), 2, 9, 166–167, 188
Romantic relationships, 30–31, 42, 81,
      90–94, 225
Rule-breaking behavior, 89

S
Salience, 158, 160, 162, 165
School
      avoiding, 164
      incidents, 108, 192–194, 210

Second Life, 2, 11, 14, 65, 171
Sedentary lifestyle, 127
Self
      -disclosure, 2, 13, 15–16, 31, 71, 82, 87,
            89–90, 99, 148, 218
      -efficacy, 151, 167
      -esteem, 20, 63, 107, 114, 130–131,
            133–136, 151, 167–168, 174,
            220–223
      -exploration, 74, 220
      -image, 61, 67, 75
      -injury, 148, 222
      -presentation, 59–77, 148, 167, 216,
            218–220, 226
      -reports, 21
Sensation seeking, 185, 217, 223
Sense
      of belonging, 75, 116, 190
      of humor, 91
Sensitive health-related questions, 147
Sex
      segregation, 94
      slang, 30, 42
Sexting, 46, 201
Sexual abuse, 148, 196
Sexual activity, 30, 41–42, 49, 148, 170–171,
      220, 226
Sexual competence, 42
Sexual experience, 47, 50, 75, 90
Sexual exploration, 41–55, 216, 218–219
Sexual harassment, 51
Sexual health, 54, 144–145
Sexuality, 12, 22, 28, 30–31, 33–34, 41–55, 69,
      81, 90, 94, 103, 145, 150, 211, 216,
      218–219, 222, 225
Sexualized nicknames, 45, 64, 219
Sexually explicit material, 47–52, 216, 219
Sexually Transmitted Diseases (STDs),
      144–145, 148, 153
Sexually violent materials, 52
Sexual maturation, 28–29, 90, 124
Sexual minority, 41, 43, 53–54
Sexual permissiveness, 51
Sexual preoccupation, 51
Sexual self, 41, 219
Sexual solicitation, 22, 54, 105, 180, 190,
      195–196, 201, 203, 217, 223–224
Sexual themes, 41
Sexual utterance, 44–45
Short-message systems (SMS), 2
Skype, 8
Slang, 15, 30, 42, 75

Sleep patterns (reduced sleep patterns,
        decreased sleep), 124, 126, 129
Sleep quantity, 124
Smart mobile devices, 2
SMS, *see* Short-message systems (SMS)
Social anxiety, 107, 132, 194
Social compensation, 74, 90
Social context, 32, 42, 62, 82, 103, 158
Social control, 72, 138, 167
Social facilitation, 74
Social identity, 62–63, 66
Social networking sites, 2, 6, 10, 14–16, 19–20,
        22, 33–36, 43, 45, 60, 63–64, 69,
        73, 81–83, 86–88, 93–94, 107, 114,
        118, 133–137, 174, 190, 195, 201,
        209–210, 215–218, 220, 225–226
Social role, 28–29, 62
Social similarity, 89
Social support, 34, 53–54, 130–131, 135–137,
        168, 170, 174, 220
Social ties, 130–131
Software, 2, 8, 75, 98, 103–104, 106, 109,
        111–113, 130, 132, 203, 206–207,
        209–210, 224
    as a public property, 113
Sports, 9, 12, 18, 68, 83, 123–124, 132,
        149, 171
Stimulants, 152
Substance abuse, 50, 129, 164–165, 217, 223
Suicide, 144, 179, 181–182, 204

T
Target audience, 116
Technological mediation, 205–206, 209
Teen smoking cessation, 144, 152
Television, 1, 3–4, 12–13, 17, 32–33, 53, 118,
        123–124, 127–129, 131, 179–184,
        189, 205, 215, 218, 221
Terrorist groups, 182
Text-based communication, 8, 14–15, 16, 218
Textercises, 125
Texting, 2, 6, 125, 201, 222
    tenosynovitis, 125, 222
Text-messenger's thumb, 125
Textspeak, 15
Theory of identity, 60
Thinspiration, 150
Time
    efficacy, 165
    measurement, 132
    restriction, 208
Tolerance of violence, 189

Torture, 181
Transgender, 53, 91
Triple A Engine, 42–43, 47
Trust, 89, 146, 150, 210
Twitter, 8

U
Unsolicited content, 105–106
Username, 62, 64, 67
User pictures, 66, 218

V
Value system, 33
Victimization, 22, 54, 137, 179–197, 201–204,
        208–210, 217, 221, 223–224
Video
    downloading, 12–13
    game, 1–3, 17, 33, 123, 125, 127–129, 158,
        179–180, 183–186, 189–190, 218
Violating the law, 113
Violence
    in online games, 188–190
    sexual, 52, 181
Violence-themed websites, impact of,
        183–185, 196
Violent content, 126, 180–184, 202, 206
Violent images, 183–184, 205
Violent video games, 180, 189
Virtual identity, 62–63, 75–76
Virtual representation, 62, 66, 74–75
Virtual sex, 47, 158, 165
Virtual worlds, 11, 14, 22, 35, 65, 70, 74,
        108–109, 164

W
Weak ties, 93, 130
Web 2.0, 202
Weight control, 145
Weight-loss advice, 151
Well-being
    physical, 124–129
    psychological, 130–137
Wellness, 143–154, 221–222
White power music, 186
Whyville, 11, 108–109
Withdrawal difficulties, 158
World of Warcraft (WoW), 2, 9, 65,
        166–167, 188

Y
Youth protection, 210
YouTube, 72, 183, 185, 191, 205

CPSIA information can be obtained at www.ICGtesting.com
Printed in the USA
LVOW070459101212

310848LV00002B/31/P